IL-12

Chemical Immunology

Vol. 68

Series Editors
Luciano Adorini, Milan
Ken-ichi Arai, Tokyo
Claudia Berek, Berlin
J. Donald Capra, Oklahoma City, Okla.
Anne-Marie Schmitt-Verhulst, Marseille
Byron H. Waksman, New York, N.Y.

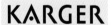

Basel · Freiburg · Paris · London · New York ·
New Delhi · Bangkok · Singapore · Tokyo · Sydney

······························

IL-12

Volume Editor   *Luciano Adorini,* Milan

33 figures, 1 in color, and 10 tables, 1997

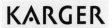

Basel · Freiburg · Paris · London · New York ·
New Delhi · Bangkok · Singapore · Tokyo · Sydney

····························
Chemical Immunology

Formerly published as 'Progress in Allergy'
Founded 1939 by Paul Kallòs

Bibliographic Indices. This publication is listed in bibliographic services, including Current Contents® and Index Medicus.

Drug Dosage. The authors and the publisher have exerted every effort to ensure that drug selection and dosage set forth in this text are in accord with current recommendations and practice at the time of publication. However, in view of ongoing research, changes in government regulations, and the constant flow of information relating to drug therapy and drug reactions, the reader is urged to check the package insert for each drug for any change in indications and dosage and for added warnings and precautions. This is particularly important when the recommended agent is a new and/or infrequently employed drug.

....

Contents

110 Initiation of T-Helper Cell Immunity to *Candida albicans* by IL-12: The Role of Neutrophils
L. Romani, F. Bistoni, Perugia; *P. Puccetti,* Rome

136 Identification and Characterization of Protozoan Products That Trigger the Synthesis of IL-12 by Inflammatory Macrophages
R.T. Gazzinelli, Belo Horizonte/Bethesda, Md.; *M.M. Camargo,* Belo Horizonte;
I.C. Almeida, Dundee; *Y.S. Morita,* Baltimore, Md.; *M. Giraldo,* Belo Horizonte;
A. Acosta-Serrano, Baltimore, Md.; *S. Hieny,* Bethesda, Md.;
P.T. Englund, Baltimore, Md.; *M.A.J. Ferguson,* Dundee; *L.R. Travassos,* São Paulo;
A. Sher, Bethesda, Md.

Preface

In the mid-1980s, IL-12 was still a factor; T-cell differentiation factor (TCDF), cytotoxic lymphocyte maturation factor (CLMF), natural killer stimulatory factor (NKSF) were some of the names given to this cytokine. Then, at the beginning of the 1990s, IL-12 was cloned almost simultaneously by two groups, one led by Giorgio Trinchieri at the Wistar Institute in collaboration with Stanley Wolf of Genetics Institute, and the other by Maurice Gately at Hoffmann-La Roche in Nutley. It is really remarkable how rapidly information on IL-12 has accumulated since then.

IL-12 is a unique cytokine in many respects. First, it is the only cytokine detected so far to have a heterodimeric structure composed of two chains, p35 and p40. Second, it is the key cytokine driving Th1 cell development, and the Th1/Th2 dichotomy appears to largely depend on cell sensitivity to IL-12 signaling. Third, it is a potent inducer of IFN-γ production by T and NK cells. This accounts for the important role of IL-12 in bridging innate and acquired cell-mediated immunity. Among its many functions, the induction of Th1 cell development is certainly what has contributed most to attract such a widespread interest in IL-12. In a sense, IL-12 is so central to Th1/Th2 cell development that they both had to be studied together. This underscores the impact of IL-12 research on the current most popular paradigm in immunology: the Th1/Th2 dichotomy. The subdivision of T cells into Th1 and Th2 subsets has been extended to suggest that allograft rejection, antitumor immunity, and most organ-specific autoimmune diseases are Th1-mediated, whereas immediate-type hypersensitivities are Th2-mediated. Although clinical situations are certainly more complex, this paradigm offers the possibility to design straightforward experiments to probe the role of IL-12 in the regulation of Th1 and Th2 cells and in the pathogenesis of immunological diseases. The goal is not only to understand the basic mechanisms induced by IL-12 which control the Th1/Th2 balance, but also to explore the possibility of using IL-12 as an inducer of protective Th1 responses capable of controlling allergies, some infectious diseases and cancer. Conversely, inhibition of endogenous IL-12 could ameliorate Th1-mediated autoimmune diseases.

The contributions collected in this volume represent the most recent findings, reviewed by leading scientists in the field, on several different aspects of IL-12 biology. The opening chapter analyzes the molecular regulation of IL-12 production and its immunomodulatory activities. This is followed by three contributions describing the structure of the IL-12 receptor and its role in determining the early events in the differentiation of T-cell subsets. The modulation of IL-12 activities by other cytokines such as TGF-β, IFN-γ and IL-4 is also addressed. IL-12 is a key cytokine that controls infectious diseases and its role in leishmania, candida, and protozoal infections is specifically examined. IL-12 is one of the most powerful anti-tumor cytokines as yet identified. In this respect, IL-12 provides a new tool to explore the regulatory role of the immune system in tumor development, and a new potential drug which is already being tested in clinical trials. Finally, the role of IL-12 in Th1-mediated autoimmune diseases and the potential for immunotherapy based on IL-12 targeting is discussed. Collectively, these contributions should give a relatively detailed account of the present knowledge on critical aspects of IL-12.

Questions still remain. An intriguing one that I am personally interested in, is whether inhibition of IL-12 may serve as a suitable target for immunointervention in autoimmune diseases. Experimental models clearly indicate the important role of IL-12 in Th1-dependent autoimmunity, but whether this approach may translate into clinical efficacy still remains to be seen.

I would like to thank my colleagues for contributing to this volume and for portraying so vividly the many facets of IL-12. I also wish to thank the dedicated staff at Karger for their assistance in bringing this volume to light.

Luciano Adorini

Adorini L (ed): IL-12. Chem Immunol. Basel, Karger, 1997, vol 68, pp 1–22

....

Immunomodulatory Functions and Molecular Regulation of IL-12

Xiaojing Ma[a], *Miguel Aste-Amezaga*[a], *Giorgia Gri*[a], *Franca Gerosa*[b], *Giorgio Trinchieri*[a]

[a] The Wistar Institute of Anatomy and Biology, Philadelphia, Pa., USA and
[b] Istituto di Immunologia e Malattie Infettive, University of Verona, Italy

Interleukin-12 (IL-12) Production by Different Cell Types

IL-12 is a unique cytokine of 70 kD, composed of two covalently linked chains of 35 kD (p35) and 40 kD (p40) [1]. Although the single p40 chain is always produced in large excess over the p70 heterodimer, only the latter has biological activity and coexpression of both the p40 and the p35 genes in the same cells is required for the production of the biologically active p70 heterodimer [2]. IL-12 was originally identified in the cultured supernatant of Epstein-Barr virus (EBV)-transformed B-cell lines such as RPMI-8866 by virtue of its ability to activate NK cells and to induce production of IFN-γ. All EBV-transformed B-cell lines constitutively produce the p40 chain ranging from negligible amounts to several nanograms per milliliter, and much lower amounts of p70. After 24–48 h stimulation with phorbol diesters, all of them produce higher amounts of the cytokines, up to more than 10 ng/ml of the p40 and 1 ng/ml of p70 for the best producer cell lines, RPMI-8866 and NC37 [1, 3, 4]. Most African Burkitt's lymphoma cell lines produced no or negligible amounts of IL-12. However, most AIDS-associated EBV-positive Burkitt's lymphoma cell lines constitutively produce very high levels of IL-12 which were enhanced by phorbol diester stimulation to levels much higher than those observed in normal B-cell lines [5]. In addition to lymphomas, chronic B-lymphocyte leukemia cells have also been shown to produce low levels of IL-12 [A. Sartori, G. Trinchieri, V. Pistoia, unpubl. results]. Although malignant or EBV-transformed B-cell lines produce IL-12, the physiological relevance of IL-12 from normal B cells remains to be established. In humans, only very low levels of IL-12 were found to be produced by *Staphylococcus aureus* (SAC)-stimulated peripheral blood B cells and by secondary follicle mantle zone B cells, whereas the more mature B cells in the germinal center appear not to produce IL-12 [A.Sartori, G. Trinchieri, V. Pistoia, unpubl. results].

Since the original identification of IL-12 in EBV B cells, it has been firmly established that phagocytic cells are the major source of IL-12 production in response to both gram-negative and gram-positive bacteria or their products such as lipopolysaccharide (LPS) and lipoteichoic acid (LTA) via the CD14 receptor [6]. Recently, bacterial DNA was also shown to be a potent inducer of IL-12 production and this activity was found to be dependent on nonmethylated CpG repeats [7, 8].

The in vivo induction of IL-12 from phagocytic/APC under pathological conditions can be either T-cell-independent or -dependent. Upon infection with bacteria or intracellular parasites, IL-12 is produced rapidly, most likely by direct stimulation of phagocytic cells through T-cell-independent pathways, as demonstrated by the ability of T-cell-deficient SCID mice to produce IL-12 upon infection [9, 10]. DeKruyff et al. [11] and Maruo et al. [12] recently demonstrated using adherent mouse splenic cells as antigen-presenting cells (APCs) that IL-12 production occurred during responses to T-cell-dependent antigens such as OVA and required triggering of CD40 molecules on the APCs. IL-12 production in this T-cell-dependent system increased in direct proportion to antigen concentration and required TCR ligation but not CD28 costimulation, whereas the LPS- or heat-killed *Listeria monocytogenes*-induced IL-12 production occurred in the absence of T cells and was completely independent of CD40 signaling. These findings are extensions of earlier observations on the role of CD40-CD40L interaction in the induction of IL-12 production [13–16]. Additionally, Kato et al. [15] showed in the mouse splenic APC system that the CD40-CD40L interaction plays a critical role in IL-12 p40 mRNA accumulation and bioactive IL-12 production but p35 mRNA accumulation is regulated via a different mechanism.

Dendritic cells (DCs) are professional APCs that have been shown to be the most powerful producers of IL-12 when triggered by the ligation of CD40 with DC40L, even in the absence of cognate antigen recognition. These effects of CD40 ligation result in an increased capacity of DCs to trigger proliferative responses and IFN-γ production by T cells [17–19]. Within the skin cell population, Langerhans' cells (LC), in particular cultured LC maturing into DCs, are the major source of IL-12 production [20].

Polymorphonuclear cells (PMN) also produce IL-12 p40 and p70 in response to LPS stimulation. On a per cell basis, PMN produce less p40 and p70 than monocytes. However, because of the large number of PMN present in the blood or in the inflammatory tissues, it is possible that IL-12 produced locally at the inflammatory site may play an important physiological role against bacterial or parasitic infection.

In addition to phagocytic cells and B lymphocytes, mast cells derived in vitro from mouse bone marrow in the presence of mast cell growth factors and considered representative of connective-type mast cells produce IL-12, whereas IL-3-derived mucosal-type mast cells produce IL-4 [21]. These data, which suggest the existence of different types of mast cells that favor Th1 or Th2 differentiation, await confirmation with data from in vivo differentiated mast cells.

Intracellular bacteria commonly stimulate IL-12 in infected monocytes/ macrophages. *L. monocytogenes*, a facultative intracellular bacterium, is a potent inducer of macrophage activation and cell-mediated immunity. IL-12 production by macrophages is stimulated by *Listeria* and is absolutely required for NK cell IFN-γ production in vitro and in vivo during an initial infection [22]. *Mycobacterium bovis* bacille Calmette-Guérin (BCG), the widely used vaccine strain against tuberculosis, causes chronic infectious disease in mice. Unlike *L. monocytogenes*, production of IL-12 by murine bone marrow-derived macrophages (BMM) in response to *M. bovis* BCG depend on prior stimulation with IFN-γ. In vivo, IL-12 production was induced in spleens of C57BL/6 mice after *M. bovis* BCG infection in a time-dependent fashion but only trace amounts were detectable in supernatants from splenocytes of IFN-γ receptor deficient mice. In addition, IL-12 production in *M. bovis* BCG-infected C57Bl/6 mice was inhibited by administration of anti-IFN-γ mAbs [23]. The mechanism of IFN-γ priming of the producer cells for higher IL-12 production is discussed in greater detail later. *Mycobacterium tuberculosis* infection of humans resulted in selectively concentrated p40 mRNA and protein in pleural fluid, compared to blood. In addition, the frequency of IL-12-producing macrophages is much greater in lymph nodes from tuberculosis patients than in normal lymph nodes [24]. Possibly as a result of the locally activated IL-12 expression, tuberculosis patients mount a strong cell-mediated immune response, restricting the growth of the pathogen. On the other hand, patients infected with *Mycobacterium leprae* showed 10- to 50-fold lower p40 mRNA in lepromatous lesions than in tuberculoid lesions while p35 mRNA levels were equal in both lesions. The percentage of IL-12 p70 positive cells as identified by immunohistology was 10-fold lower in lepromatous granulomas than in tuberculoid lesions, suggesting that the weak cell-mediated immunity and strong humoral responses manifested by lepromatous patients may be due to the lower levels of locally produced IL-12. *Salmonella* spp. causes typhoid fever in humans. Chong et al. [25] have shown that murine macrophages produced IL-12 p40 mRNA differentially in response to viable or killed *Salmonella* spp., correlating with protection of mice that produced higher levels of IL-12 p40 in response to viable organisms.

Infection of macrophages by intracellular parasites generally induce IL-12 production which plays a pivotal role in determining the outcome of the infection. When *Leishmania major* promastigotes were analyzed for their ability to induce IL-12 production in human PBMC, metacyclic promastigotes were found to be very poor inducers of IL-12. Moreover, these promastigotes and the factors they secreted into the supernatant fluid strongly inhibited IL-12 production induced by other stimuli. IFN-γ priming of PBMC, however, resulted in quite elevated IL-12 production upon addition of metacyclic promastigotes. Unlike the more mature metacyclic parasite, procyclic promastigotes, collected after 2 days' expansion in culture, were very efficient inducers of IL-12 production and were much less inhibitive of IL-12 production induced by other stimuli [A. Sartori, P. Scott, G. Trinchieri, submitted for publication]. In addition, tissue-phase amastigote forms of *Leishmania* also induced PCR-detectable p40 mRNA expression in macrophage cultures [26]. Interestingly, a recombinant *Leishmania braziliensis* antigen derived from the ribosomal protein eIF4A induces IL-12 and IFN-γ production in PBMC [27].

Toxoplasma gondii stimulates macrophages to produce IL-12 during infection. The potent induction of IL-12 by *T. gondii* can be mimicked by the use of a soluble tachyzoite extract (STAg) in cultures of thioglycolate-elicited macrophages from LPS nonresponsive C3H/HeJ mice, and the induction is dramatically enhanced in the presence of IFN-γ [9]. The effect of STAg on the induction of IL-12 can be recapitulated in an in vitro transient transfection system using the human IL-12 p40 promoter linked to the luciferase gene and the murine macrophage-derived cell line RAW264.7, suggesting that the regulation of IL-12 by STAg is exerted primarily at the transcriptional level [pers. unpubl. results]. Nevertheless, co-culture of *T. gondii* antigen and macrophages from IFN-γ-deficient mice also resulted in augmented IL-12 production, thus, *T. gondii* is capable of triggering IL-12 synthesis both in vitro and in vivo in the absence of IFN-γ [28].

Coutelier et al. [29] analyzed IL-12 message expression after infection of mice with lactase dehydrogenase-elevating virus (LDV), mouse hepatitis virus, and mouse adenovirus, and found that the p40 message was transiently induced shortly after infection. Biron and Orange [30] examined the induction of IL-12 expression in C57BL/6 mice infected with mouse cytomegalovirus (MCMV) or lymphocyte choriomeningitis virus (LCMV). IL-12 p40 evaluated by ELISA and p70 heterodimer measured by a capture biological assay were not detectable in samples from LCMV-infected mice but were expressed at significant levels in MCMV-infected mice, peaking on day 2 after infection which correlated with the emergence of the production of IFN-γ. Influenza virus induces

IL-12 p40 production in the bronchoalveolar lavage of the lungs beginning at day 3 postinfection and peaking at around day 5. By day 10, the level of IL-12 p40 returns to the preinfection level. Live virus is needed for the induction. The endogenous IL-12 is critical for the initial IFN-γ production up to day 5 postinfection and for the protection of infected mice by, possibly, a CTL-related mechanism. However, IL-12 appears to have no effect on viral titer or virally induced lung pathology [31]. Herpes simplex virus (HSV) has been shown to induce IL-12 p40 production upon infection of the mouse eye [32]. There is an early induction and maintenance of IL-12 p40 mRNA in the cornea and draining lymph node upon ocular infection with HSV. Inflammatory cells including DCs, macrophages and neutrophils that infiltrate the cornea in response to HSV infection appear to be the main source of IL-12 p40 production.

HIV-infected individuals have decreased production of SAC-stimulated IL-12 in PBMC. The reduced IL-12 production was also observed in monocytes infected in vitro with HIV [34, 35]. This deficiency of IL-12 production in HIV-seropositive individuals can be overcome by priming PBMC with IFN-γ [36] and, even more efficiently, with IL-4 or IL-13 [J. Marshall, G. Trinchieri, J. Chehimi, submitted for publication]. Another study also reported a decreased p40 expression in PBMC from HIV+ patients, as well as decreased Th1 responses, after stimulation by *T. gondii* antigens [37]. The mechanism(s) by which HIV infection results in the suppressed IL-12 production has not been determined although it appears that infection of all producer cells is not required for this effect, suggesting that HIV may cause the inhibition of IL-12 production through an indirect route, e.g. by the secretion of either host or virally encoded factor(s).

Similarly to HIV infection, infection with measles virus and vaccination with high titer measles vaccines are also associated with immunodepression, although transient, characterized by expression of Th2 cytokines and defective T-cell proliferation and DTH. In vitro infection of monocyte cultures with measles results in a profound inhibition of both IL-12 p70 and p40 production, with minimal effect on the production of other proinflammatory cytokines [38]. This inhibitory effect on IL-12 production is most likely due to the interaction of the measles virus with its receptor on monocytes, CD46 or membrane cofactor protein (MCP), because monoclonal antibodies against CD46 or another of its ligands, polymerized C3b, also selectively depress IL-12 production in human monocytes [38], and this inhibition occurs at the transcriptional level [pers. unpubl. data]. The presence of the regulatory linkage between the complement system and cell-mediated immunity (CMI) provided by CD46 implies the possibility of its subversion by other macrophage-tropic pathogens. For example, infection with HIV is associated with profound defects in mononuclear cell-derived IL-12 production and CMI [34, 35]. HIV efficiently activates complement, and virions as well as productively infected cells are coated with C3 activation fragments. The data presented by Karp et al. [37] suggest the hypothesis that such complement opsonization of pathogens may lead to suppression of CMI through the inhibition of IL-12 production by monocytes.

Molecular Regulation of IL-12 Gene Expression

The production of IL-12 is regulated by both positive and negative feedback mechanisms involving Th1 cytokines such as IFN-γ and Th2 cytokines such as IL-10 and IL-4, respectively, as central players in the regulatory pathways [38]. The ability of IFN-γ to enhance the production of IL-12 by phagocytic cells [39, 40] is of particular interest because IL-12 is a potent inducer of IFN-γ production by T and NK cells [41]. Thus, IL-12-induced IFN-γ acts as a potent positive feedback mechanism in inflammation by enhancing IL-12 production. Also, because IL-12 is the major cytokine responsible for the differentiation of T-helper type 1 cells which are potent producers of IFN-γ [42], the enhancing effect of IFN-γ on IL-12 production may represent a mechanism by which Th1 responses are maintained in vivo. In both monocytes and PMN, the enhancing effect of IFN-γ on IL-12 production is observed when IFN-γ is added simultaneously to the stimulus (e.g. LPS), but it is more effective when the producer cells are primed for 12–18 h in the presence of IFN-γ [43, 44]. In addition to IFN-γ, GM-CSF has a modest enhancing effect on IL-12 production by phagocytic cells [39]. Unlike IFN-γ which enhances the expression of the IL-12 p40 and p35 genes, GM-CSF priming only enhances the production of p40 [43, pers. unpubl. observation]. The ability of IFN-γ to enhance IL-12 production is particularly evident in the case of certain infectious agents, e.g. mycobacteria, which are rather poor inducers of IL-12 production. In in vitro or in vivo infections with these microorganisms, IFN-γ production appears to precede and to be required for IL-12 production [45]. However, with many other inducers, such as LPS, toxoplasma, and SAC, IL-12 production in vivo and in vitro both precedes and is required for IFN-γ production. For example, following injection of LPS, IL-12 is induced at 2–3 h, simultaneously with the induction of expression of IL-12 receptors and it is followed by IFN-γ production at 5–7 h [46 pers. unpubl. results]. Neutralizing anti-IL-12 antibodies inhibit IFN-γ production, but anti-IFN-γ antibodies do not inhibit IL-12 production. With potent inducers such as LPS or *T. gondii*, IL-12 production is also observed in mice that lack functional IFN-γ or IFN-γ receptor genes.

A detailed molecular analysis examining simultaneously the nuclear transcription, steady-state mRNA and secreted protein levels established that the human IL-12 p40 gene is primarily regulated by IFN-γ and LPS at the transcriptional level in monocytic cells [44]. Both the human and mouse IL-12 p40 gene promoters have been cloned [44, 47]. The 3.3 kb human p40 promoter, when linked to a luciferase reporter gene and transfected transiently into various IL-12-producing and nonproducing cell lines, largely recapitulated the tissue specificity of the endogenous p40 gene in that it is constitutively active in EBV-transformed B-cell lines (e.g. RPMI-8866, CESS), and inducible in myeloid cell lines (e.g. THP-1 and RAW264.7), but inactive in T-cell lines (e.g. Molt-13 and Jurkat) [44]. Moreover, this promoter construct responds to IFN-γ priming in monocytic cells, much like the endogenous p40 gene transcription, suggesting that it contains sufficient sequence elements to reconstitute the in vivo response.

A comparison of the human and mouse IL-12 p40 promoters revealed some interesting features. The promoters are well conserved up to approximately –400 with respect to the transcription start site, where the homology breaks down with large gaps between them. Within the –400 proximal promoter region, several putative transcription factor-binding motifs are very well conserved: ets at –211/–206, PU.1 and NFκB between –124 and –105. Functional characterization of the human p40 promoter in myeloid cell lines has identified the ets element, TTTCCT (AGGAAA for the complement), as a major response region. This element interacts with a large nuclear complex named F1 that binds to a region between –196 and –292. By electrophoretic mobility shift assay (EMSA) and DNAse I footprint/methylation interference assays, we have established that F1: (1) is induced by LPS or IFN-γ in RAW264.7; (2) interacts with the ets-2 element within the –211/–206 region in a complex way, i.e. the interaction requires substantial flanking 'anchoring' space; (3) may function as a transcription activator in response to IFN-γ and LPS stimulation since loss of binding results in dramatic decrease in promoter activity; (4) is consisted of multiple factors including ets-2, IRF-1, c-Rel, and a novel, 109-kD protein that is highly induced by either IFN-γ or LPS (hence named Glp109 for its IFN-γ and LPS inducibility), and (5) its induction appears to be closely correlated with the expression of the IL-12 p40 gene in various cell lines and primary human monocytes [48]. A second factor that also interacts with this region but requires less physical space is a complex formed with a fragment derived from –196 to –243 of the p40 promoter, named F2. F2 seems to respond more to IFN-γ stimulation than to LPS, yet its identity remains to be established. An interesting observation is that the ets element in unstimulated RAW264.7 cells is occupied by PU.1 which becomes displaced by F1 upon IFN-γ or LPS stimulation [48].

The regulation of IL-12 p40 gene transcription in the EBV-B cell line RPMI-8866 appears to be somewhat divergent from that of monocytic cells. The transfected p40 promoter is constitutively active, paralleling the endogenous gene. The nuclear complex F1 is also constitutively present but its role in the regulation of the p40 gene transcription does not seem to be as prominent as it is in monocytic cells in that elimination of the F1-binding element resulted in a decrease of the promoter activity by only 30%. The composition of F1 in RPMI cells differs also from that of monocytic cells in that IRF-2, instead of IRF-1, is present. The implication of the differing composition of F1 is not clear at the present time. Another region of potential transcriptional regulation is the 'NFκB half site' located between –116 and –106, TGAAATTCCCC (or GGGGAATTTCA for the complement). This site has been reported by Murphy et al. [47] in the mouse IL-12 p40 promoter to bind NFκB (p50/p65 and p50/c-Rel) in macrophages activated by a number of IL-12-activating pathogens including LPS and SAC. In EBV-B cells, NFκB constitutively binds to this site. The NFκB complex is composed of c-Rel and p50 heterodimers [pers. unpubl. observation]. Base substitutions at this site, which abolishes the NFκB binding, results in about 70% decrease in the constitutive promoter activity in B-cell lines. Our preliminary data in cotransfection experiments with various combinations of expression vectors containing cDNAs for NFκB p65, p50, c-Rel, and ets-2 demonstrated that ets-2 and c-Rel can synergistically activate the transfected p40 promoter in both IL-12 p40-expressing cells (RPMI-8866), and non-expressing cells such as Bjab (EBV-negative B-cell line) and Jurkat (T-cell line), strongly suggesting that c-Rel and ets-2 may be the transcription factors essential and sufficient to determine the cell type-specific expression of the p40 gene.

Study of expression of the IL-12 p35 gene is hindered by the fact that this gene is not highly active and inducible, in addition to the complication by the ubiquity of its expression. Comparative studies with cycloheximide (CHX) demonstrated fundamental differences in mRNA regulation of IL-12 p40 and p35 genes. The increase in SAC- or LPS-induced IL-12 p40 mRNA level was abrogated when the cells were pretreated with CHX, suggesting that the regulation of IL-12 p40 gene requires the induction of a CHX-sensitive, transcription activator(s). Conversely, IL-12 p35 mRNA was further up-regulated indicating that the activation of IL-12 p35 mRNAs requires only presynthesized activator(s) that can be activated either by SAC or LPS at posttranslational level. Superinduction of some cytokine genes such as TNF-α, IL1-β [49], IFN-γ, and IL-2, [50, 51] is observed when the cells are induced in the absence of CHX for about 2 h, followed by addition of CHX. IL-12 p40 and p35 steady-state mRNA levels underwent superinduction when CHX was added 2 h after SAC [M. Aste-Amezaga, X. Ma, G. Trinchieri, manuscript in preparation].

The promoters of the mouse p35 gene contains putative elements including Sp1, AP1, ISRE, ICSBP, NFκB, GATA-1, and GAS [52, 53]. Unlike the p40 gene, the p35 gene appears to initiate its transcription from multiple sites. It is of great interest to investigate the nature of these alternatively initiated transcripts with respect to their cell-type distribution and response to different stimuli. Based on the increasing number of observations, it appears that under certain conditions the p35 chain may be a rate-limiting factor and may play a critical role in determining the level of IL-12 p70 production via either altering its level of expression or its posttranslational modification which would affect its association with the p40 chain, in response to specific inducers in IL-12-producing cells [54].

The positive feedback amplification of IL-12 production mediated by IFN-γ obviously represents a potentially dangerous mechanism leading to uncontrolled cytokine production and possibly shock. There are, however, potent mechanisms of down-regulation of IL-12 production and of the ability of T and NK cells to respond to IL-12. The Th2 cytokine IL-10 is a potent inhibitor of IL-12 production by phagocytic cells; the ability of IL-10 to suppress production of IFN-γ and other Th1 cytokines is primarily due to its inhibition of IL-12 production from APCs as well as by inhibition of expression of other costimulatory surface molecules (e.g. B7) and soluble cytokines (e.g. TNF-α, ILβ) [55–57]. Note that IL-12 is able to induce IL-10 production and to prime T-cell clones for high IL-10 production both in vivo [58] and in vitro [59–63], indicating that IL-12 can induce factors that enhance (via IFN-γ) or suppress (via IL-10) its own production. Our studies on the effect of IL-10 on SAC- or LPS-induced IL-12 p40 and p35 gene expression in PBMCs and monocytes demonstrate that IL-10 inhibition of IL-12 production is accompanied by reduced steady-state mRNA levels of the two components of the heterodimeric cytokine, i.e. p40 and p35. The mechanism(s) of IL-10 suppression of IL-12 p40 appears to be mainly at the level of transcription, without significant modulation of mRNA stability. The transcriptional activity of IL-12 p35, primed by IFN-γ and induced by LPS, was also substantially inhibited by IL-10. The $t_{1/2}$ of SAC-induced IL-12 p40, was 4 h and not altered by IL-10. We also observed that CHX abolished the inhibitory effect of IL-10 on the induction of IL-12 p40, IL-12 p35 and TNF-α mRNAs. This, together with other reports [64–66], suggests that IL-10 may exert its negative effect through a newly synthesized repressor protein(s).

Another powerful inhibitor of IL-12 production is TGF-β [67]. IL-4 and IL-13 can also partially inhibit IL-12 production, suggesting the hypothesis that Th2 cells, by producing cytokines such as IL-10, IL-4 and IL-13, suppress IL-12 production and prevent the emergence of a Th1 response. However, if monocytes are primed with IL-4 or IL-13 for 24 h or longer, IL-12 production is not inhibited, and instead is significantly enhanced [67]. The mechanism of enhancement of IL-12 production by IL-4 and IL-13 may be secondary to a differentiation effect on monocytes, which requires prolonged incubation and exposure to the cytokine, unlike the inhibitory effect observed when the cytokines are added simultaneously to the IL-12 inducers. In this context, it is of interest to note that the inhibitory effects of Th2 cytokines IL-10, IL-6, and IL-4 on the regulation of IL-12 production induced through the T-cell-dependent and -independent pathways were further examined by Takenaka et al. [68] using murine macrophage/DCs. IL-10 inhibited IL-12 production induced through both pathways. IL-6 inhibited only IL-12 production induced through the T-cell independent pathway. IL-4 inhibited T-cell independent IL-12 production while potentiating the T-cell-dependent IL-12 production. Interestingly, treatment of PBMC from HIV(+) patients with IL-4 or IL-13 almost completely corrects their inability to produce IL-12 in response to SAC [J. Marshall, G. Trinchieri, J. Chehimi, submitted for publication].

Induction of IFN-γ Production by IL-12 in Both Resting and Activated T Lymphocytes and NK Cells

IL-12 induces IFN-γ production from resting and activated NK and T cells, with a similar dose-response relationship and half-maximal activity at 3.5 pM [1, 41]. Within T cells, $CD4^+/CD8^+$ T cells with αβ T-cell receptor (TCR) and T cells with γδ TCR are induced to produce IFN-γ [41]. The induction of IFN-γ by IL-12 is characterized by a powerful synergistic effect with other IFN-γ inducers, in particular IL-2 and phorbol diesters [1, 41]. On T cells, IL-12 also synergizes with mitogenic lectins, with stimulation of the TCR-CD3 complex by anti-CD3 antibodies or alloantigens [41], and with stimulation of the CD28 receptor by anti-CD28 antibodies or its ligand B7 [56, 57]; and on NK cells with stimulation by ligands of the CD16 receptor for IgG-Fc (anti-CD16 antibodies or immunocomplexes) and by target cells [69]. IL-12 rapidly increases the transcriptional rate of the IFN-γ gene; however, when IL-12 and IL-2 are added together to the cells, most of the synergistic effects of the two inducers is observed at the posttranscriptional level, with an increase of more than 2-fold of the half-life of the IFN-γ mRNA in the cells treated with the two inducers together [70, 71]. Both resting and activated NK and T cells are induced by IL-12 to produce IFN-γ, although maximal IFN-γ mRNA accumulation is reached in 2–4 h in activated T or NK cells and in 18–24 h in resting peripheral blood lymphocytes (PBL) [41]. Within PBL, IL-12 induces mRNA accumulation, as detected by in situ hybridization, in a proportion of both NK and T cells [41], although NK cells might be a major contributor to the early production of IFN-γ in response to IL-12 or IL-2 [72]. Although NK and T cells are the IFN-γ producers in PBL preparations stimulated by IL-12, an accessory cell type (MHC class II-positive, nonmonocyte, non-B cells) is required for optimal IFN-γ production by resting PBL [41]. These accessory cells might provide costimulatory molecules for IFN-γ production. In murine spleen cells, it has been shown that IL-12 synergizes with TNF-α in inducing IFN-γ production [73, 74]. This synergistic effect of TNF-α was not demonstrated with human lymphocytes, but antibodies to TNF-α or IL-1β efficiently inhibited IL-12-induced IFN-γ production suggesting that these two cytokines endogenously produced in the PBL cultures, possibly by the class II-positive accessory cells, act as constimulatory molecules for IFN-γ production together with IL-12 [55]. Another costimulatory signal possibly provided by the accessory cells is the B7 molecule, ligand for the CD28 receptors on T cells. Stimulation of T cells with B7-transfected cells or with anti-CD28 antibodies strongly synergized with IL-12 for induction of IFN-γ production [56, 57] and blocking of B7-CD28 interaction with the hybrid recombinant molecule CTLA4-Ig significantly inhibited the ability of PBL to produce IFN-γ in response to IL-12 [56]. These results suggest that TNF-α, IL-1β, and B7, possibly at least in part provided by the class II accessory cells, are important costimulators for IFN-γ production in response to IL-12. The ability of IL-10 to inhibit IFN-γ production in T and NK cells is primarily due to its ability to suppress IL-12 production, but also, in part, to its ability to suppress expression of these costimulatory molecules on accessory cells [55–57].

The ability of IL-12 to induce a rapid production of IFN-γ in vivo has been clearly shown in several experimental models of infectious diseases. A very informative experimental model for the understanding of the role of IL-12 in inducing IFN-γ in vivo is provided by the endotoxic shock in BCG-primed mice [46]. Several cytokines, in particular TNF-α and IFN-γ, have been shown to be responsible for pathologic reactions which may lead to shock and death observed in infection with Gram-negative bacteria and in response to endotoxins. Priming of mice with the avirulent BCG vaccine strain of *M. bovis* increases the sensitivity of mice to the lethal effect of LPS and results in an efficient priming for cytokine production in response to LPS. Mice injected with LPS produced IL-12 which induced IFN-γ production, as demonstrated by the ability of neutralizing anti-IL-12 which induced IFN-γ production, as demonstrated by the ability of neutralizing anti-IL-12 antibodies to suppress IFN-γ production [46]. However, the concentration of biologically active IL-12 was similar in the serum of both BCG-primed or unprimed mice, reaching levels of 1–3 ng/ml at 3–6 h after LPS injection, whereas IFN-γ production was observed only in BCG-primed mice [46]. TNF-α and other

LPS-induced cofactors were required in cooperation with IL-12 to induce optimal IFN-γ production. The priming effect of BCG on IFN-γ production appears to be mostly due to its ability to increase TNF-α production, which acts as cofactor with LPS-induced IL-12 in inducing IFN-γ production [46]. Neutralizing anti-IL-12 antibodies, in addition to inhibiting the in vivo LPS-induced IFN-γ production, also protected mice from septic shock-induced death [46]. Thus, IL-12 is required for IFN-γ production and lethality in an endotoxic shock model in mice.

Induction of Th1 and Th2 Cell Differentiation by IL-12 and IL-4, Respectively

The requirement of IL-4 for the generation of IL-4-producing Th2 cells has been a well-established concept for several years [75–77]. More recently, the role of IL-12 for the efficient generation of IFN-γ production Th1 cells has become evident, and it has been proposed that the balance between the levels of IL-4 and IL-12 early during an immune response may be responsible to bias the generation of Th2 and Th1 cells, respectively [78], although the presence of other cytokines and various other factors regulating the immune response also play a major role. Furthermore, the synergistic/antagonistic interaction between IL-4 and IL-12 in regulating such responses is complex and not yet fully understood [59, 79].

Stimulation in vitro of PBL from atopic patients with allergens such as *Dermatophagoides pteronyssinus* Group 1 (Der p1) results in the generation of T-cell lines and clones with the high IL-4 and low IFN-γ production typical of Th2-cells, whereas PBL stimulation with bacterial products (e.g. purified protein derivative, PPD) generate Th1-type T-cell lines and clones that produce IFN-γ but not IL-4. When PBL are stimulated with Der p1 in the presence of IL-12, T-cell lines and clones are generated that exhibited a reduced ability to produce IL-4 and an increased ability to produce IFN-γ [42]. This Th1-inducing effect of IL-12 was not inhibited by anti-IFN-γ, but was reduced by removal of NK cells from the PBL preparation. PPD-specific T-cell lines generated in the presence of anti-IL-12 antibodies during the initial antigenic stimulation produced significant levels of IL-4, unlike the cell lines generated in the absence of antibodies, and gave rise to PPD-specific CD4$^+$ cell clones showing a Th0/Th2 phenotype rather than a Th1 phenotype [42]. These results indicate not only that IL-12 is able to facilitate proliferation and activation of Th1 cells in a memory response in vitro, but also that, as shown by the effect of anti-IL-12 antibodies, endogenously produced IL-12 is an obligatory factor for Th1 generation.

The ability of IL-12 to directly initiate Th1 cell development in naive T cells was shown by Hsieh et al. [79] who reported that naive CD4$^+$ T cells derived from mice transgenic for an antiovalbumin TCR are induced by ovalbumin to develop into Th1 cells in the presence of IL-12, whereas they develop into Th2 cells in the presence of IL-4. The effect of IL-4 in that system is, however, dominant over that of IL-12. Since these early studies, the ability of IL-12 to induce Th1 cell generation was demonstrated in many models, in humans and in experimental animals, both in vitro and in vivo [38]. The originally reported dominance of IL-4 action over IL-12 [80] was observed to be a much more complex interaction, with the two cytokines antagonizing or synergizing each other, depending on the function analyzed [59, 79, 81].

The experimental system used for studying Th response have not permitted determination of whether the different cytokines affecting Th cell development, induce differentiation of bipotential Th precursors or rather a selective priming and/or expansion of already committed Th1 and Th2 precursor cells [82–85]. This question is particularly relevant in human studies analyzing clonal expansion of memory Th cells [42, 86]. However, once a Th1 or Th2 response has been established, it appears to be relatively stable, and no factors capable of inducing qualitative changes in the cytokine profile of established murine or human T-cell clones have been reported.

In the analysis of cytokine production from human T cells stimulated with recall antigens (PPD) or allergens (Der p1), the expansion of the small proportion of memory T cells was first obtained in polyclonal T-cell cultures, from which single antigen-specific clones were obtained only after several weeks of culture of the polyclonal cell line [42, 86]. During this culture period, emergence of Th cell subsets with characteristic cytokine production profiles could be due to differentiation of precursor Th cells, as well as to positive selection (growth advantage) of certain Th subsets or negative selection (apoptosis, cytotoxicity, antiproliferative effects) of other subsets.

When human T-cell cultures were stimulated by a polyclonal stimulus such as PHA or anti-CD3, in the presence or absence of IL-12, similar results were obtained as in antigen-stimulated cultures, i.e. IFN-γ production by the cells was enhanced and IL-4 production was almost completely abolished [87]. However, very different results were obtained when freshly islolted human peripheral blood T cells were immediately cloned by limiting dilution in cultures stimulated by PHA and IL-2, in the presence or absence of IL-12 [88]. When restimulated with anti-CD3 and TPA after 5 weeks of culture, the clones generated in the presence of IL-12 produced on average 5- to 20-fold higher levels of IFN-γ than the clones generated in the absence of IL-12. This priming for IFN-γ production required the addition of IL-12 within the first week, but its presence for maximal priming was required only for 1 or 2 weeks [59].

Once the clones were established for 2 or 3 weeks, removal or additon of IL-12 from the culture medium did not significantly affect their ability to produce IFN-γ [88]. Because the cloning efficiency in these experiments was close to 100%, the priming effect of IL-12 was not due to selection of high IFN-γ-producing clones, but was exerted on each single T cell, naive or memory. Furthermore, this effect was observed on both $CD4^+$ and $CD8^+$ cells, suggesting that IL-12 affects the differentiation of Th1-type clones from both subsets. Thus, the presence of IL-12 during the initial clonal proliferation of T cells induces an irreversible priming for high IFN-γ production, which is maintained even when the clones are cultured for several weeks in the absence of IL-12. However, unlike what is consistently observed in vivo in polyclonal cultures and their derivative clones, the clones originated by limiting dilution in the presence or absence of IL-12 did not show any significant difference in their average ability to produce IL-4 [87, 88]. These results suggested that the ability of IL-12 to prime $CD4^+$ cells for high IFN-γ production is due to a differentiation effect acting at the level of $CD4^+$ T-cell clone precursors. The ability of IL-12 to down-regulate IL-4 production, however, was not observed at the clonal level, and is likely due to selective processes operative on polyclonal cultures and not to a direct effect on single clonal progenitors [88]. The nature of these mechanisms remains to be investigated, although a possible selective proliferative effect of IL-12 on Th1 clones or on IFN-γ-mediated negative selection against IL-4-producing clones can be postulated. Alternatively, the down-regulation of IL-4 production might be a differentiation effect that requires cellular interaction or cell crowding (e.g. for the production Th2-suppressing factors such as IFN-γ) during the initial phase of proliferation of the T cells; such interactions are not obtained in limiting dilution cultures, even in the presence of irradiated feeder cells.

CD4$^+$ and CD8$^+$ clones obtained by limiting dilution in the presence of IL-12 produced significantly more IL-10 than clones generated in the absence of IL-12 [59]. We also observed that stimulation of human T-cell clones in the presence of IL-12 results in a severalfold increase in IL-10 production, in both high or low IL-10-producing clones [D. Peritt, G. Trinchieri, in preparation]. However, in allergen-stimulated polyclonal T-cell culture, IL-12 was shown to down-regulate both IL-10 and IL-4 [89]. These apparently contradictory results are, however, consistent with the conclusion that IL-12 directly up-regulates Th1 cytokine production, but suppresses Th2 cytokine production by an indirect, possibly selective mechanism. These data also put in a new light the observation that IL-12 treatment in vivo induces accumulation of IL-10 mRNA [58]: although that finding was attributed to production of IL-10 by macrophages, the possibility that IL-12 also induces IL-10 production from T cells must now be investigated.

Exogenously added or endogenously produced IL-4 was necessary in the limiting dilution cultures to prime T-cell clones generated from 'naive' CD45RO$^-$CD4$^+$ T cells for IL-4 production. Although IL-12 is a major and probably necessary inducer of a Th1 response, it was also shown to potentiate IL-4 production and the development of Th2 cells from naive CD4$^+$ murine T cells [90] and from neonatal CD4$^+$ human T cells [91], and to potentiate a Th2 response to *Schitosoma mansoni* in IFN-γ knockout mice [92]. We [59] showed that IL-12 does not prevent IL-4 production from CD4$^+$ clones derived from limiting dilutions of 'naive' adult peripheral blood CD45RO$^-$ cells and, in fact, significantly enhances the ability of IL-4 to prime the clones for high IL-4 production, thus extending the previous results [90–92] by demonstrating the IL-12 can enhance IL-4 production at the single clonal level via a differentiation effect. Furthermore, when T cells were cloned in the simultaneous presence of IL-12 and IL-4, the IFN-γ priming effect of IL-12 was only partially and often not significantly inhibited by IL-4, whereas the priming for IL-10 production was reproducibly and almost completely blocked by IL-4 [59]. Thus, paradoxically, IL-4 is more potent in inhibiting priming of Th cells for production of a Th2-type cytokine than for the typical Th1-type cytokine, IFN-γ.

Acute Induction versus Priming for Cytokine Production

From the studies of the generation of Th1 and Th2 cells, including those of our group reviewed above, it is becoming apparent that production of lymphokines, both type 1 and type 2, can be regulated with two different mechanisms. The first mechanism, observed particularly in preactivated lymphocytes, but also in resting T cells and NK cells, is the ability of various stimuli, including TCR stimulation and other stimuli or costimuli, including cytokines, acting alone or in combination, to rapidly induce gene expression and cytokine production. For example, IL-12, alone or in synergy with other stimuli, induces accumulation of mRNA for IFN-γ within a few hours of treatment of either resting or activated T or NK cells, followed by secretion of IFN-γ. This acute induction of IFN-γ subsides within a couple of days (or, in vivo, even within less than 12 h [46]) and does not induce a permanent alteration in the ability of the cells to produce IFN-γ in response to IL-12 or other stimuli.

The phenomenon of priming of the cytokine genes is quite different from acute induction. When T cells (and NK cells) are clonally expanded in the presence of IL-12 during the first few days of expansion, the clones are primed for high production of IFN-γ and IL-10 even when cultured for several more weeks in the absence of IL-12 and then restimulated in its absence; conversely, the exposure of T cells to IL-4 during clonal expansion induces priming for IL-4 production and generation of IL-4-producing cells. IL-12 is particularly potent in mediating both acute induction of the IFN-γ gene and in stably priming it for response to other stimuli; however, although IL-12 similarly primes the IL-10 gene, its ability to acutely induce this gene is modest and difficult to demonstrate. Analogously, whereas IL-4 is necessary and extremely potent for the priming of the IL-4 and the generation of IL-4-producing cells, its ability to acutely induce the expression of the IL-4 gene has not been demonstrated. The IL-2 effect on lymphokine production is different from that of IL-12 and IL-4: IL-2, alone or in synergy with other stimuli, is a potent inducer of acute expression of the several lymphokines, including IFN-γ, IL-4, and IL-10; however, although the presence of IL-2 may be required in the priming phenomena of all three genes, IL-2 by itself does not determine the specificity of the priming, that is instead dictated by IL-12 and IL-4 [41, 72, 93].

The priming of lymphokine genes represents a stable modification of the inducibility of the genes which is analogous to the stable phenotype in the pattern of cytokine production typical of Th subsets. Thus, it is likely that this priming mechanism plays a role in the determination of the Th phenotype of activated T cells. However, certain effects of IL-12 and IL-4 on Th generation are not observed when the ability of these cytokines to induce differentiation is analyzed at the single clonal level (for example, in this clonal analysis, the powerful ability of IL-12 to block IL-4 production is not reproduced and IL-12, paradoxically, induces T-cells priming for production of IL-10, a prevalently type 2 cytokine). Thus, although the priming of lymphokine genes is most likely the predominant mechanism by which IL-12 and IL-4 induce differentiation of Th cells, the finall generation of cells with Th1 and Th2 phenotype, both in vivo and in vitro, also depends on complex indirect effects of the cytokines, including selective mechanisms, in addition to a direct differentiative effect at the single cell level.

The molecular mechanisms of both the acute induction and the priming effects, still remain largely undetermined. The major signal transduction mechanisms for IL-4 and IL-12 have recently been elucidated, with the former cytokine inducing activation of STAT-6 [94] and the latter of STAT-1, -3 and -4 [95, 96]; however, the role of these transcription factors in the induction of expression of the IL-4, IFN-γ , and the IL-10 genes still remains to be investigated. The priming effects may depend on induction of a constitutive or facilitated expression of the transcription factors responsible for the expression of the lymphokine genes or in a stable alteration of the genes in a transcriptionally-prone conformation. For example, the IFN-γ gene has been shown to be differentially methylated in Th1 and Th2 clones [97]. Post-transcriptional mechanisms could also be responsible for the priming effect.

Conclusions

IL-12 is a unique heterodimeric cytokine with important immunoregulatory activities in both the innate and adaptive immunities. Its main sources are APCs which produce IL-12 in response to pathogenic and antigenic stimulation in either the T-cell-independent (via CD14) or -dependent (through CD40-CD40L interactions) pathways. The production of IL-12 is regulated also by both positive and negative feedback mechanisms, depending on the specific pathological conditions. IFN-γ on the one hand, IL-10 and IL-4 on the other, represent some of the key players in the loops. The mechanisms by which IFN-γ and LPS induce IL-12 p40 and p35 gene expression in monocytic cells are beginning to be understood. Our data suggest that there may be protein-protein interactions between members of the ets and NFκB family at specific sites of the p40 promoter which result in synergistic activation of p40 gene transcription in response to certain stimuli in monocytic cells or constitutively in EBV-B cells.

IL-12, a potent inducer of IFN-γ production in T and NK cells, induces the differentiation of type 1 cytokine-producing T cells primarily through its ability to prime them for high IFN-γ production. However, paradoxically, IL-12 also primes T cells for high production of the type 2 cytokine IL-10. The ability of IL-12 to induce generation of Th1 cells is most likely mediated by direct differentiation effects acting at the single cell level and indirect selective mechanisms. IL-4, which has a very powerful effect in priming T cells for IL-4 production, does not appear to have a significant ability to directly and acutely activate the expression of the IL-4 gene. Thus, two mechanisms appear to be involved in the regulation of the expression of type 1 and type 2 cytokine genes by IL-12 and IL-4: a rapid and reversible acute induction of gene expression, and a priming of the genes to a highly responsive state to restimulation, a state that is stable, maintained through repeated cell divisions, and probably irreversible.

References

1   Kobayashi M, Fitz L, Ryan M, Hewick RM, Clark SC, Chan S, Loudon R, Sherman F, Perussia B, Trinchieri G: Identification and purification of natural killer cell stimulatory factor, a cytokine with multiple biologic effects on human lymphocytes. J Exp Med 1989;170:827–846.
2   Wolf SF, Temple PA, Kobayashi M, Young D, Dicig M, Lowe L, Dzialo R, Fitz L, Ferenz C, Hewick RM, Kelleher K, Herrmann SH, Clark SC, Azzoni L, Chan SH, Trinchieri G, Perussia B: Cloning of cDNA for natural killer cell stimulatory factor, a heterodimeric cytokine with multiple biologic effects on T and natural killer cells. J Immunol 1991;146:3074–3081.
3   Stern AS, Podlaski FJ, Hulmes JD, Pan YE, Quinn PM, Wolitzky AG, Familletti PC, Stremlo DL, Truitt T, Chizzonite R, Gately MK: Purification to homogeneity and partial characterization of cytotoxic lymphocyte maturation factor from human B-lymphoblastoid cells. Proc Natl Acad Sci USA 1990;87:6808–6812.

4   D'Andrea A, Regaraju M, Valiante NM, Chehimi J, Kubin M, Aste-Amezaga M, Chan SH, Kobayashi M, Young D, Nickbarg E, Chizzonite R, Wolf SF, Trinchieri G: Production of natural killer cell stimulatory factor (NKSF/IL-12) by peripheral blood mononuclear cells. J Exp Med 1992; 176:1387–1398.

5   Benjamin D, Sharma V, Kubin M, Klein JL, Sartori A, Holliday J, Trinchieri G: IL-12 expression in AIDS-related lymphoma B cell lines. J Immunol 1996;156:1626–1637.

6   Cleveland MG, Gorham JD,Murphy TL, Tuomanen E, Murphy KM: Lipoteichoic acid preparations of gram-positive bacteria induce interleukin-12 through a CD14-dependent pathway. Infect Immun 1996;64:1906–1912.

7   Halpern MD, Kurlander RJ, Pisetsky DS: Bacterial DNA induces murine interferon-gamma production by stimulation of interleukin-12 and tumor necrosis factor-alpha. Cell Immunol 1996;167:72–78.

8   Ballas ZK, Rasmussen WL, Krieg AM: Induction of natural killer activity in murine and human cells by CpG motifs in oligodeoxynucleotides and bacterial DNA. J Immunol 1996;157:1840–1845.

9   Gazzinelli RT, Wysocka M, Hayashi S, Deukers EY, Hieny S, Caspar P, Trinchieri G, Sher A: Parasite-induced IL-12 stimulates early IFN-γ synthesis and resistance during acute infection with *Toxoplasma gondii*. J Immunol 1994;153:2533–2543.

10   Tripp CS, Gately MK, Hakimi J, Ling P, Unanue ER: Neutralization of IL-12 decreases resistance to *Listeria* in SCID and CB-17 mice. J Immunol 1994;152:1883–1887.

11   DeKruyff RH, Gieni RS, Umetsu DT: Antigen-driven but not lipopolysaccharide-driven IL-12 production in macrophages requires triggering of CD40. J Immunol 1997;158:359–366.

12   Maruo S, Oh-Hora M, Ahn H, Ono S, Wysocka M, Kaneko Y, Yagita H, Okumura K, Kikutani H, Kishimoto T, Kobayashi M, Hamaoka T, Trinchieri G, Fujiwara H: B cells regulate CD40 ligand-induced IL-12 production in antigen-presenting cells (APC) during T cell/APC interactions. J Immunol 1997;158:120–126.

13   Shu U, Kiniwa M, Wu CY, Maliszewski C, Vezzio N, Hakimi J, Gately M, Delespesse G: Activated T cells induce interleukin-12 production by monotypes via CD40-CD40 ligand interaction. Eur J Immunol 1995;25:1125–1128.

14   Hino A, Nariuchi H: Negative feedback mechanism suppresses interleukin-12 producion by antigen-presenting cells interacting with T-helper 2 cells, Eur J Immunol 1996;26:623–628.

15   Kato T, Hakamada R, Yamane H, Nariuchi H: Induction of IL-12 p40 messenger RNA expression and IL-12 production of macrophages via CD40-CD40 ligand interaction. J Immunol 1996;156:3932–3938.

16   Kennedy MK, Picha KS, Fanslow WC, Grabstein KH, Alderson MR, Clifford KN, Chin WA, Mohler KM: CD40/CD40 ligand interactions are required for T-cell-dependent production of interleukin-12 by mouse macrophages. Eur J Immunol 1996;26:370–378.

17   Cella M, Scheidegger D, Plamer-Lehmann K, Lane P, Lanzavecia A, Alber G: Ligation of CD-40 on dendritic cells triggers production of high levels of interleukin-12 and enhances T cell stimulatory capacity: T-T help via APC activation. J Exp Med 1996;184:747–752.

18   Koch F, Stanzl U, Jennewein P, Janke K, Heufler C, Kämpgen E, Romani N, Schuler G: High level IL-12 production by murine dendritic cells: Upregulation via MHC class II and CD40 molecules and downregulation by IL-4 and IL-10. J Exp Med 1996;184:741–746.

19   Heufler C, Koch F, Stanzl U, Topar G, Wysocka M, Trinchieri G, Enk A, Steinman RM, Romani N, Schuler G: Interleukin-12 is produced by dendritic cells and mediates Th1 development as well as IFN-γ production by Th1 cells. Eur J Immunol 1996;26:659–668.

20   Kang K, Kubin M, Cooper KD, Lessin SR, Trinchieri G, Rook AH: IL-12 synthesis by human Langerhans' cells. J Immunol 1996;156:1402–1407.

21   Smith TJ, Ducharme LA, Weis JH: Preferential expression of interleukin-12 or interleukin-4 by murine bone marrow mast cells derived in mast cell growth factor or interleukin-3. Eur J Immunol 1994;24:822–826.

22   Tripp CS, Unanue ER: Macrophage production of IL-12 is a critical link between the innate and specific immune responses to *Listeria*. Res Immunol 1995;146:515–519.

23   Flesch IEA, Kaufmann SHE: Differential induction of IL-12 synthesis by *Mycobacterium bovis* BCG and *Listeria monocytogenes*. Res Immunol 1995;146:520–526.

24   Modlin RL, Barnes PF: IL-12 and the human immune response to mycobacteria. Res Immunol 1995;146:527–531.

25   Chong C, Bost KL, Clements JD: Differential production of interleukin-12 mRNA by murine macrophages in response to viable or killed Salmonella spp. Infect Immun 1996;64:1154–1160.

26   Reiner LS, Zheng S, Wang Z, Stowring L, Locksley RM: Leishmania promastigotes evade interleukin-12 induction by macrophages and stimulate a broad range of cytokines from CD4+ T cells during initiation of infection. J Exp Med 1994;179:447–456.

27   Skeiky YAW, Guderian JA, Benson DR, Bacelar O, Carvalho EM, Kubin M, Badaro R, Trinchieri G, Reed SG: A recombinant Leishmania antigen that stimulates human peripheral blood mononuclear cells to express a Th1-type cytokine profile and to produce interleukin-12. J Exp Med 1995; 181:1527–1537.

28   Khan IA, Matsuura T, Fonseka S, Kasper LH: Production of nitric oxide is not essential for protection against acute Toxoplasma gondii infection in IRF-1-/- mice. J Immunol 1996;156:636–643.

29   Coutelier JP, Van Broeck J, Wolf SF; Interleukin-12 gene expression after viral infection in the mouse. J Virol 1995;69:1955–1958.

30   Biron CA, Orange JS: IL-12 in acute viral infectious disease. Res Immunol 1995;146:590–599.

31   Montiero J, Trinchieri G: Does IL-12 play a role in the viral immune response? Ann N Y Acad Sci 1996;795:366–367.

32   Kanangat S, Thomas J, Gangappa S, Babu JS, Rouse BT: Herpes simplex virus type 1-mediated up-regulation of IL-12 (p40) mRNA expression. Implications in immunopathogenesis and protection. J Immunol 1996;156:1110–1116.

33   Chehimi J, Starr S, Frank I, D'Andrea A, Ma X, MacGregor RR, Sennelier J, Trinchieri G: Impaired interleukin-12 production in human immunodeficiency virus-infected patients. J Exp Med 1994; 179:1361–1366.

34   Chougnet C, Clerici M, Shearer GM: Role of IL-12 in HIV disease/AIDS. Res Immunol 1995;146: 615–621.

35   Harrison TS, Levitz SM: Priming with IFN-γ restores deficient IL-12 production by peripheral blood mononuclear cells from HIV-seropositive donors. J Immunol 1997;158:459–463.

36   Gazzinelli RT, Bala S, Stevens R, Baseler M, Wahl L, Kovacs J, Sher A: HIV infection suppresses type 1 lymphokine and IL-12 responses to Toxoplasma gondii but fails to inhibit the synthesis of other parasite-induced monokines. J Immunol 1995;155:1565–1574.

37   Karp CL, Wysocka M, Wahl LM, Ahearn JM, Cuomo PJ, Sherry B, Trinchieri G, Griffin DE: Mechanism of suppression of cell-mediated immunity by measles virus. Science 1996;273:228–231.

38   Trinchieri G: Interleukin-12: A proinflammatory cytokine with immunoregulatory functions that bridge innate resistance and antigen-specific adaptive immunity. Annu Rev Immunol 1995;13:251–276.

39   Kubin M, Chow JM, Trinchieri G: Differential regulation of interleukin-12, tumor necrosis factor-α, and IL-1β production in human myeloid leukemia cell lines and peripheral blood mononuclear cells. Blood 1994;83:1847–1855.

40   Cassatella MA, Meda L, Gasperini S, D'Andrea A, Ma X, Trinchieri G: Interluekin-12 production by human polymorphonuclear leukocytes. Eur J Immunol 1995;25:1–5.

41   Chan SH, Perussia B, Gupta JW, Kobayashi M, Popísil M, Young HA, Wolf SF, Young D, Clark SC, Trinchieri G: Induction of IFN-γ production by NK cell stimulatory factor: Characterization of the responder cells and synergy with other inducers. J Exp Med 1991;173:869–879.

42   Manetti R, Parronchi P, Giudizi MG, Piccinni M-P, Maggi E, Trinchieri G, Romagnani S: Natural killer cell stimulatory factor (NKSF/IL-12) induces Th1-type specific immune responses and inhibits the development of IL-4 producing Th cells. J Exp Med 1993;177:1199–1204.

43   Hayes MP, Wang J, Norcross MA: Regulation of interleukin-12 expression in human monocytes: Selective priming by IFN-γ of LPS-inducible p35 and p40 genes. Blood 1995;86:646–650.

44   Ma X, Chow JM, Gri G, Carra G, Gerosa F, Wolf SF, Dzialo R, Trinchieri G: The interleukin-12 p40 gene promoter is primed by interferon-γ in monocytic cells. J Exp Med 1996;183:147–157.

45   Flesch IEA, Hess JH, Huang S, Aguet M, Rothe J, Bluethmann H, Kaufmann SHE: Early interleukin-12 production by macrophages in response to mycobacterial infection depends on interferon-γ and tumor necrosis factor-α. J Exp Med 1995;181:1615–1621.

46   Wysocka M, Kubin M, Vieira LQ, Ozmen L, Garotta G, Scott P, Trinchieri G: Interleukin-12 is required for interferon-γ production and lethality in lipopolysaccaride-induced shock in mice. Eur J Immunol 1995;25:672–676.

47   Murphy TL, Cleveland MG, Kulesza P, Magram J, Murphy KM: Regulation of interleukin-12 p40 expression through an NF-κB half-site. Mol Cell Biol 1995;15:5258–5267.

48   Ma X, Neurath M, Gri G, Trinchieri G: Identification and characterization of a novel ets-2-related nuclear complex implicated in the activation of the human IL-12 p40 gene promoter. J Biol Chem 1997;272:10389–10395.

49   Osipovich O, Fegeding K, Misuno N, Kolesnikova T, Savostin I, Sudarikov A, Viotenok N: Differential action of cycloheximide and activation stimuli on transcription of tumor necrosis factor-α, IL-1β, IL-8, and p53 genes in human monocytes. J Immunol 1993;150:4958–4965.

50   Shaw J, Meerovitch K, Elliot JF, Bleackley RC, Paetkau V: Induction, suppression and superinduction of lymphokine mRNA in T lymphocytes. Mol Immunol 1987;24:409–419.

51   Zubiaga A, Muñoz E, Huber B: Superinduction of IL-2 gene transcription in the presence of cycloheximide. J Immunol 1991;146:3857–3863.

52   Yoshimoto T, Kojima K, Funakoshi T, Endo Y, Fujita T, Nariuchi H: Molecular cloning and characterization of murine IL-12 genes. J Immunol 1996;156:1082–1088.

53   Tone Y, Thompson SA, Babik JM, Nolan KF, Tone M, Raven C, Waldmann H: Structure and chromosomal location of the mouse interleukin-12 p35 and p40 subunit genes. Eur J Immunol 1996;26:1222–1227.

54   Snidjers A, Hilkens CM, van der Pouw Kraan TC, Engel M, Aarden LA, Kapsenberg ML: Regulationn of bioactive IL-12 production in lipopolysaccharide-stimulated human monocytes is determined by the expression of the p35 subunit. J Immunol 1996;156:1207–1212.

55   D'Andrea A, Aste-Amezaga M, Valiante NM, Ma X, Kubin M, Trinchieri G: Interleukin-10 inhibits human lymphocyte IFN-γ production by suppressing natural killer cell stimulatory factor/ interleukin-12 synthesis in accessory cells. J Exp Med 1993;178:1041–1048.

56   Kubin M, Kamoun M, Trinchieri G: Interleukin-12 synergizes with B7/CD28 interaction in inducing efficient proliferation and cytokine production of human T cells. J Exp Med 1994;180:211–222.

57   Murphy EE, Terres G, Macatonia SE, Hsieh C, Mattson J, Lanier L, Wysocka M, Trinchieri G, Murphy K, O'Garra A: B7 and IL-12 cooperate for proliferation and IFN-γ production by mouse T-helper clones that are unresponsive to B7 costimulation. J Exp Med 1994;180:223–231.

58   Finkelman FD, Madden KB, Cheever AW, Katona IM, Morris SC, Gately MK, Hubbard BR, Gause WC, Urban JF, Jr: Effects of interleukin-12 on immune responses and host protection in mice infected with intestinal nematode parasites. J Exp Med 1994;179:1563–1572.

59   Gerosa F, Paganin C, Peritt D, Paiola F, Scupoli MT, Aste-Amezaga M, Frank I, Trinchieri G: Interleukin-12 primes human CD4 and CD8 T-cell clones for high production of both interferon-γ and interleukin-10. J Exp Med 1996;183:2559–2569.

60   Daftarian PM, Kumar A, Kryworuchko M, Diaz-Mitoma F: IL-10 production is enhanced in human T cells by IL-12 and IL-6 and in monocytes by tumor necrosis factor-α. J Immunol 1996; 157:12–20.

61   Meyaard L, Hovenkamp E, Otto SA, Miedema F: IL-12-induced IL-10 production by human T cells as a negative feedback for IL-12-induced immune reponses. J Immunol 1996;156:2776 – 2782.

62   Jeannin P, Delneste Y, Seveso M, Life P, Bonnefoy J: IL-12 synergizes with IL-2 and other stimuli in inducing IL-10 production by human T cells. J Immunol 1996;156:3159–3165.

63   Windhagen A, Anderson DE, Carrizosa A, Williams RE, Hafler DA: IL-12 induces human T cells secreting IL-10 with IFN-γ. J Immunol 1996;157:1127–1131.

64   Bogdan C, Paik J, Vodovotz Y, Nathan C: Contrasting mechanisms for suppression of macrophage cytokine release by transforming growth factor-beta and interleukin-10. J Biol Chem 1992;267: 23301–23308.

65   Wang P, Wu P, Siegel MI, Egan RW, Billah MM: IL-10 inhibits transcription of cytokine genes in human peripheral blood mononuclear cells. J Immunol 1994;153:811–816

66   Kasma T, Strieter RM, Lukacks NW, Burdick MD, Kunkel SL: Regulation of neutrophil-derived chemokine expression by IL-10. J Immunol 1994;152:3559–3569.

67   D'Andrea A, Ma X, Aste-Amezaga M, Paganin C, Trinchieri G: Stimulatory and inhibitory effects of IL-4 and IL-13 on production of cytokines by human peripheral blood mononuclear cells: Priming for IL-12 and TNF-α production. J Exp Med 1995;181:537–546.

68   Takenaka H, Maruo S, Yamamoto N, Wysocka M, Ono S, Kobayashi M, Yagita H, Okumura K, Hamaoka T, Trinchieri G, Fujiwara H: Regulation of T-cell-dependent and -independent IL-12 production by three Th2-type cytokines IL-10, IL-6 and IL-4. J Leuk Biol 1997;61:80–87.

69   Aste-Amezaga M, D'Andrea A, Kubin M, Trinchieri G: Cooperation of natural killer cell stimulatory factor/interleukin-12 with other stimuli in the induction of cytokines and cytotoxic cell-associated molecules in human T and NK cells. Cell Immunol 1994;156:480–492.

70   Chan SH, Kobayashi M, Santoli D, Perussia B, Trinchieri G: Mechanisms of IFN-γ induction by natural killer cell stimulatory factor (NKSF/IL-12): Role of transcription and mRNA stability in the synergistic interaction between NKSF and IL-2. J Immunol 1992;148:92–98.

71   Trinchieri G, Matsumoto-Kobayashi M, Clark SC, Sheehra J, London L, Perussia B: Response of resting human peripheral blood natural killer cells to interleukin-2. J Exp Med 1984;160:1147–1169.

72   Gazzinelli RT, Heiny S, Wynn TA, Wolf S, Sher A: Interleukin-12 is required for the T-lymphocyte independent induction of interferon-γ by an intracellular parasite and induces resistance in T-deficient hosts. Proc Natl Acad Sci USA 1993;90:6115–6119.

73   Tripp CS, Wolf SF, Unanue ER: Interleukin-12 and tumor necrosis factor-alpha are costimulators of interferon-gamma production by natural killer cells in severe combined immunodeficiency mice with listeriosis, and interleukin-10 is a physiologic antagonist. Proc Natl Acad Sci USA 1993;90:3725–3729.

74   Le Gros G, Ben-Sasson SZ, Seder R, Finkelman FD, Paul WE: Generation of interleukin-4 (IL-4)-producing cells in vivo and in vitro: IL-2 and IL-4 are required for in vitro generation of IL-4-producing cells. J Exp Med 1990;172:921–929.

75   Swain SL, Weinberg AD, English M, Huston G: IL-4 directs the development of Th2-like helper effectors. J Immunol 1990;145:3796–3806.

76   Seder RA, Paul WE, Davis MM, Fazekas de St Groth B: The presence of interleukin-4 during in vitro priming determines the lymphokine-producing potential of CD4+ T cells from T-cell receptor transgenic mice. J Exp Med 1992;176:1091–1098.

77   Trinchieri G: Interleukin-12 and its role in the generation of T_H1 cells. Immunol Today 1993;14:335–338.

78   Trinchieri G, Scott P: Interleukin-12: A proinflammatory cytokine with immunoregulatory functions. Res Immunol 1995;146:423–431

79   Hsieh C, Macatonia SE, Tripp CS, Wolf SF, O'Garra A, Murphy KM: Listeria-induced Th1 development in αβ-TCR transgenic CD4+ T cells occurs through macrophage production of IL-12. Science 1993;260:547–549.

80   Seder RA, Gazzinelli R, Sher A, Paul WE: IL-12 acts directly on CD4+ T cells to enhance priming for IFNγ production and diminishes IL-4 inhibition of such priming. Proc Natl Acad Sci USA 1993;90:10188–10192.

81   Swain SL, McKenzie DT, Weinberg AD, Hancock W: Characterization of T helper 1 and 2 cell subsets in normal mice. Helper T cells responsible for IL-4 and IL-5 production are present as precursors that require priming before they develop into lymphokine-secreting cells. J Immunol 1988;141:3445–3455.

82   Street NE, Schumacher JH, Fong AT, Bass H, Fiorentino DF, Leverah JA, Mosmann TR: Heterogeneity of mouse helper T cells: Evidence from bulk cultures and limiting dilution cloning for precursors of Th1 and Th2 cells. J Immunol 1993;144:1629–1639.

83   Gajewski TF, Joyce J, Fitch FW: Antiproliferative effect of IFN-γ in immune regulation. III. Differential selection of Th1 and Th2 murine helper T lymphocyte clones using recombinant IL-2 and recombinant IFN-γ. J Immunol 1989;143:15–22.

84   Wu CY, Demeure C, Kiniwa M, Gately M, Delespesse G: IL-12 induces the production of IFN-gamma by neonatal human CD4 T cells. J Immunol 1993;151:1938–1949.

85   Del Prete GF, De Carli M, Mastromauro C, Biagiotti R, Macchia D, Falagiani P, Ricci M, Romagnani S: Purified protein derivative of Mycobacterium tuberculosis and excretory-secretory antigen(s) of Toxocara canis expand in vitro human T cells with stable and opposite (type 1 T helper or type 2 T helper) profile of cytokine production. J Clin Invest 1991;88:346–350.

86   Gerosa F, Trinchieri G: Mechanisms of T helper cell differentiation induced by interleukin-12; in Romagnani S (ed): Cytokines: Basic Principles and Practical Applications. Rome, Ares-Serono Symposia Publications. 1994, pp 251–263.

87   Manetti R, Gerosa F, Giudizi MG, Biagiotti R, Parronchi P, Piccinni M, Sampognaro S, Maggi E, Romagnani S, Trinchieri G: Interleukin-12 induces stable priming for interferon-γ (IFN-γ) production during differentiation of human T helper (Th) cells and transient IFN-γ production in established Th2 cell clones. J Exp Med 1994;179:1273–1283.

88   Marshall J, Secrist H, DeKruyff RH, Wolf SF, Umetsu DT: IL-12 inhibits the production of IL-4 and IL-10 in allergen-specific human CD4+ T lymphocytes. J Immunol 1995;155:111–117.

89   Schmitt E, Hoehn P, Germann T, Rüde E: Differential effects of interleukin-12 on the development of naive mouse CD4+ T cells. Eur J Immunol 1994;24:343–347.

90   Wu CY, Demeure CE, Gately M, Podlaski F, Yssel H, Kiniwa M, Delespesse G: In vitro maturation of human neonatal CD4 T lymphocytes. I. Induction of IL-4-producing cells after long-term culture in the presence of IL-4 plus either IL-2 or IL-12. J Immunol 1994;152:1141–1153.

91   Wynn TA, Jankovic D, Heiny S, Zioncheck K, Jardieu P, Cheever AW, Sher A: IL-12 exacerbates rather than suppresses T helper 2-dependent pathology in the absence of endogenous IFN-γ. J Immunol 1995;154:3999–4009.

92   Van der Pouw-Kraan T, Van Kooten C, Rensuik I, Aarden L: Interleukin (IL)-4 production by human T cells: Differential regulation of IL-4 vs. IL-2 production. Eur J Immunol 1992;22:1237–1241.

93   Quelle FW, Shimoda K, Thierfelder W, Fischer C, Kim A, Ruben SM, Cleveland JL, Pierce JH, Keegan AD, Nelms K: Cloning of murine Stat6 and human Stat6, Stat proteins that are tyrosine phosphorylated in responses to IL-4 and IL-3 but are not required for mitogenesis. Mol Cell Biol 1995;15:3336–3343.

94   Jacobson NG, Szabo SJ, Weber-Nordt RM, Zhong Z, Schreiber RD, Darnell JE Jr, Murphy KM: Interleukin-12 signaling in T helper type 1 cells involves tyrosine phosphorylation of signal transducer and activator of transcription (Stat)3 and Stat.4 J Exp Med 1995;181:1755–1762.

95   Bacon CM, Petricoin EF III, Ortaldo JR, Rees RC, Larner AC, Johnston JA, O'Shea JJ: IL-12 induces tyrosine phosphorylation and activation of STAT4 in human lymphocytes. Proc Natl Acad Sci USA 1995;92:7307–7311.

96   Young HA, Ghosh P, Ye J, Lederer J, Lichtman A, Gerard JR, Penix L, Wilson CB, Melvin AJ, McGurn ME, Lewis DB, Taub DD: Differentiation of the T helper phenotypes by analysis of the methylation state of the IFN-γ gene. J Immunol 1994;153:3603–3610.

Giorgio Trinchieri, The Wistar Institute of Anatomy and Biology, 3601 Spruce Street, Philadelphia, PA 19104 (USA)
Tel. (215) 898-3992, Fax (215) 898-2357, E-mail: trinchieri@wista.wistar.upenn.edu

Adorini L (ed): IL-12. Chem Immunol. Basel, Karger, 1997, vol 68, pp 23–37

....

Structural and Functional Aspects of the IL-12 Receptor Complex

Alvin S. Stern, Ueli Gubler, David H. Presky, Jeanne Magram

Hoffmann-La Roche Inc., Nutley, N.J., USA

IL-12 is an important regulator of the immune response and exerts its effects through binding to specific IL-12 receptors (IL-12R) that are expressed on T and NK cells [1]. Binding studies using labeled IL-12 have identified at least two classes of IL-12 binding sites on PHA-activated human lymphoblasts with K_d values of 5–20 pM (100–1,000 sites/cell) and 2–6 nM (1,000–5,000 sites/cell), as well as an additional third class of medium affinity binding sites ($K_d = 50$–200 pM, 200–1,000 sites/cell) [2]. Analogous to the human system, three affinity classes of IL-12 binding sites on concanavalin (ConA)-stimulated mouse splenocytes have been observed. Dissociation constants were determined to be 40 pM (100–500 sites/cell), 200 pM (600-800 sites/cell) and 7 nM (1,000–2,000 sites/cell) [3]. Thus, the IL-12 binding characteristics of the IL-12R as it is naturally expressed on human and mouse T cells are similar.

The molecular cloning of two IL-12R subunits from human and mouse cells has led to an improved understanding of several aspects of IL-12 binding and signalling. Despite the similarities in binding affinities to human and mouse cells, significant differences between the subunits which provide these affinities are observed between the two species. It has also become clear that both the naturally expressed IL-12R and recombinant IL-12R can use the JAK-STAT signalling pathway, although there are indications that IL-12 is also capable of activating other pathways.

This review describes the molecular cloning and characterization of the two known IL-12R subunits. Furthermore, studies aimed at understanding the biology of the receptor by analyzing mice deficient in one subunit of the receptor are summarized. Lastly, a short summary of the properties of natural IL-12 antagonists is presented.

Molecular Cloning of IL-12R cDNAs

Two different IL-12R subunits have been identified, cloned and characterized from human and murine T cells [4–6]. Both chains contain a cytoplasmic region ranging in size from about 100 to 200 amino acids, including the box 1 and 2 motifs that occur in other cytokine receptors. Receptors containing this type of cytoplasmic region have been classified as β-type cytokine receptors by Stahl and Yancopoulos [7]. Thus, the two known IL-12R subunits were designated IL-12Rβ1 and IL-12Rβ2, respectively [6]. An expression cloning approach using panning with an antibody directed against human PHA-activated lymphoblasts was successful in isolating the cDNA encoding the first subunit of the IL-12R, human IL-12Rβ1 [4]. The corresponding murine cDNA was isolated by cross-hybridization techniques [5]. When expressed in COS cells, the human IL-12Rβ1 protein binds IL-12 with only a low affinity ($K_d = 2$–5 nM) unlike the three sites observed on PHA blasts including a high affinity site ($K_d = 5$–20 pM). Thus it was likely that, similar to other cytokine receptor systems, an additional IL-12R subunit existed. It was postulated that when coexpressed with IL-12Rβ1 on the cell surface, this additional subunit would yield the high affinity site similar to that expressed on PHA blasts. Based on this premise, a second expression cloning strategy was subsequently undertaken with the specific aim of isolating cDNAs that upon coexpression with the cDNA for IL-12Rβ1 would yield IL-12 binding sites with picomolar affinity. This approach led to the isolation of cDNAs encoding the human IL-12Rβ2 [6]. The corresponding murine IL-12Rβ2 cDNA was isolated by cross-hybridization techniques [6]. Each human IL-12R subunit binds IL-12 with low affinity ($K_d = 2$–5 nM). However, upon coexpression of IL-12Rβ1 with β2, both high ($K_d = 20$ pM) and low ($K_d = 2$–10 nM) affinity sites are formed.

Structural Features of IL-12Rβ1 and β2

Both IL-12Rβ1 and IL-12Rβ2 subunits are members of the gp130 subgroup of the cytokine receptor superfamily [4–6]. A general structural scheme is depicted in figure 1, with the amino acid sequence alignment of the human and murine receptor subunits shown in figure 2. The extracellular domains (ECDs) are made up of a number of different structural domains. The N-terminus of IL-12Rβ1 consists of the cytokine receptor homology or CRH domain. This domain is about 200 amino acids long and contains the N-terminal Cys-Cys pair and C-terminal WSXWS motif that are characteristic for all cytokine receptors. The remainder of the ECD of IL-12Rβ1 is made

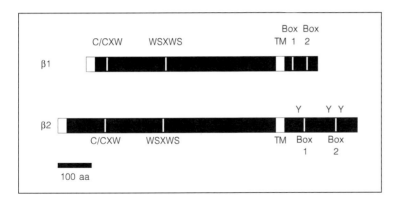

Fig. 1. Schematic illustration of the structural features of IL-12Rβ1 and IL-12Rβ2. The white box at the left end represents the signal peptide. The amino acid sequence motifs characteristic of the cytokine receptor superfamily are indicated (C/CXW, WSXWS). TM = Transmembrane region. Approximate positions of the box 1 and box 2 motifs are indicated. Y = Cytoplasmic tyrosine residues in IL-12Rβ2. [Reprinted with permission from the New York Academy of Science, 1996.]

Table 1. Number of amino acids in different regions of IL-12R subunits

Receptor	ECD	TM	CYTO	Total amino acids	Predicted MW kD	Observed MW kD
Human IL-12Rβ1	516	31	91	638	70.4	100
Mouse IL-12Rβ1	542	31	146	719	81.7	100
Human IL-12Rβ2	595	24	216	835	94.1	130
Mouse IL-12Rβ2	614	24	213	851	95.5	ND

ECD = Extracellular domains; TM = transmembrane domain; CYTO = cytoplasmic region; Predicted MW = deduced molecular size of the protein backbone of the mature proteins; Observed MW = molecular size estimated experimentally by reducing SDS-PAGE; ND = not determined.

up of three fibronectin type III repeats, each about 100 amino acids in length. The ECD of the IL-12Rβ2 subunit is about 100 amino acids longer than the β1 ECD, due to the presence of an N-terminal immunoglobulin domain. This immunoglobulin domain is followed by a 200 amino acid CRH domain and three fibronectin type III repeats. A summary of the lengths of the different regions of the IL-12R subunits is shown in table 1. All characterized receptor

```
                1                                                      50
HuIL-12Rβ2      MAHTFRGCSL AFMFIITWLL IKAKIDACKR GDVTVKPSHV ILLGSTVNIT
MsIL-12Rβ2      MAQTVRECSL ALLFLFMWLL IKANIDVCKL GTVTVQPAPV IPLGSAANIS
HuIL-12Rβ1      .......... .......... .......... .......... ..........
MsIL-12Rβ1      .......... .......... .......... .......... ..........
Consensus       ---------- ---------- ---------- ---------- ----------

                51                                                     100
                CSLKPRQGCF HYSRRNKLIL YKF....... ...DRRINFH HGHSLNSQVT
                CSLNPKQGCS HYPSSNELIL LKFVNDVLVE NLHGKKVHDH TGHSSTFQVT
                .......... .......... .......... .......... ...MEPL.VT
                .......... .......... .......... .......... ...MDMMGLP
                ---------- ---------- ---------- ---------- ----------

                101                                                    150
                GLPLGTTLF. VCKLACINSD E...IQICGA EIFVGVAPEQ PQNLSCIQKA
                NLSLGMTLF. VCKLNCSNSQ KKPPVPVCGV EISVGVAPEP PQNLSCVQEG
                WVVPLLFLFL LSRQGAACRT SECCFQDPPY PDADSGSASG PRDLRCYRIS
                GTSKHITFLL LCQLGASGPG DGCCVEKTSF PEGASGSPLG PRNLSCYRVS
                ---------- ---------- ---------- ---------- ----P----

                151                                                    200
                EQGTVACTWE .RGRDTHLYT EYTLQLSGPK NL.TWQKQC. ..KDIYCDYL
                ENGTVACSWN .SGKVTYLKT NYTLQLSGPN NL.TCQKQCF SDNRQNCNRL
                .SDRYECSWQ YEGPTAGVSH FLRCCL.... ...SSGRCC YFAAGSATRL
                .KTDYECSWQ YDGPEDNVSH VLWCCFVPPN HTHTGQERCR YFSSGPDRTV
                ------C-W- --G------- ---------- ---------- -------C--

                201                                                    250
                DFGINLTPES PESNFTAKVT AVNSLGSSSS LPSTFTFLDI VRPLPPW.DI
                DLGINLSPDL AESRFIVRVT AINDLGNSSS LPHTFTFLDI VIPLPPW.DI
                QFS.DQAGVS VLYTVTLWVE SWARNQTEKS PEVTLQLYNS VKYEPPLGDI
                QFW.EQDGIP VLSKVNFWVE SRLGNRTHKS QKISQYLYNW TKTTPPLGHI
                ---------- --------V- --------S- ---------- ----PP---I

                251                                                    300
                RIKFQKASVS RCTLYWRDEG LVLLNRLRYR .PSNSRLWNM VNVTKAKGRH
                RINFLNASGS RGTLQWEDEG QVVLNQLRYQ .PLNSTSWNM VNATNAKGKY
                KVS.KLAGQL RMEWETPDNQ VGAEVQFRHR TPSSPWKLGD CGPQDDDT..
                KVS.QSHGQL RMDWNVSE.E AGAEVQFRRR MPTTNWTLGD CGPQVNSGSG
                ---------- R--------- -------R-- -P-------- ----------

                301                                                    350
                DLLDLKPFTE YEFQISSKLH LYKGSWSDWS ESLRAQTPEE EPTGMLDVWY
                DLRDLRPFTE YEFQISSKLH LSGGSWSNWS ESLRTRTPEE EPVGILDIWY
                .......... ESCLCPLEMN VAQEFQL.RR RQLGS..QGS SWSKWSSPVC
                VLGDICGSMS ESCLCPSE.N MAQEIQIRRR RRLSSGAPGG PWSDWSMPVC
                ---------- ---------- ------L--- ---------- ----------

                351                                                    400
                MKRHIDYSRQ QISLFWKNLS VSEARGKILH ...YQVTLQE LTGGKAMTQN
                MKQDIDYDRQ QISLFWKSLN PSEARGKILH ...YQVTLQE VT.KKTTLQN
                VPPENP.PQP QVRFSVEQLG QDGRRRLTLK EQPTQLELPE GCQGLAPGTE
                VPPEVL.PQA KIKFLVEPLN QGGRRRLTMQ GQSPQLAVPE GCRG.RPGAQ
                ---------- --------L- ----R----- ----Q----E ----------

                401                                                    450
                ITGHTSWTTV IP.RTGNWAV AVSAANSKG. .SSLPTRINI M..NLCEAGL
                TTRHTSWTRV IP.RTGAWTA SVSAANSKG. .ASAPTHINI V..DLCGTGL
                VTYRLQL.HM LSCPCKAKAT RTLHLGKMPY LSGAAYNVAV ISSNQFGPGL
                VKKHLVLVRM LSCRCQAQTS KTVPLGKKLN LSGATYDLNV LAKTRFGRST
                ---------- ---------- ---------- ---------- ----------

                451                                                    500
                LAPRQVSAN. .SEGMD.NIL VTWQPP...R KDPSAVQEYV VEWREL.HPG
                LAPHQVSAK. .SENMD.NIL VTWQPP...K KADSAVREYI VEWRAL.QPG
                NQTWHIPADT HTEPVALNIS VGTNGTTMYW PARAQSMTYC IEWQPVGQDG
                IQKWHLPAQE LTETRALNVS VGGNMTSMQW AAQAPGTTYC LEWQPWFQHR
                -------A-- --E----N-- V--------- --------Y- -EW-------

                501                                                    550
                GDTQVPLNWL RSR.PYNVSA LI....SENI KSYICYEIRV YALSGDQGGC
                SITKFPPHWL RIP.PDNMSA LI....SENI KPYICYEIRV HALSESQGGC
                GLATCSLTAP QDPDPAGMAT SYWSRESGAM GQEKCYYITI FASAHPEKLT
                NHTHCTLIVP EEEDPAKMVT HSWSSKP.TL EQEECYRITV FASKNPKNPM
                ---------- ----P----- ---------- ----CY-I-- -A--------

                551                                                    600
                ..SSILG... .NSKHKAPLS GPHINAITEE KGSILISWNS IPVQEQMGCL
                ..SSIRG... .DSKHKAPVS GPHITAITEK KERLFISWTH IPFPEQRGCI
                LWSTVLSTYH FGGNASAAGT PHHVSVKNHS LDSVSVDWAP SLLSTCPGVL
                LWATVLSSYY FGGNASRAGT PRHVSVRNQT GDSVSVEWTA SQLSTCPGVL
                ---------- ---------- --H------- -----W---- -------G--

                601                                                    650
                LHYRIYWKER DSNSQPQLCE IPYRVSQNSH PINSLQPRVT YVLWMTALTA
                LHYRIYWKER DSTAQPELCE IQYRRSQNSH PISSLQPRVT YVLWMTAVTA
                KEY.VVRCRD EDSKQ..VSE HPVQPTETQV TLSGLRAGVA YTVQVRADTA
                TQY.VVRCEA EDGAW..ESE WLVPPTKTQV TLDGLRSRVM YKVQVRADTA
                ----Y----- ---------E ---------- ----L---V- Y-----A-TA

                651                                                    700
                AGESSHGNER EFCLQGKANW MAFVAPSIC. .IAIIMVGIF STHYFQQKVF
                AGESPQGNER EFCPQGKANW KAFVISSIC. .IAIITVGTF SIRYFRQKAF
                WLRGVWSQPQ RFSIEVQVSD WLIFFASLGS FLSILLVGVL GYLGLNRAAR
                RLPGAWSHPQ RFSFEVQISR LSIIFASLGS FASVLLVGSL GYIGLNRAAW
                ---------- -F-------- --------S-- -------VG-- ----------

                701                                                    750
                VLLAALRPQ. .WCSREIPDP .ANSTCAKKY PIAEEKTQLP LDRLLIDWP.
                TLLSTLKPQ. .WYSRTIPDP .ANSTWVKKY PILEEKIQLP TDNLLMAWP.
                HLCPPLPTPC ASSAIEFPG. .GKETWQWIN PVDFQEEASL QEALVVEMSW
                HLCPPLPTPC GSTAVEFPGS QGKQAWQWCN PEDFPEVLYP RDALVVEMPG
                -L---L---- -------P-- ---------- P--------- ---L------

                751                                                    800
                .TPEDPEPLV ISEVLHQVTP VFRHPPCSNW PQREKGIQGH QASEKDMMHS
                .TPEEPEPLI IHEVLYHMIP VVRQPYYFKR GQ...GFQGY STSKQDAMYI
                DKGERTEPLE KTELPEGAPE LALDTELSLE DGDRCKAKMX ..........
                DRGDGTES.. ....PQAAPE CALDTRRPLE TQRQRQVQAL SEARRLGLAR
                ------E--- ---------- ---------- ---------- ----------

                801                                                    850
                ASSPPPPRAL QAESRQLVDL YKVLESRGSD PKPENPACPW TVLPAGDLPT
                A.NPQATGTL TAETRQLVNL YKVLESRDPD SKLANLTSPL TVTPVNYLPS
                .......... .......... .......... .......... ..........
                EDCPRGDLAH VTLPLLLGGV TQGASVLDDL WRTHKTAEPG PPTLGQEA*.
                ---------- ---------- ---------- ---------- ----------

                851                                                    900
                HDGYLPSNID DLPSHEAPLA DSLEELEPQH ISLSVFPSSS LHPLTFSCGD
                HEGYLPSNIE DLPSHEADPT DSF.DLEHQH ISLSIFASSS LRPLIFG.GE

                901               919
                KLTLDQLKMR CDSLML...
                RLTLDRLKMG YDSLMSNEA
```

Fig. 2. Amino acid sequence alignment of the human and mouse IL-12Rβ1 and IL-12Rβ2 subunits. The alignment was generated using the GCG program PILEUP (gap creation penalty = 1.5, gap extension penalty = 0.8). Shaded amino acids highlight (i) the residues defining the cytokine receptor superfamily (CXW, WSXWS); (ii) the transmembrane regions, and (iii) the cytoplasmic tyrosines conserved between human and mouse IL-12Rβ2.

subunits are glycoproteins based on their molecular weights, estimated by reducing SDS-PAGE, which are consistently higher than the molecular weights calculated on the basis of the predicted amino acid sequence (table 1). The cytoplasmic domains of both β1 and β2 subunits contain the characteristic box 1 and box 2 motifs that are located within the first 100 amino acids from the transmembrane region and have been found in other cytokine receptors. Interestingly, only the β2 cytoplasmic region contains tyrosine residues. The three tyrosine residues found in the human IL-12Rβ2 are all conserved in the murine IL-12Rβ2. However, the murine β2 cytoplasmic region contains an additional seven tyrosine residues (fig. 2). Some of these tyrosines likely play a role in signalling within the cell (see below). The overall amino acid sequence identity between the complete human and murine IL-12Rβ1 is 54%, while the β2 chains of the two species appear to be more conserved, with 68% identity. Each recombinant receptor subunit forms dimers/oligomers at the surface of transfected COS cells [4, 6]; the formation of these higher-order structures does not depend on the presence of the IL-12 ligand [4, 6].

Studies on Expression of IL-12R Subunit mRNAs and Proteins

Induction of IL-12Rβ1 and β2 mRNAs following polyclonal activation using either PHA or ConA has been studied. Transcript levels are generally very low or undetectable in unactivated T cells. Upon activation in vitro for 2–3 days, transcript levels increase dramatically for both receptor subunits. Transcripts of 2.3 and 3 kb for human IL-12Rβ1, 3 and 6 kb for mouse IL-12Rβ1, 4.5 and 6 kb for human IL-12Rβ2 and 4.5 kb for mouse IL-12Rβ2 are induced under these conditions [4, 6].

Studies of IL-12R subunit protein expression have thus far mostly concentrated on IL-12Rβ1. Expression of IL-12Rβ1 protein was shown to be upregulated by PHA, anti-CD3 monoclonal antibody, IL-2, IL-7 or IL-15 [8]. The effects of anti-CD3 treatment were augmented by anti-CD28 treatment. Upon treatment of resting PBMC with anti-CD3 and either TGF-β2 or IL-10, the cells failed to proliferate or secrete IFN-γ in response to IL-12. This lack of responsiveness correlated with decreased levels of IL-12R expression. Therefore, Th2 cell-derived cytokines can inhibit IL-12 biological functions by inhibiting IL-12R expression [8].

More extensive studies on IL-12R distribution using flow cytometry and RT-PCR have shown that human IL-12Rβ1 is not only expressed on T and NK cells, but surprisingly, also on B cells [9, 10]. Intriguingly however, the IL-12Rβ1 receptor chain expressed on human B cells or on resting human PBMC does not bind IL-12, even though it is recognized by receptor-specific antibodies [10]. It is not clear at this time what the basis is for the differences in IL-12 binding between the IL-12Rβ1 subunit expressed on T cells and that expressed on B cells.

Analysis of IL-12 Binding to Recombinant IL-12R

Binding experiments using cDNA expression constructs for human IL-12Rβ1 and β2 demonstrated that COS-7 cells singly transfected with either human IL-12Rβ1 or β2 bind ^{125}I-huIL-12 with a K_d of about 2–5 nM, corresponding to the low affinity human ^{125}I-IL-12 binding sites observed on PHA-activated lymphocytes [4, 6]. In contrast to the low affinity binding observed with singly transfected COS-7 cells, coexpression of both human IL-12Rβ1 and β2 yields two classes of human ^{125}I-IL-12 binding sites with apparent affinities (K_ds of about 50 pM and 5 nM) that correspond to the high and low affinity binding sites measured on PHA-activated lymphoblasts [6]. Interestingly, when huIL-12Rβ1 is expressed in either the mouse cytolytic T-cell line CTLL or the mouse pro-B-cell line Ba/F3 rather than in COS-7 cells, human ^{125}I-IL-12 binds with only very low affinity ($K_d > 50$ nM). This suggests that the COS-7 cells are providing either an additional protein or a posttranslational modification not present in CTLL or Ba/F3 cells that enables low affinity (K_d of 5 nM) human ^{125}I-IL-12 binding by human IL-12Rβ1 [4, 6, 11].

In contrast to human IL-12Rβ1-expressing Ba/F3 cells, human IL-12Rβ2-expressing Ba/F3 cells bind human ^{125}I-IL-12 with a K_d of about 5 nM, similar to that observed when human IL-12Rβ2 is expressed in COS-7 cells [6]. Coexpression of human IL-12Rβ1 and β2 in Ba/F3 cells results in both high (K_d of about 50 pM) and low (K_d of about 5 nM) affinity human ^{125}I-IL-12 binding [6]. The binding characteristics of the human IL-12R proteins, when expressed in COS-7 or Ba/F3 cells, are summarized in table 2.

Although the mouse and human IL-12Rβ1 and β2 subunits share significant similarity on the amino acid sequence level, they differ in their IL-12 binding characteristics. ConA-activated mouse splenocytes exhibit three classes of mouse ^{125}I-IL-12 binding sites with K_ds of about 40 pM, 200 pM and 7 nM, and expression levels of 100–500, 600–800 and 1,300–2,000 sites/cell, respectively, similar to the human ^{125}I-IL-12 binding characteristics of PHA-activated human lymphocytes [2]. Expression of mouse IL-12Rβ1 in COS-7 cells has been reported to yield a single class of mouse ^{125}I-IL-12 binding sites, with a K_d of about 1 nM [5]. Recent experiments have shown that a small number of high affinity (K_d of about 100 pM) mouse ^{125}I-IL-12 binding sites are occasionally observed in mouse IL-12Rβ1-transfected COS-7 cells as well [Wilkinson and Presky, unpubl. data], although it is not clear why these high

Table 2. IL-12 binding affinities (K_d)

Cell type	Receptor type					
	human IL-12Rβ1	human IL-12Rβ2	human IL-12Rβ1 + β2	mouse IL-12Rβ1	mouse IL-12Rβ2	mouse IL-R12β1 + β2
Transfected						
COS	2 nM	5 nM	55 pM; 8 nM	120 pM; 2 nM	> 50 nM	40 pM; 5 nM
Ba/F3	> 50 nM	3 nM	50 pM; 10 nM	100 pM; 2 nM	> 50 nM	100 pM; 2 nM
Native T cells			10 pM; 200 pM; 5 nM			40 pM; 200 pM; 7 nM

affinity binding sites are not reproducibly detected. However, mouse IL-12Rβ1-expressing Ba/F3 cells reproducibly bind mouse ^{125}I-IL-12 with both high (K_d of 50–100 pM) and low (K_d of about 0.5–2 nM) affinities [5]. It is possible that the Ba/F3 cells allow more efficient oligomerization or other post-translational processing of mouse IL-12Rβ1 than COS-7 cells. Alternatively, the mouse Ba/F3 cells might be contributing an additional mouse-specific protein component that enables more efficient high affinity binding of mouse ^{125}I-IL-12 by the mouse IL-12Rβ1 subunit. Nevertheless, it is clear that in contrast to human IL-12Rβ1, mouse IL-12Rβ1 can mediate both high and low affinity IL-12 binding.

Unlike Ba/F3 cells expressing human IL-12Rβ2, Ba/F3 cells expressing mouse IL-12Rβ2 bind mouse ^{125}I-IL-12 with only very low affinity ($K_d > 50$ nM) [Wilkinson et al., manuscript in preparation]. Coexpression of mouse IL-12Rβ1 and β2 in Ba/F3 cells yields high and low affinity binding sites, with K_ds of about 100 pM and 2 nM, similar to the human system [Wilkinson et al., manuscript in preparation]. The binding characteristics of the mouse IL-12R proteins, when expressed in COS-7 or Ba/F3 cells, are summarized in table 2.

Therefore, although coexpression of IL-12Rβ1 and IL-12Rβ2 yields high and low affinity IL-12 binding sites in both the human and mouse systems, the relative contribution of the various IL-12R subunits in binding IL-12 appears to differ significantly between the two species. When expressed in Ba/F3 cells, human IL-12Rβ2 binds IL-12 with low (K_d of about 5 nM) affinity. Expression of both human IL-12R subunits is required for high affinity IL-12 binding in Ba/F3 cells. In contrast, it appears that the mouse IL-12Rβ1 subunit alone can mediate both high and low affinity IL-12 binding, especially when expressed in Ba/F3 cells. However, the IL-12Rβ2 subunit is required for IL-12 signalling in both the mouse and human system (see below). Therefore, it appears that the mouse IL-12Rβ2 subunit functions primarily as a signal-transducing subunit, with a minor role, if any, in contributing additional IL-12 binding affinity to the mouse IL-12R complex. It appears as if low affinity binding of IL-12 to mouse IL-12Rβ2 in cells lacking mouse IL-12Rβ1 (from IL-12Rβ1$^{-/-}$ mice) is insufficient to trigger a response (see below). Similarly, Ba/F3 cells expressing only mouse IL-12Rβ2 do not exhibit long-term growth in IL-12-containing medium [Wilkinson et al., manuscript in preparation].

In contrast to the mouse system, both human IL-12R subunits contribute significantly to IL-12 binding affinity in the human IL-12R complex, with human IL-12Rβ2 also functioning as the signal-transducing subunit. The idea that the human IL-12Rβ2 subunit has both an important binding as well as signalling function is further supported by the fact that Ba/F3 cells expressing only human IL-12Rβ2 proliferate in IL-12-containing medium. However, a higher ED_{50} for huIL-12 is observed for these cells, commensurate with the reduced binding affinity of human IL-12Rβ2-expressing Ba/F3 cells as compared to huIL-12Rβ1/β2 cotransfected Ba/F3 cells [6].

IL-12 Signalling

Early reports described the IL-12-induced phosphorylation of p56 lck in purified NK cells [12]. A subsequent report from the same group described the IL-12-induced phosphorylation and activation of MAP kinase in normal mitogen-activated human T cells [13]. In addition, activation in normal T cells of STATs 3 and 4 and JAK2/Tyk2 has also been described [14–17]. STAT3 is activated by many different cytokines. In contrast, STAT4 has thus far only been found to be activated through IL-12 [15, 16] and IFN-α [18]. This rather tight link between STAT4 and IL-12 has also been demonstrated in STAT4 knockout mice. These mice are completely unresponsive to IL-12 [19, 20] and therefore have a phenotype essentially identical to IL-12 knockout mice [21]. It is possible that IL-12 signals through both the RAS/Raf pathway as well as the JAK/STAT pathway. It is not known at this time whether the different activities of IL-12 (i.e., induction of secretion of IFN-γ and induction of proliferation) use different signalling pathways.

It has also been shown that CD2 stimulation can synergize with the induction of IL-12-mediated T-cell responses (i.e., induction of secretion of IFN-γ and proliferation) [22]. This mechanism operates independently of the IL-12R, since CD2-specific antibodies do not block binding of IL-12 to its receptor.

Ba/F3 cells transfected with both cloned human IL-12R subunits become responsive to IL-12 (see above) and long-term growth of such cell clones in IL-12 has been achieved [6]. Interestingly, Ba/F3 cells transfected with huIL-12Rβ2 alone are also capable of long-term growth in IL-12. As expected from the lower K_d value measured for IL-12Rβ2 expressed in Ba/F3 cells (see above), the corresponding EC_{50} value for IL-12 in these cells is also higher. The importance of the cytoplasmic region of the IL-12Rβ2 in signalling was further emphasized in a study in which a receptor chimera consisting of the extracellular domain of the EGF receptor fused to the cytoplasmic domain of the IL-12Rβ2 was shown to render Ba/F3 cells responsive to EGF [23]. The same study also presented evidence for differential interactions between the cytoplasmic regions of IL-12Rβ1 and β2 and JAK2/Tyk2. Thus, based on the above evidence, a current model for IL-12 signalling may be that the IL-12Rβ2 subunit represents the signalling subunit, while the IL-12Rβ1 chain acts as an affinity converter and possibly also as a docking site for JAK2 and Tyk2.

IL-12 Antagonists

Experimental data have identified the p40 subunit of IL-12 as an IL-12 antagonist. Supernatant solutions containing p40 from cultures of COS-7 cells transfected with the mouse IL-12 p40 cDNA have been demonstrated to specifically inhibit IL-12-stimulated Th1 cell proliferation, IFN-γ production and leukocyte function-associated molecule 1 (LFA-1)- and intercellular adhesion molecule 1 (ICAM-1)-dependent homotypic aggregation [24]. However, the mouse p40 in such supernatant fluids exists in two forms: p40 monomer and a disulfide-linked p40 homodimer [(p40)$_2$] [25, 26]. The mouse p40 was purified by immunoaffinity chromatography on an affinity resin prepared by cross-linking an anti-mouse IL-12 antibody to protein G-Sepharose [25]. To separate (p40)$_2$ from p40 monomer, the immunoaffinity-purified sample was resolved into two components by anion exchange chromatography [25, 26]. By SDS-PAGE, the two proteins were of greater than 95% purity and revealed molecular weights of 40 and >97 kD. Under reducing conditions, the electrophoretic mobility of the >97 kD protein was identical to that of the reduced monomer p40 indicating that the high molecular weight protein is an oligomer of p40. Size exclusion chromatography [25] and time of flight mass spectrometry [25, 26] indicated that the protein consists of two p40 subunits and that this protein migrates anomalously in SDS-PAGE [25, 26].

The purified (p40)$_2$ was found to be 25- to 50-fold more effective than the p40 monomer in competing with mouse ^{125}I-IL-12 for binding to mouse ConA-activated lymphoblasts and in causing specific, dose-dependent inhibition of IL-12-induced mouse ConA blast proliferation, IFN-γ secretion, and activation of mouse NK cells [25]. However, (p40)$_2$ has also been shown to stimulate, rather than inhibit, CD8$^+$ Th1 development in vitro [27]. Mouse (p40)$_2$ was equivalent to mouse IL-12 in competing with mouse ^{125}I-IL-12 for binding to high affinity IL-12R on mouse ConA blasts [25] and was, in fact, more effective than mouse IL-12 in competing for binding to COS cells which had been transfected with mouse IL-12Rβ1 cDNA [28]. This suggests that (p40)$_2$ may interact primarily with the β1 subunit of the IL-12R. In addition, preliminary experiments have demonstrated that ^{125}I-(p40)$_2$ binds to Ba/F3 cells transfected with the β1 subunit and not to those transfected with the β2 subunit [Wang et al., unpubl. data]. Although mouse and human IL-12 bind with similar affinity to PHA-activated human lymphoblasts that bear high affinity IL-12R, mouse (p40)$_2$ did not compete with human ^{125}I-IL-12 for binding to human PHA blasts under high affinity binding conditions nor did it inhibit huIL-12-induced proliferation of human PHA blasts [25]. Nonetheless, mouse (p40)$_2$ was effective in competing with human ^{125}I-IL-12 for binding to transfected COS cells expressing the huIL-12Rβ1 subunit [25]. It could also synergistically inhibit huIL-12 induced human PHA blast proliferation when combined with the heterodimer-specific anti-huIL-12 monoclonal antibody 20C2 [28] which previously had been shown not to compete with human ^{125}I-IL-12 for binding to human IL-12Rβ1-transfected COS cells [2]. Therefore, mouse (p40)$_2$ and 20C2 appear to have very different mechanisms of inhibition of IL-12 binding with mouse (p40)$_2$ interfering with interactions of IL-12 with the IL-12Rβ1 subunit, and 20C2 blocking IL-12 interactions with IL-12Rβ2.

Studies have revealed that a human congener of the mouse p40 also exists in a monomeric and dimeric form [29]. Additionally, human (p40)$_2$ was at least 20-fold more effective than the human monomer at inhibiting either the activity of human IL-12 in proliferation of PHA-activated human lymphoblasts or its binding to a human IL-12R-expressing T-cell line. However, in contrast to mouse (p40)$_2$, which binds to mouse IL-12R with similar affinity as heterodimeric mouse IL-12 itself, the affinity of human (p40)$_2$ for the human IL-12R is only 10–20% of that of human IL-12 [29]. Likewise, human (p40)$_2$ has approximately 10% of the potency of mouse (p40)$_2$ in its ability to inhibit bioactivity.

If (p40)$_2$ is a physiologic antagonist of IL-12 activity in vivo is presently unclear. However, it has been observed that in vitro stimulation of IL-12 production by human B-lymphoblastoid cell lines, human PBMC, or mouse peritoneal exudate cells results in the secretion of p40 in $\geq$ 5-fold excess over IL-12 [30]. Furthermore, p40 has also been shown to be present in excess over IL-12 in sera from mice injected with endotoxin [31, 32] and in pleural fluid from humans with tuberculous pleuritis [33]. Moreover, in situ hybridization studies on sections of mouse spleen showed that the spatial distribution of p40 mRNA expression was distinct from that of p35 mRNA expression, suggesting that some cells may produce p40 independent of IL-12 [34]. If the excess p40 produced in vivo contains (p40)$_2$ independent of IL-12 or after IL-12 production, then this may serve as a regulatory mechanism of the heterodimer. Further evidence for p40 regulation of IL-12 is that administration of (p40)$_2$ to mice causes dose-dependent inhibition in vivo of endotoxin-induced IFN-γ and of the development of Th1 cells in response to immunization with a protein antigen and *Corynebacterium parvum* [35]. Finally, when a murine myoblast cell line was transplanted into allogeneic recipients, survival was substantially prolonged when the cells were transduced with the p40 gene [34]. Cytokine (IL-2 and IFN-γ) production and cytotoxic T-lymphocyte induction against allogeneic cells were impaired in the recipients transplanted with the p40 transfectant [36]. Delayed-type hypersensitivity response against the cells was also diminished in the p40 recipients [36].

The distinct possibility that the p40 subunit, in some form, exerts a physiologic effect for limiting the actions of IL-12 may be useful for clinical treatment of Th1-dependent autoimmune diseases such as multiple sclerosis and autoimmune uveitis.

IL-12R-Deficient Mice

To investigate the role of IL-12Rβ1 in IL-12-mediated signalling events, we generated mice lacking this receptor chain [37]. Furthermore, due to its homology to gp130, it was postulated that IL-12Rβ1 could be a signalling component for additional receptor pathways. Therefore, comparing mice deficient in IL-12Rβ1 with mice deficient in IL-12 ligand would provide insight into this hypothesis.

The genomic organization of the IL-12Rβ1 gene consists of 16 exons spanning approximately 13.2 kb of DNA (fig. 3). Using the targeting vector and strategy outlined in figure 3, homologous recombination would result in the replacement of the first three coding exons with a neomycin resistance gene. These exons contain the ATG translation initiation codon as well as the signal sequence. Therefore, this mutation would be expected to result in a null phenotype. Four correctly targeted clones were identified and two of these clones were used to generate chimeric animals which were subsequently bred to obtain mice homozygous for the mutant allele, referred to as IL-12Rβ1$^{-/-}$ mice.

IL-12Rβ1$^{-/-}$ mice were obtained in the expected mendelian frequency indicating that IL-12Rβ1 was not required for embryonic development. This was of interest as a mutation in the homologous gp130 receptor subunit was

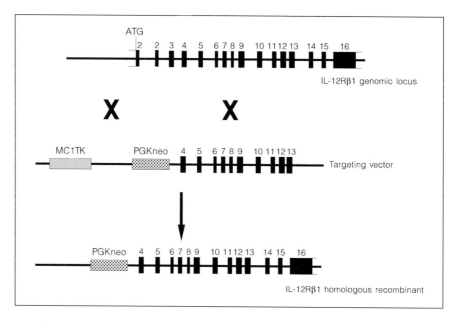

Fig. 3. Targeting strategy for the IL-12Rβ1 gene. Introduction of the targeting vector into ES cells and subsequent homologous recombination will result in the generation of a mutant IL-12Rβ1 gene. The IL-12Rβ1 genomic structure is indicated; numbered black boxes indicate coding exons, ATG depicts the location of the translation initiation codon. The MC1TK gene is drawn as a gray box; the PGK*neo* gene is drawn as a stippled box.

embryonically lethal [38]. Furthermore, IL-12Rβ1$^{-/-}$ mice had comparable T- and B-cell subset distributions to wild-type mice in the thymus, spleen and lymph nodes indicating that this receptor subunit was not required for development of immune cells. These results are consistent with those reported for the IL-12 p40-deficient mice [21] and suggest that IL-12-mediated signalling is not required for B- and T-cell development in vivo.

Binding studies using labeled IL-12 and splenocytes obtained from IL-12Rβ1$^{-/-}$ or wild-type control mice demonstrated the presence of only low affinity bindings sites ($K_d = 5.5$ nM) on IL-12Rβ1$^{-/-}$ splenocytes, whereas wild-type splenocytes demonstrated both high ($K_d = 4.5$ pM) and low affinity binding sites ($K_d = 17$ nM) [37]. The absence of high affinity sites is consistent with the binding observed in Ba/F3 cells transfected with only the IL-12Rβ2 receptor subunit chain [Wilkinson et al., manuscript in preparation], although the K_d for mouse ^{125}I-IL-12 binding determined using IL-12Rβ1$^{-/-}$ cells is lower than on the IL-12Rβ2-transfected cells where the K_d is difficult to quantitate. It was further demonstrated that these low affinity binding sites were not sufficient to mediate a biological response to IL-12 by a number of lines of evidence. First, ConA-activated splenocytes derived from IL-12Rβ1$^{-/-}$ mice failed to proliferate or induce IFN-γ production in response to IL-12, but proliferated normally in response to IL-2 or IL-7. In contrast, splenocytes from IL-12Rβ1$^{+/+}$ mice proliferated in response to all three cytokines and secreted large amounts of IFN-γ in response to IL-12. Second, intra-peritoneal administration of IL-12 or LPS failed to induce IFN-γ secretion in IL-12Rβ1$^{-/-}$ mice as compared to IL-12Rβ1$^{+/+}$ control mice. Third, measurements of both in vitro and in vivo Th1 responses are impaired in IL-12Rβ1$^{-/-}$ mice, similar to that observed in IL-12-deficient mice. Lastly, evaluation of IL-12-enhanced NK cell lytic activity also demonstrated a deficiency in IL-12Rβ1$^{-/-}$ mice when compared to IL-12Rβ1$^{+/+}$ mice. However, IL-2-enhanced NK activity was comparable in both types of mice. These data, taken together, demonstrate the requirement for IL-12Rβ1 for IL-12 signalling in both mouse T and NK cells, and suggest that IL-12Rβ1 and/or IL-12Rβ2 are potential targets for the development of IL-12 antagonists.

Conclusions

In conclusion, the identification and characterization of human and mouse IL-12R subunits has been reviewed. Although very similar with respect to their molecular properties, significant differences exist between the two species with respect to IL-12 binding. These differences should be considered when evaluating potential therapeutic IL-12 antagonists directed against these receptors in mouse models of human disease. Our study using IL-12$^{-/-}$ and IL-12Rβ1$^{-/-}$ mice demonstrate that IL-12 plays an important role in the generation of Th1-type immune responses in vivo, and suggest that antagonists directed against IL-12Rβ1 or IL-12Rβ2 may be useful in treating Th1-mediated immune pathologies. The intriguing idea that the IL-12 p40 homodimer may be a physiologic regulator of IL-12 function suggests that this molecule may be useful in studying the impact of IL-12 antagonism on various disease processes.

References

1   Chizzonite R, Truitt T, Desai BB, Nunes P, Podlaski FJ, Stern AS, Gately MK: IL-12 receptor-I. Characterization of the receptor on phytohemagglutinin-activated human lymphoblasts. J Immunol 1992;148:3117–3124.
2   Chizzonite R, Truitt T, Nunes P, Desai BB, Chua AO, Gately MK, Gubler U: High and low affinity receptors for interleukin-12 (IL-12) on human T cells: Evidence for a two subunit receptor by IL-12 and anti-receptor antibody binding. Cytokines 1994;6:A82a.

3   Chizzonite R, Truitt T, Griffin M, Nickbarg E, Hubbard B, Desai BB, Stern AS, Gubler U, Gately MK: Initial characterization of the IL-12 receptor on concanavalin-A activated mouse splenocytes. J Cell Biochem 1993;17B:A73.

4   Chua AO, Chizzonite R, Desai BB, Truitt TP, Nunes P, Minetti LJ, Warrier RR, Presky DH, Levine JF, Gately MK: Expression cloning of a human IL-12 receptor component. A new member of the cytokine receptor superfamily with strong homology to gp130. J. Immunol 1994;153:128–136.

5   Chua AO, Wilkinson VL, Presky DH, Gubler U: Cloning and characterization of a mouse IL-12 receptor-β component. J Immunol 1995;155:4286–4294.

6   Presky DH, Yang H, Minetti LJ, Chua AO, Nabavi N, Wu CY, Gately MK, Gubler U: A functional interleukin-12 receptor complex is composed of two β-type cytokine receptor subunits. Proc Natl Acad Sci USA 1996;93:14002-14007.

7   Stahl N, Yancopoulos GD: The alphas, betas, and kinases of cytokine receptor complexes. Cell 1993;74:587–590.

8   Wu C-Y, Warrier RR, Wang X, Presky DH, Gately MK: Regulation of IL-12 receptor β1 chain expression and interleukin-12 binding by human peripheral blood mononuclear cells. Eur J Immunol 1997;27:147–154.

9   Vogel LA, Lester TL, Van Cleave VH, Metzger DW: Inhibition of murine B1 lymphocytes by interleukin-12.Eur J Immunol 1996;26:219–223.

10   Wu C-Y, Warrier RR, Cavajal DM, Chua AO, Minetti LJ, Chizzonite R, Mongini PKA, Stern AS, Gubler U, Presky DH, Gately MK: Biological function and distribution of human interleukin-12 receptor β chain. Eur J Immunol 1996;26:345–350.

11   Presky DH, Gubler U, Chizzonite RA, Gately MK: IL-12 receptors and receptor antagonists. Res Immunol 1995;146:439–445.

12   Pignata C, Prasad KVS, Robertson MJ, Levine H, Rudd CE, Ritz J: FcγRIIIA-mediated signaling involves src-family lck in human natural killer cells. J Immunol 1993;151:6794-6800.

13   Pignata C, Sanghera JS, Cossette L, Pelech SL, Ritz J: Interleukin-12 induces tyrosine phosphorylation and activation of 44-kDa mitogen-activated protein kinase in human T cells. Blood 1994;83:184–190.

14   Bacon CM, McVicar DW, Ortaldo JR, Rees RC, O'Shea JJ, Johnston JA: Interleukin-12 (IL-12) induces tyrosine phosphorylation of JAK2 and TYK2: Differential use of Janus family tyrosine kinases by IL-2 and IL-12. J Exp Med 1995;181:399–404.

15   Bacon CM, Petricoin EF, Ortaldo JR, Rees RC, Larner AC, Johnston JA, O'Shea JJ: Interleukin-12 induces tyrosine phosphorylation and activation of STAT4 in human lymphocytes. Proc Natl Acad Sci USA 1995;92:7307–7311.

16   Jacobson NG, Szabo SJ, Weber-Nordt RM, Zhong Z, Schreiber RD, Darnell JE Jr, Murphy KM: Interleukin-12 signaling in T helper 1 (Th1) cells involves tyrosine phosphorylation of signal transducer and activator of transcription (Stat)3 and Stat4. J Exp Med 1995;181:1755–1762.

17   Szabo SJ, Jacobson NG, Dighe AS, Gubler U, Murphy KM: Developmental commitment to the Th2 lineage by extinction of IL-12 signaling. Immunity 1995;2:665–675.

18   Cho SS, Bacon CM, Sudarshan C, Rees RC, Finbloom D, Pine R, O'Shea JJ: Activation of STAT4 by IL-12 and IFNα. J Immunol 1996;157:4781–4789.

19   Thierfelder WE, van Deursen JM, Yamamoto K, Tripp RA, Sarawar SR, Carson RT, Sangster MY, Vignali DA, Doherty PC, Grosveld GC, Ihle JN: Requirement for Stat4 in interleukin-12-mediated responses of natural killer and T cells. Nature 1996;82:171–174.

20   Kaplan MH, Sun YL, Hoey T, Grusby MJ: Impaired IL-12 responses and enhanced development of Th2 cells in Stat4-deficient mice. Nature 1996;382:174–177.

21   Magram J, Connaughton SE, Warrier RR, Carvajal DM, Wu C-Y, Ferrante J, Stewart C, Sarmiento U, Faherty DA, Gately MK: IL-12 deficient mice are defective in IFN-γ production and type 1 cytokine responses. Immunity 1996;4:471–481.

22   Gollob JA, Li J, Reinherz EL, Ritz J: CD2 regulates responsiveness of activated T cells to interleukin-12. J Exp Med 1995;182:721–731.

23   Zou J, Presky DH, Wu C-Y, Gubler U: Differential association between the cytoplasmic regions of the IL-12 receptor subunits β1/β2 and JAK kinases. J Biol Chem 1997;272:6073–6077.

24   Mattner F, Fischer S, Guckes S, Jin S, Kaulen H, Schmitt E, Rüde E, Germann T: The interleukin-12 subunit p40 specifically inhibits effects of the interleukin-12 heterodimer. Eur J Immunol 1993; 23:2202–2208.

25   Gillessen S, Carvajal D, Ling P, Podlaski FJ, Stremlo DL, Familletti PC, Gubler U, Presky DH, Stern AS, Gately MK: Mouse interleukin-12 (IL-12) p40 homodimer: A potent IL-12 antagonist. Eur J Immunol 1995;25:200–206.

26   Nickbarg EB, Vath JE, Pittman DD, Leonard JE, Waldburger KE, Bond MD: Structural characterization of the recombinant p40 heavy chain subunit monomer and homodimer of murine IL-12. Bioorg Chem 1995;23:380–396.

27   Piccotti JR, Chan SY, Li K, Eichwald EJ, Bishop DK: Differential effects of IL-12 receptor blockade with IL-12 p40 homodimer on the induction of CD4[+] and CD8[+] IFN-gamma-producing cells. J Immunol 1997;158:643–648.

28   Presky DH, Minetti LJ, Gillessen S, Gubler U, Chizzonite R, Stern AS, Gately MK: Evidence for multiple sites of interaction between IL-12 and its receptor. Ann N Y Acad Sci 1996;795:390–393.

29   Ling P, Gately MK, Gubler U, Stern AS, Lin P, Hollfelder K, Su C, Pan Y-CE, Hakimi J: Human IL-12 p40 homodimer binds to the IL-12 receptor but does not mediate biologic activity. J Immunol 1995;154:116–127.

30   D'Andrea A, Rengaraju M, Valiante NM, Chehimi J, Kubin M, Aste M, Chan SH, Kobayashi M, Young D, Nickbarg E, Chizzonite R, Wolf SF, Trinchieri G: Production of natural killer cell stimulatory factor (interleukin-12) by peripheral blood mononuclear cells. J Exp Med 1992;176: 1387–1398.

31   Heinzel FP, Rerko DM, Ling P, Hakimi J, Schoenhaut DS: Interleukin-12 is produced in vivo during endotoxemia and stimulates synthesis of gamma interferon. Infect Immun 1994;62:4244–4249.

32   Wysocka M, Kubin M, Vieira LQ, Ozmen L, Garotta G, Scott P, Trinchieri G: Interleukin-12 is required for interferon-γ production and lethality in lipopolysaccharide-induced shock in mice. Eur J Immunol 1995;25:672–676.

33   Zhang M, Gately MK, Wang E, Gong J, Wolf SF, Lu S, Modlin RL, Barnes PF: Interleukin-12 at the site of disease in tuberculosis. J Clin Invest 1994;93:1733–1739.

34   Bette M, Jin S-C, Germann T, Schäfer MK-H, Weihe E, Rüde E, Fleischer B: Differential expression of mRNA encoding interleukin-12 p35 and p40 subunits in situ. Eur J Immunol 1994;24:2435–2440.

35   Gately MK, Carvajal DM, Connaughton SE, Gillessen S, Warrier RR, Kolinsky KD, Wilkinson VL, Dwyer CM, Higgins GF, Podlaski FJ, Faherty DA, Familletti PC, Stern AS, Presky DH: Interleukin-12 antagonist activity of mouse interleukin-12 p40 homodimer in vitro and in vivo. Ann N Y Acad Sci 1996;795:1–12.

36   Kato K, Shimozato O, Hoshi K, Wakimoto H, Hamada H, Yagita H, Okumura K: Local production of the p40 subunit of interleukin-12 T-helper 1-mediated immune responses and prevents allogeneic myoblast rejection. Proc Natl Acad Sci USA 1996;93:9085–9089.

37   Wu C-Y, Ferrante J, Gately MK, Magram J: Characterization of IL-12 receptor β1 chain (IL-12Rβ1) deficient mice: IL-12Rβ1 is an essential component of the functional mouse IL-12R. J Immunol 1997, in press.

38   Yoshida K, Taga T, Saito M, Suematsu S, Kumanogoh A, Tanaka T, Fujiwara H, Hirata M, Yamagami T, Nakahata T, Hirbayashi T, Yoneda Y, Tanaka K, Wang WZ, Mori C, Shiota K, Yoshida N, Kishimoto T: Targeted disruption of gp130, a common signal transducer for the interleukin-6 family of cytokines, leads to a myocardial and hematological disorders. Proc Natl Acad Sci USA 1996;93:407–411.

Dr. Alvin S. Stern, Hoffmann-La Roche Inc., Building 123/3,
Nutley, NJ 07110-1199 (USA)
Tel. (201) 235 5129, Fax (201) 235 3805, E-mail: Alvin_S.Stern@Roche.COM

Adorini L (ed): IL-12. Chem Immunol. Basel, Karger, 1997, vol 68, pp 38–53

....

Early Events Controlling T-Helper Cell Differentiation: The Role of the IL-12 Receptor

Lars Rogge, Francesco Sinigaglia

Roche Milano Ricerche, Milano, Italy

In a seminal study a decade ago, Mosmann et al. [1] showed that murine CD4$^+$ T-helper (Th) cells can be classified into two major subsets, termed Th1 and Th2, according to the pattern of lymphokines they produce. Th1 cells secrete IFN-γ and predominantly promote cell-mediated immune responses, while Th2 cells, which produce IL-4, IL-5 and IL-13, provide help for some B-cell responses. IL-4 in particular is the major inducer of B-cell switching to IgE production [2], and therefore plays a crucial role in allergic reactions involving IgE and mast cells. Th cells producing cytokines typical of both Th1 and Th2 clones have also been described in both the murine and human system, and they have been named Th0 [3]. The concept of polarized Th cell subsets was later extended to the human system [4], and the balance between Th1 and Th2 subsets was shown to be a major determinant of the outcome of physiological as well as pathological immune responses, including autoimmune, allergic and infectious diseases [5, 6]. Thus, understanding the mechanisms underlying Th cell differentiation could prove to be essential for therapeutic manipulation of the cytokine phenotype in disease conditions.

The role of various factors influencing the development of Th cells has been studied using $\alpha\beta$ T-cell receptor (TCR) transgenic mice as a source of antigen-specific naive CD4$^+$ T cells [7–11] and with purified naive (Mel-14$^+$) T cells stimulated in vitro with plate-bound anti-CD3 antibodies [12]. In the human system, Th cell development has been studied by analyzing T-cell clones obtained either from peripheral blood specific for a variety of bacterial and parasite antigens or allergens, or from target organs of patients with immunopathological disorders [13–17]. Important results have also been obtained with T-cell lines generated by stimulation of cord blood derived neonatal (CD45RA$^+$) T cells [18–20]. These results suggest that the dose and route of antigen administration, the type of antigen-presenting cell (APC), and the costimulatory pathways, could influence Th cell differentiation [21–26]. However, the cytokines present at the time of priming play the most prominent role in inducing polarized Th cell responses. In particular, IL-4 promotes Th2 development [8, 10], whereas IL-12 produced by APCs is a potent inducer of Th1 cells [9, 11, 27]. Consistent with the importance of IL-12 for induction of Th1 cell differentiation is the finding that IL-12 p40$^{-/-}$ mice are defective in IFN-γ production and almost completely lack the ability to generate a Th1 response [28]. In contrast, knockout of the IL-4 gene resulted in deficient Th2 responses [29, 30].

Here we review recent data on the mechanisms by which IL-12 and other cytokines control the differentiation of naive CD4$^+$ T cells into Th1 or Th2 effector cells.

Differential Signaling in Response to IL-12 in Th1 and Th2 Cells

IL-12 is a powerful inducer of Th1 cells producing high levels of IFN-γ [31]. We have therefore analyzed the mechanisms by which this cytokine exerts its biological effects on the target cells. The IL-12 signaling pathway has been studied by analyzing the molecules that become phosphorylated on tyrosine residues when T cells are exposed to IL-12. These studies revealed that IL-12 induces tyrosine phosphorylation of the Janus kinases Tyk2 and Jak2 [32] and the signal transducer and activator of transcription 4 (STAT4) in mitogen-activated peripheral blood mononuclear cells (PBMC) [33], and in a murine Th1 clone [34]. These phosphorylation events are necessary for functional activation of both Janus kinases [35, 36] and STAT proteins [37, 38]. Upon phosphorylation on specific tyrosine residues, STAT proteins dimerize and translocate to the nucleus, where they act as transcriptional activators by binding specific DNA sequences in the promoters of cytokine-inducible genes [39, 40].

Using a murine TCR transgenic system, Szabo et al. [41] have recently described a novel mechanism controlling the stable commitment to a Th2 lineage. While IL-4 could reverse early Th1 differentiation, IL-12 failed to reverse early Th2 development. To examine the reasons for the irreversibility of early Th2 responses, the ability of Th1 and Th2 cells to induce tyrosine phosphorylation of STATs in response to several cytokines was analyzed. While IFN-α and IL-4 activated STAT-containing complexes to a similar extent in both Th1 and Th2 cells, IL-12 selectively activated Jak2, STAT3, and STAT4 in Th1 cells, but not in differentiated Th2 cells. Thus, reversibility of early Th1 responses results from the maintenance of the IL-4 signaling pathway in the Th1 subset, whereas commitment to the Th2 phenotype results from the rapid loss of IL-12-induced signaling in early developing Th2 cells [41]. The question whether IL-12 can reverse established Th2 responses into Th1/Th2 responses was also addressed in human allergen-specific CD4+ T-cell clones generated from the peripheral blood of atopic patients. This study showed that human allergen-specific Th cells with a strongly polarized Th2 cytokine profile are not able to phosphorylate STAT4 in response to IL-12, and cannot be induced to produce IFN-γ [42].

To characterize the role of IL-12 and other cytokines in the differentiation of Th cell subsets, we have generated Th1 and Th2 lines by stimulating human cord blood leukocytes with mitogen in the presence of IL-12 and neutralizing anti-IL-4 monoclonal antibody (mAb) or IL-4 and neutralizing anti-IL-12 mAb, respectively. This protocol allows the establishment of human T-cell lines with strongly polarized cytokine production. To ascertain whether early developing human Th1 and Th2 subsets also differ in IL-12 signaling, we examined STAT4 expression and tyrosine phosphorylation in response to IL-12 in Th1 and Th2 lines. IL-12 treatment induced tyrosine phosphorylation of STAT4 selectively in Th1 but not in Th2 cells, although both cell types expressed comparable amounts of the STAT4 protein. Similarly, Jak2, which was also expressed at comparable levels in Th1 and Th2 cells, was phosphorylated only in Th1 cells following IL-12 stimulation [20].

Expression of IL-12 Receptors during Th Cell Development

A possible explanation for the observed failure of human and mouse Th2 cells to respond to IL-12 could be a differential expression of IL-12 receptors on Th1 and Th2 cells. This question was addressed in parallel studies in the human system in our laboratory [20] and using a murine TCR transgenic system in Ken Murphy's laboratory [43] (see also Ken Murphy's review in this book [44]).

We examined whether the defect in IL-12 signaling observed in Th2 cells was due to a differential expression of IL-12 receptors in the two Th subsets. To date, two IL-12R subunits, termed β1 and β2, have been identified. Human IL-12R β1 or β2, independently expressed in COS cells, bind human IL-12 with low affinity, whereas coexpression of IL-12R β1 and β2 in COS cells gives rise to high affinity binding sites, suggesting that both chains are sufficient and necessary to reconstitute a functional receptor [45, 46]. These studies have also shown that IL-12R β2 is the signaling component of the IL-12R, in accord with the fact that IL-12R β2, in contrast to IL-12R β1, contains tyrosine residues in its cytoplasmic domain [46]. These tyrosine residues, when phosphorylated upon receptor activation, constitute docking sites for STAT proteins [47–49]. We have analyzed the mRNA expression levels for the IL-12R β1 and β2 subunits in both Th1 and Th2 lines at different time-points after priming. While IL-12R β1 transcripts were expressed in similar amounts in both Th1 and Th2 cells, the transcripts coding for the IL-12R β1 subunit were selectively expressed in established Th1 but not Th2 lines. Maximum expression in Th1 cells was seen between day 3 and day 8 and declined thereafter. Th2 cells, in contrast, expressed little IL-12R β2 transcripts on day 3; none were detected after day 8.

A key question is whether cytokine signaling is required for IL-12R induction or whether stimulation via the TCR/CD3 complex is sufficient to induce IL-12 receptors in naive T cells. IL-12R transcripts were therefore analyzed in CD45RA$^+$ T cells purified from PBMC of healthy individuals before and after stimulation with plate-bound anti-CD3. IL-12R transcripts were not found in naive T cells, but could be detected as early as 24 h after T-cell activation. Priming of naive T cells in the presence of IL-12 resulted in enhanced expression of IL-12R β2 transcripts in this population; priming of cells in the presence of IL-4, in contrast, resulted in very low levels of IL-12R β2. Thus, antigen receptor triggering is sufficient to induce expression of a functional IL-12 receptor, and to make naive T cells susceptible to IL-12 signaling. IL-12R expression was also analyzed by radioligand binding assays. Scatchard analysis of specific ^{125}I-IL-12 binding to human cord blood derived Th1 and Th2 cell lines revealed both high and low ^{125}I-IL-12 binding sites in Th1 cell lines. In contrast, Th2 cells lines exhibited only low affinity ^{125}I-IL-12 binding sites. The absence of measurable high affinity ^{125}I-IL-12 binding to the human Th2 cell lines is in accord with the observed lack of IL-12R β2 expression in these cells [20]. In contrast, similar levels of high and low affinity IL-12 binding were measured in mouse Th1 and Th2 cell lines [41]. This difference in IL-12 binding behavior in the mouse and human systems may reflect the dominant role mouse IL-12R β1 plays in binding IL-12 [50], while in human both IL-12R β1 and β2 appear to contribute equally to IL-12 binding [46]. These results demonstrate that the IL-12R β2 subunit is selectively expressed in Th1 cells where it is induced upon T-cell activation. Moreover, these findings suggest that the lack of IL-12R β2 chain expression is the reason underlying the inability of IL-12 to activate the Jak2-STAT4 pathway in either human or mouse Th2 cells.

Regulation of IL-12R β2 mRNA Expression during Th Cell Differentiation

Earlier studies have demonstrated that IL-4 blocks the development of naive murine CD4$^+$ T cells into Th1 effectors. The block is complete in the absence of IL-12 in the priming culture, but incomplete if IL-12 is also present [11]. Consistent with these data, it was observed that naive T cells primed in the presence of IL-4 and IL-12 together developed into cells secreting both IL-4 and IFN-γ. These cells phosphorylate STAT4 in response to IL-12 and accordingly express the IL-12R β2 mRNA, although to a lower level, as compared to Th1 cells. In contrast, naive T cells primed in the presence of IL-4 and neutralizing anti-IL-12 mAb completely lost IL-12R β2 expression and, consequently, IL-12-mediated signaling [20, 43]. Although the mechanism by which IL-4 induces the generation of IL-12 nonresponsive Th2 cells remains to be clarified, these results are consistent with a model in which IL-12 prevents the gradual extinction of the IL-12R β2 subunit that appears to follow exposure to IL-4. Alternatively, the presence of IL-12 or IL-4 could result in the preferential expansion of IL-12-responsive Th1 cells or IL-12 nonresponsive Th2 cells, respectively.

Since the expression of several cytokine receptors has been shown to be regulated according to a positive or negative feedback pathway, we asked whether IL-12 could directly influence expression of the IL-12R β2 transcripts. IL-12 added to quiescent Th1 and Th2 cells resulted in a 7-fold increase in IL-12R β2 transcripts in Th1 lines and a 2-fold increase in Th2 lines. Time-course experiments revealed that the IL-12-induced up-regulation of the IL-12R β2 mRNA in primed Th cells was transient: maximal induction was seen 24–48 h after the addition of IL-12 but returned to the level of the control cultures after 96 h. Similar results were obtained with established Th1 and Th2 clones [20]. The IL-12-induced transient up-regulation of the IL-12R β2 transcripts in Th2 clones may account for the transient period of IL-12-induced IFN-γ production in cells with an established Th2 phenotype [51, 52].

Analysis of the IL-4 and IL-12 Signaling Pathways in vivo

The crucial role of IL-4 and IL-12 signaling in the differentiation of Th subsets has also been analyzed more recently in STAT6- and STAT4-deficient mice. These proteins are thought to mediate functional responses to IL-4 and IL-12, respectively. Although no significant differences in cell numbers or composition of T- and B-lymphocyte subsets were detectable between wild-type and STAT-deficient mice, STAT6-deficient T lymphocytes fail to differentiate into Th2 cells in response to IL-4 [53–55]. In contrast, the analysis of STAT4$^{-/-}$ T cells revealed an impaired production of IFN-γ upon antigen receptor triggering, indicative of a defect in Th1 differentiation [56, 57]. It had been shown previously, that STAT1$^{-/-}$ cells are solely deficient in IFN-mediated biological responses [58, 59]. Taken together, these data indicate that, despite the fact that cytokines activate multiple signaling pathways, STAT proteins are specific, nonredundant, and therefore essential components of the cytokine signaling apparatus. The availability of mice deficient in STAT proteins might therefore prove useful to further analyze the roles of cytokines and their signaling pathways in the differentiation of Th subsets in vivo.

The Role of IFNs in the Generation of Th1 Cells

In addition to IL-12, IFNs act as cofactors for Th1 cell development. It has been shown that in the mouse, IFN-γ but not IFN-α induces Th1 cell development [60]. Neutralization of endogenous IFN-γ in cultures of murine naive CD4$^+$ T cells differentiated in the presence of IL-12 resulted in a significantly reduced IFN-γ production upon restimulation [12, 61], indicating that IFN-γ acts as an important cofactor for Th1 development in mouse cells. These data are consistent with the recent observation, that IFN-γ can rescue IL-12R β2 mRNA expression even in the presence of IL-4 and restore IL-12 responsiveness in early developing mouse Th2 cells [43]. This regulatory mechanism appears not to be true in the development of human Th1 subsets. As a matter of fact, addition of IFN-γ at the time of Th2 priming, or the addition of neutralizing anti-IFN-γ mAb at Th1 priming has no significant effect either on the pattern of Th cell development or on the expression of the IL-12R β2 chain [20]. In contrast, stimulation of purified resting human T cells in the presence of IFN-α increases the frequency of IFN-γ secreting CD4$^+$ T cells [62]. In addition, allergen-specific T-cell clones generated in the presence of IFN-α from the peripheral blood of atopic patients show a skewing towards the Th0/Th1 phenotype [63]. Importantly, human cord blood leukocytes primed in the presence of IFN-α or IFN-β develop into IFN-γ-producing Th1 cells, even when cultured in the presence of the Th2-inducing cytokine IL-4 and of neutralizing anti-IL-12 antibodies. The Th1 cells generated in this manner express the IL-12R β2 mRNA and are responsive to IL-12 [20]. These experiments provide the first evidence that Th1 development is possible in the absence of IL-12. Taken together, these results suggest that type I IFNs induce IL-12R β2 expression and Th1 development in human T cells, whereas in mouse T cells the same effect is obtained with IFN-γ. Interestingly, IFNs dominate and override the functional effects of IL-4 in both human and mouse T cells.

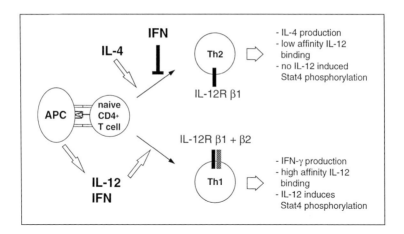

Fig. 1. The role of cytokines in the differentiation of naive T cells into polarized Th subsets. TCR triggering induces initial expression of functional IL-12 receptors on primed T cells. The further developmental fate of the T cells depends on the cytokine environment at the time of priming. IL-12 and IFNs activate specific STAT proteins in primed T cells which up-regulate expression of the IL-12R β2 subunit, the signaling component of the IL-12R. These cells will differentiate into IL-12-responsive Th1 cells, secreting primarily IFN-γ. In contrast, T cells developing in the presence of IL-4 lose their capacity to bind and respond to IL-12 but will differentiate into IL-4-producing Th2 cells. The extinction of the IL-12 signaling pathway in Th2 cells is due to the loss of IL-12R β2 expression mediated directly or indirectly by a STAT protein activated in response to IL-4. IFNs dominantly block IL-4-induced differentiation of Th2 cells.

The divergent effect that type I and type II IFNs have on Th1 development in the human as compared to the mouse system could be explained by their ability to activate different signaling pathways within the cell. Indeed, preliminary results from our laboratory indicate that in human Th2 cells, both IFN-α and IFN-β are able to induce a much stronger phosphorylation of STAT1 as compared to IFN-γ. In addition, it has recently been demonstrated that IFN-α efficiently induces phosphorylation of STAT4 in human activated T cells [64]. Thus, both IL-12 and type I IFNs appear to activate STAT4, a protein critically involved in the generation of Th1 responses [56, 57]. In contrast, a previous report has shown that IFN-α is unable to activate STAT4 in murine T cells [34], while IFN-γ induces strong phosphorylation of STAT1 in murine Th2 cells [65, 66]. These quantitative and qualitative differences in IFN-induced signaling in human and mouse cells may explain the differential effects of type I and type II IFNs on human and mouse Th cell development. Figure 1 summarizes the role of cytokines in the development of polarized T helper subsets.

IL-6 Induces Th2 Development

The early events leading to Th1 differentiation in mice infected by various intracellular pathogens are fairly well understood. Microbial products or direct infection induces production of IL-12 by macrophages, which, in turn, activates IFN-γ production by NK cells. This event creates a cytokine environment dominated by IL-12 and IFN-γ. Naive CD4$^+$ T cells migrating to the site of infection and initiating a specific immune response to the pathogen in this micro-environment will preferentially develop into Th1 effector cells. Therefore, the effector functions of the innate response that are most efficient to control this type of infectious microorganism are the same that subsequently direct a polarized antigen-specific Th1 response necessary to eliminate the pathogen [67].

The source of IL-4 required to induce Th2 differentiation is less clear. Potential sources include conventional CD4$^+$ memory T cells, NK1.1$^+$ T cells (an atypical population of CD4$^+$ T cells expressing several markers characteristic of NK cells), mast cells, basophils, and eosinophils [68]. A recent report suggests that IL-6 is able to initiate the polarization of naive CD4$^+$ T cells to effector Th2 cells by inducing the production of endogenous IL-4 [69]. IL-6 is produced by a wide spectrum of cells including fibroblasts, endothelial cells, neuronal cells, macrophages, mast cells, and CD4$^+$ Th2 cells. It constitutes an important component of inflammatory and acute-phase responses, but has not previously been implicated in the generation of polarized Th cell responses. Rincon et al. [69] stimulated in vitro purified mouse CD4$^+$ T cells in the presence or absence of IL-6 and other cytokines. The production of IL-4 and IFN-γ upon restimulation was measured as a readout for Th1 or Th2 differentiation. The addition of either IL-6 or IL-4 to the primary cultures directed differentiation of the CD4$^+$ T cells to a Th2 phenotype. Development towards a Th2 phenotype is obtained also without the addition of exogenous cytokines, when IL-6 producing APCs are present in the culture. IL-6 did not induce Th2 differentiation in the presence of neutralizing antibodies to IL-4, indicating that its effect is mediated by IL-4 production in the primary cultures. This study suggests that IL-6 produced by APCs may trigger the Th2 pathway by acting directly on the naive CD4$^+$ T cells and by inducing endogenous IL-4 production. This initial production of IL-4 might act as an autocrine differentiation factor for the development of a Th2 response.

Transcriptional Events Controlling Th Cell Differentiation

The effector functions of Th1 and Th2 cells are mainly mediated by the cytokines they secrete. It is therefore not only important to analyze the mechanisms that induce polarized Th cell responses, but also how cytokine production by the Th1/Th2 effector cells is controlled. The mechanism by which expression of the IFN-γ and IL-4 genes is restricted to the appropriate Th subset appears to be fairly complex. Considerable efforts were made to identify nuclear factors that are either selectively present or active in Th1 or Th2 cells. Recent evidence may provide some insight into this important question.

Previous studies have demonstrated that the nuclear factor of activated T cells (NF-AT) is critically involved in the induction of IL-2 gene expression in response to TCR ligation [70]. NF-AT is a multisubunit transcription factor consisting of a pre-existing cytoplasmic subunit and an inducible nuclear component containing the AP-1 family members Fos and Jun [71]. It has been shown that the immunosuppressive drugs cyclosporin A and FK-506 block nuclear translocation of the pre-existing cytoplasmic subunit of NF-AT which occurs in response to antigen receptor triggering [72]. The genes encoding NF-AT family members have been cloned and sequenced [73–75]. Interestingly, all NF-AT family members have a region of sequence homology with the Rel homology domain of the NF-κB transcription factors. The NF-AT Rel homology domain is believed to interact with polypeptides of the basic region-leucine zipper families, such as Fos and Jun [76]. Even though NF-AT has initially been described as a transcription factor critically involved in the expression of the IL-2 gene, detailed studies of the protein-DNA interactions in the murine IL-4 promoter revealed cooperative binding of NF-AT and AP-1 family members to specific sites within the proximal IL-4 promoter [77, 78]. These findings, however, cannot explain Th2-specific expression of the IL-4 gene, since the same factors are involved in the regulation of the IL-2, granulocyte-macrophage colony-stimulating factor (GM-CSF), and tumor necrosis factor-α (TNF-α) genes [77, 79–81], some of which are also expressed in Th1 cells. Thus, it appears that both Th1 and Th2-specific cytokine genes encoding IL-2 and IL-4, respectively, are regulated by the same transcription factors [82]. In addition, the analysis of anti-CD3 activated T cells derived from NF-ATp$^{-/-}$ mice revealed not only dysregulation of the IL-4 gene, but also impaired expression of the genes encoding IL-2, IFN-γ, GM-CSF, IL-13, and TNF-α [83].

To discriminate between Th1- and Th2-specific gene regulation, Lederer et al. [84] analyzed the activation of the NF-κB transcription factor in murine Th1 and Th2 clones. They showed that nuclear extracts prepared from TCR-stimulated Th2 clones contained significantly less p65(RelA)-p50 NF-κB transcription complexes than nuclear extracts prepared in parallel from Th1 or Th0 clones. Interestingly, both Th1/Th0 and Th2 cells expressed similar amounts of cytoplasmic p65(RelA), however TCR ligation failed to induce nuclear translocation of p65(RelA) in Th2 clones, which is necessary for the formation of an active NF-κB transcription factor. A subsequent study was performed with Th1 and Th2 cell lines generated by stimulating T cells from TCR-transgenic animals with APCs and the corresponding peptide in the presence of IL-12 or IL-4, respectively. No significant differences in the nuclear presence of NF-κB could be observed [85]. The discrepancy could be explained by the fact that IL-2 production, which also depends on active nuclear NF-κB, is detectable in early developing Th1 and Th2 lines, but not in Th2 clones that had been restimulated many times, and which lack the active nuclear form of the transcription factor.

The same study also addressed the important question of when T cells acquire cytokine transcription profiles characteristic of Th1 and Th2 subsets during in vitro differentiation. The kinetics of IL-2, IL-4, and IFN-γ mRNA expression in early developing Th1 and Th2 cells were determined at different time-points after stimulating naive T cells in the presence of IL-12 or IL-4, respectively. IL-2 transcripts were detectable 6 h after stimulation in both Th1 and Th2 cultures and expression of the IL-2 gene was not significantly affected by the presence of IL-12 or IL-4. IFN-γ mRNA expression was induced as early as 6 h after initial stimulation in the presence of IL-12, and IL-12-treated cultures expressed significantly higher levels of IFN-γ transcripts than control or IL-4-treated cultures. In contrast, IL-4 transcripts were not detected until 48 h after priming in the IL-4-treated cultures [85]. These results suggest that regulation of IFN-γ and IL-4 gene expression are temporally distinct events and may be regulated by independent mechanisms. This study also indicates that IL-2 expression is not restricted to the Th1 subset.

STAT6 and c-Maf as Regulators of the IL-4 Gene

In an attempt to identify factors that interact with the Rel-homology domain of NF-ATp with the yeast two-hybrid system, Ho et al. [86] recently isolated, among other clones, a cDNA excoding the proto-oncogene c-*maf*. c-*maf* is expressed in murine Th2, but not in Th1 clones after restimulation with anti-CD3 antibodies. Expression of c-*maf* was also detected in Th2 lines 8 days after initial stimulation of naive T cells in the presence of IL-4. c-*maf* encodes a basic region-leucine zipper protein and shares homology with c-*fos* and c-*jun*. In analogy to other AP-1 family members, c-Maf can form homodimers and heterodimers with Fos and Jun. The evidence that c-Maf is functionally involved in the regulation of the IL-4 gene stems from experiments in which the cDNA encoding c-Maf was introduced into a murine Th1 clone and a B-cell line. Ectopic expression of c-Maf induced IL-4 gene expression in Th1 and B cells. In addition, overexpression of both c-Maf and NF-ATp revealed a synergistic effect on the transactivation of the IL-4 gene [86]. c-Maf represents the first subset-specific transcription factor identified to date. An additional factor interacting with the Rel-homology domain of NF-ATp was recently published by the same laboratory. This factor, designated NIP45 (for **N**F-ATp **I**nteracting **P**rotein), potentiates transactivation by NF-AT family members and synergizes with c-Maf in the induction of IL-4 mRNA expression [87]. Even though these results may explain nicely Th2-specific expression of the IL-4 gene, further studies are required to determine whether c-Maf is involved in the early polarization of naive T cells towards the Th2 subset, or whether the Th2-specific expression of c-Maf is a consequence of Th2 differentiation.

Lederer et al. [85] recently reported the identification of a transcription factor that appears to be selectively activated in early developing Th2 cells and which binds to a novel *cis*-element in the IL-4 promoter. Sequence analysis of the IL-4 promoter revealed the presence of a potential binding site for STAT6. Gel-shift assays were performed with an oligonucleotide encompassing this potential STAT6 binding element. Nuclear extracts prepared from T-cell lines as early as 24 h after priming of naive T cells in the presence of IL-4 contained an activity that formed a specific protein-DNA complex with the STAT6 binding site. Supershift assays showed that this complex consisted of STAT6. Importantly, no STAT6-DNA binding activity was detected in T-cell lines generated in the presence of IL-12. This study showed that STAT6, a factor which, as discussed above, is critically involved in Th2 differentiation, binds to the IL-4 promoter in early developing Th2 cells. This event precedes IL-4 gene transcription. Even though the functional role of STAT6 in the induction of IL-4 gene expression remains to be investigated in greater detail, the authors suggest that the observed constitutive activation of STAT6 in developing Th2 cells may be induced by the autocrine effect of secreted IL-4.

STAT Multimers May Activate the IFN-γ Gene

Transcriptional activation by STAT factors may also explain Th1-specific expression of the IFN-γ gene. Xu et al. [88] analyzed the mechanisms of STAT regulation in response to IL-12. Since IL-12 induces IFN-γ production in activated T and NK cells, they searched for natural STAT binding sites near the IFN-γ gene. DNase I footprinting analysis revealed binding of purified recombinant STAT1, 4, 5, and 6 to multiple sites within the first intron of the IFN-γ gene. Each of the STAT proteins protected distinct sites within this region which does not contain any perfect STAT consensus binding elements. Given the multiple binding sites occupied by STATs, it was analyzed whether cooperative interactions between the adjacently bound STAT dimers might stabilize binding of STAT factors to degenerate sites. Gel shift assays performed with oligonucleotides encompassing two adjacent STAT4 binding sites from the first intron of the IFN-γ gene revealed strong binding of STAT4. Mutation of either site abrogated STAT4 binding, suggesting that STAT4 bound cooperatively to this element. The domain mediating tetramerization was subsequently mapped to the amino-terminal part of STAT4. The functional relevance of these findings for the regulation of IFN-γ gene expression is not yet proven, however, the evidence that STATs are capable of interacting with other factors not only through their SH2 domain and thus may form higher order structures, suggests they may bind to other sites than the canonical STAT consensus sequences. This may have important implications in the analysis of the specific and redundant effects mediated by cytokines.

Conclusions

The regulation of the IL-12 signaling pathway appears to be of critical importance for the developmental commitment of Th cells. Expression of the IL-12R β2 subunit appears to be restricted to the Th1 subset and is therefore the first Th1 subset-specific noncytokine gene to be identified to date. Recent data indicate the presence of two major signaling pathways influencing IL-12R β2 expression. Triggering of the antigen receptor on naive T cells is sufficient for the initial expression of functional IL-12 receptors on activated T cells. Depending on the cytokines present during the differentiation, T cells will then develop into IL-12-responsive Th1 cells or IL-12 nonresponsive Th2 cells. Analysis of the IL-12R β2 promoter should provide insights into the molecular mechanisms by which TCR triggering and signals mediated by IL-12, IFN-α, IL-4 and other cytokines are integrated to regulate IL-12R β2 chain expression.

The selective expression and regulation of the IL-12R β2 subunit may help to understand the molecular events controlling Th cell development and may provide therapeutic options for altering the Th1/Th2 balance in several immunopathological conditions.

References

1   Mosmann TR, Cherwinski H, Bond MW, Giedlin MA, Coffman RL: Two types of murine T helper T cell clone. I. Definition according to profiles of lymphokine activities and secreted proteins. J Immunol 1986;136:2348–2357.
2   Coffman RL, Lebman DA, Rothman P: The mechanism and regulation of immunoglobulin isotype switching. Adv Immunol 1993;54:228–269.

3   Seder RA, Paul WE: Acquisition of lymphokine-producing phenotype by CD4$^+$ T cells. Annu Rev Immunol 1994;12:635–673.
4   Romagnani S: Human Th1 and Th2: Doubt no more. Immunol Today 1991;12:256–257.
5   Romagnani S: Lymphokine production by human T cells in disease states. Annu Rev Immunol 1994;12:227–257.
6   Abbas AK, Murphy KM, Sher A: Functional diversity of helper T lymphocytes. Nature 1996;383:787–793.
7   Kaye J, Hsu M-L, Sauron M-E, Jameson SC, Gascoigne NRJ, Hedrick SM: Selective development of CD4$^+$ T cells in transgenic mice expressing a class II MHC-restricted antigen receptor. Nature 1989;341:746–749.
8   Hsieh CS, Heimberger AB, Gold JS, O'Garra A, Murphy KM: Differential regulation of T helper phenotype development by interleukins 4 and 10 in an alpha beta T cell-receptor transgenic system. Proc Natl Acad Sci USA 1992;89:6065–6069.
9   Hsieh C-S, Macatonia SE, Tripp CS, Wolf SF, O'Garra A, Murphy KM: Development of T_H1 CD4$^+$ T cells through IL-12 produced by *Listeria*-induced macrophages. Science 1993;260:547–549.
10   Seder RA, Paul WE, Davis MM, Fazekas de St Groth B: The presence of interleukin-4 during in vitro priming determines the lymphokine-producing potential of CD4$^+$ T cells from T cell receptor transgenic mice. J Exp Med 1992;176:1091–1098.
11   Seder RA, Gazzinelli R, Sher A, Paul WE: IL-12 acts directly on CD4$^+$ T cells to enhance priming for interferon-γ production and diminishes interleukin-4 inhibition of such priming. Proc Natl Acad Sci USA 1993;90:10188–10192.
12   Schmitt E, Hoehn P, Huels C, Goedert S, Palm N, Rüde E, Germann T: T helper type 1 development of naive CD4$^+$ T cells requires the coordinate action of interleukin-12 and interferon-γ and is inhibited by transforming growth factor-β. Eur J Immunol 1994;24:793–798.
13   Wierenga EA, Snoek M, de Groot C, Chretien I, Bos JD, Jansen HM, Kapsenberg M: Evidence for compartmentalization of functional subsets of CD4$^+$ T lymphocytes in atopic patients. J Immunol 1990;144:4651–4656.
14   Del Prete GF, De Carli M, Mastromaura C, Macchia D, Biagiotti R, Ricci M, Romagnani S: Purified protein derivative of *Mycobacterium tuberculosis* and excretory/secretory antigen(s) of *Toxocara canis* expand in vitro human T cells with stable and opposite (type 1 T helper or type 2 T helper) profile of cytokine production. J Clin Invest 1991;88:346–350.
15   Parronchi P, Macchia D, Piccini M-P, Biswas P, Simonelli C, Maggi E, Ricci M, Ansari AA, Romagnani S: Allergen- and bacterial antigen-specific T-cell clones established from atopic donors show a different profile of cytokine production. Proc Natl Acad Sci USA 1991;88:4538–4543.
16   Yssel H, Shanafelt MC, Soderberg C, Schneider PV, Anzola J, Peltz G: *Borrelia burgdorferi* activates a T helper type 1-like T cell subset in Lyme arthritis. J Exp Med 1991;174:593–601.
17   Salgame P, Abrams JS, Clayberger C, Goldstein H, Convitt J, Modlin RL, Bloom BR: Differing lymphokine profiles and functional subsets of human CD4+ and CD8+ T cell clones. Science 1991;254:279–281.
18   Demeure CE, Wu CY, Shu U, Schneider PV, Heusser C, Yssel H, Delespesse G: In vitro maturation of human neonatal CD4 T lymphocytes. II. Cytokines present at priming modulate the development of lymphokine production. J Immunol 1994;152:4775–4782.
19   Sornasse T, Larenas PV, Davis DA, de Vries JE, Yssel H: Differentiation of T helper 1 and 2 cells derived from naive human neonatal CD4$^+$ T cells, analyzed at the single cell level. J Exp Med 1996;184:473–483.
20   Rogge L, Barberis-Maino L, Biffi M, Passini N, Presky DH, Gubler U, Sinigaglia F: Selective expression of an interleukin-12 receptor component by human T helper 1 cells. J Exp Med 1997;185:825–832.
21   Bretscher PA, Wei G, Menon JN, Bielefeldt-Ohmann H: Establishment of stable, cell-mediated immunity that makes 'susceptible' mice resistant to *Leishmania major*. Science 1992;257:539–542.
22   Pfeiffer C, Stein J, Southwood S, Keterlaar H, Sette A, Bottomly K: Altered peptide ligands can control CD4 T lymphocyte differentiation in vivo. J Exp Med 1995;181:1569–1574.
23   Constant S, Pfeiffer A, Woodard T, Pasqualini T, Bottomly K: Extent of T cell receptor ligation can determine the functional differentiation of naive CD4$^+$ T cells. Exp Med 1995;182:1591–1596.

24   Kuchroo VK, Das MP, Brown JA, Ranger AM, Zamvil SS, Sobel RA, Weiner HL, Nabavi N, Glimcher LH: B7-1 and B7-2 costimulatory molecules activate differentially the Th1/Th2 developmental pathways: Application to autoimmune disease therapy. Cell 1995;80:707–718.

25   Lenschow DJ, Walunas TL, Bluestone JA: CD28/B7 system of T cell costimulation. Annu Rev Immunol 1996;14:233–258.

26   Guéry JC, Galbiati F, Smiroldo S, Adorini L: Selective development of T helper (Th)2 cells induced by continuous administration of low dose soluble proteins to normal and beta(2)-microglobulin-deficient BALB/c mice. J Exp Med 1996;183:485–497.

27   Manetti R, Parronchi P, Giudizi MG, Piccinni M-P, Maggi E, Trinchieri G, Romagnani S: Natural killer cell stimulatory factor (interleukin 12 [IL-12]) induces T helper 1 type (Th1)-specific immune responses and inhibits the development of IL-4-producing Th cells. J Exp Med 1993;177:1199–1204.

28   Magram J, Connaughton SE, Warrier RR, Carvajal DM, Wu C-Y, Ferrante J, Stewart C, Sarimiento U, Faherty DA, Gately MK: IL-12 deficient mice are defective in IFNγ production and type I cytokine responses. Immunity 1996;4:471–481.

29   Kühn R, Rajewsky K, Müller W: Generation and analysis of interleukin-4-deficient mice. Science 1991;254:707–710.

30   Kopf M, Le Gros G, Bachmann M, Lamers MC, Bluethmann H, Köhler G: Disruption of the murine IL-4 gene blocks Th2 cytokine responses. Nature 1993;362:245–248.

31   Trinchieri G: Interleukin-12: A proinflammatory cytokine with immunoregulatory functions that bridge innate resistance and antigen-specific adaptive immunity. Annu Rev Immunol 1995;13:251–276.

32   Bacon CM, McVicar DW, Ortaldo JR, Rees RC, O'Shea JJ, Johnston JA: Interleukin-12 (IL-12) induces tyrosine phosphorylation of Jak2 and Tyk2: Differential use of Janus family tyrosine kinases by IL-2 and IL-12. J Exp Med 1995;181:399–404.

33   Bacon CM, Petricoin EF III, Ortaldo JR, Rees RC, Larner AC, Johnston JA, O'Shea JJ: Interleukin-12 induces tyrosine phosphorylation and activation of STAT4 in human lymphocytes. Proc Natl Acad Sci USA 1995;92:7307–7311.

34   Jacobson NG, Szabo SJ, Weber-Nordt RN, Zhong Z, Schreiber RD, Darnell JE, Murphy KM: Interleukin-12 signaling in T helper type 1 (Th1) cells involves tyrosine phosphorylation of signal transducer and activator of transcription (Stat) 3 and 4. J Exp Med 1995;181:1755–1762.

35   Müller M, Briscoe J, Laxton C, Guschin D, Ziemiecki A, Silvennoinen O, Harpur AG, Barbieri G, Witthun BA, Schindler C, Pellegrini S, Wilks AF, Ihle JN, Stark GR, Kerr IA: The protein tyrosine kinase JAK1 complements defects in interferon-α/β and -γ signal transduction. Nature 1993;366:129–135.

36   Darnell JE, Kerr IM, Stark GS: Jak-STAT pathways and transcriptional activation in response to IFNs and other extracellular signaling proteins. Science 1994;264:1415–1421.

37   Fu X-Y: A transcription factor with SH2 and SH3 domains is directly activated by an interferon-α-induced cytoplasmic protein tyrosine kinase. Cell 1992;70:323–335.

38   Schindler C, Darnell JE: Transcriptional responses to polypeptide ligands: The JAK-STAT pathway. Annu Rev Biochem 1995;64:621–651.

39   Shuai K, Horvath CM, Tsai Huang LH, Qureshi SA, Cowburn D, Darnell JE: Interferon activation of the transcription factor Stat91 involves dimerization through SH2-phosphotyrosyl peptide interactions. Cell 1994;76:821–828.

40   Ihle JN: STATs: Signal transducers and activators of transcription. Cell 1996;84:331–334.

41   Szabo SJ, Jacobson NG, Dighe AS, Gubler U, Murphy KM: Developmental commitment to the Th2 lineage by extinction of IL-12 signaling. Immunity 1995;2:665–675.

42   Hilkins CMU, Messer G, Tesselaar K, van Rietschoten AGI, Kapsenberg ML, Wierenga EA: Lack of IL-12 signaling in human allergen-specific Th2 cells. J Immunol 1996;157:4316–4321.

43   Szabo SJ, Dighe AS, Gubler U, Murphy KM: Regulation of the interleukin-12R β2 subunit expression in developing T helper 1 (Th1) and Th2 cells. J Exp Med 1997;185:817–824.

44   Murphy KM, Murphy T, Szabo SJ, Jacobson NG, Guler ML, Gorham JD, Gubler U: Regulation of IL-12 receptor expression in early T helper responses implies two phases of Th1 differentiation: Capacitance and development; in Adorini L (ed): IL-12. Chem Immunol. Basel, Karger, 1997, vol 68, pp 54–69.

45   Chua AO, Chizzonite R, Desai BB, Truitt TP, Nunes P, Minetti LJ, Warrier RR, Presky DH, Levine JF, Gately MK, Gubler U: Expression cloning of a human IL-12 receptor component: A new member of the cytokine receptor superfamily with strong homology to gp130. J Immunol 1994; 153:128–136.

46   Presky DH, Yang H, Minetti LJ, Chua AO, Nabavi N, Wu C-Y, Gately MK, Gubler U: A functional interleukin-12 receptor complex is composed of two β type cytokine receptor subunits. Proc Natl Acad Sci USA 1996;93:14002–14007.

47   Greenlund AC, Farrar MA, Viviano BL, Schreiber RD: Ligand-induced IFNγ receptor tyrosine phosphorylation couples the receptor to its signal transduction system (p91). EMBO J 1994;13: 1591–1600.

48   Greenlund AC, Morales MO, Viviano BL, Yan H, Krolewski J, Schreiber RD: Stat recruitment by tyrosine-phosphorylated cytokine receptors: An ordered reversible affinity-driven process. Immunity 1995;2:677–687.

49   Ivashkiv LB: Cytokines and STATs: How can signals achieve specificity? Immunity 1995;3:1–4.

50   Chua AO, Wilkinson VL, Presky DH, Gubler U: Cloning and characterization of a mouse IL-12 receptor-beta component. J Immunol 1995;155:4286–4294.

51   Manetti R, Gerosa F, Giudizi MG, Biagiotti R, Parronchi P, Piccinni M-P, Sampognaro S, Maggi E, Romagnani S, Trinchieri G: Interleukin-12 induces stable priming for interferon γ (IFN-γ) production during differentiation of human T helper (Th) and transient IFN-γ production in established Th2 cell clones. J Exp Med 1994;179:1273–1283.

52   Yssel H, Fasler S, de Vries JE, de Waal Malefyt R: IL-12 transiently induces IFN-γ transcription and protein synthesis in human CD4+ allergen-specific Th2 T cell clones. Int Immunol 1994;6: 1091–1096.

53   Kaplan MH, Schindler U, Smiley ST, Grusby MJ: Stat6 is required for mediating responses to IL-4 and for the development of Th2 cells. Immunity 1996;4:313–319.

54   Takeda K, Tanaka T, Shi W, Matsumoto M, Minami M, Kashiwamura S-I, Nakanishi K, Yoshida N, Kishimoto T, Akira S: Essential role of Stat6 in IL-4 signalling. Nature 1996;380:627–630.

55   Shimoda K, van Deursen J, Sangster MY, Sarawar SR, Carson RT, Tripp RA, Chu C, Quelle FW, Nosaka T, Vignalli DAA, Doherty PC, Grosveld G, Paul WE, Ihle JN: Lack of IL-4-induced Th2 response and IgE class switching in mice with disrupted Stat6 gene. Nature 1996;380:630– 633.

56   Thierfelder WE, van Deursen JM, Yamamoto K, Tripp RA, Sarawar SR, Carson RT, Sangster MY, Vignali DAA, Doherty PC, Grosveld GC, Ihle JN: Requirement for Stat4 in interleukin-12-mediated responses of natural killer and T cells. Nature 1996;382:171–174.

57   Kaplan MH, Sun Y-L, Hoey T, Grusby MJ: Impaired IL-12 responses and enhanced development of Th2 cells in Stat4-deficient mice. Nature 1996;382:174–177.

58   Meraz MA, White JM, Sheehan KCF, Bach EA, Rodig SJ, Dighe AS, Kaplan DH, Riley JK, Greenlund AC, Campbell D, Carver-Moore K, DuBois RN, Clark R, Aguet M, Schreiber RD: Targeted disruption of the Stat1 gene in mice reveals unexpected physiologic specificity in the JAK-STAT signaling pathway. Cell 1996;84:431–442.

59   Durbin JE, Hackenmiller R, Simon MC, Levy DE: Targeted disruption of the mouse Stat1 gene results in compromised innate immunity to viral disease. Cell 1996;84:443–450.

60   Wenner CA, Güler ML, Macatonia SE, O'Garra A, Murphy KM: Roles of IFN-γ and IFN-α in IL-12-induced T helper cell-1 development. J Immunol 1996;1156:1442–1447.

61   Bradley LM, Dalton DK, Croft M: A direct role for IFN-γ in regulation of Th1 cell development. J Immunol 1996;157:1350–1358.

62   Brinkmann V, Geiger T, Alkan S, Heusser CH: Interferon-α increases the frequency of interferon-γ-producing CD4+ T cells. J Exp Med 1993;178:1655–1663.

63   Parronchi P, Mohapatra S, Sampognaro S, Giannarini L, Wahn U, Chong P, Mohapatra S, Maggi E, Renz H, Romagnani S: Effects of interferon-α on cytokine profile, T cell receptor repertoire and peptide reactivity of human allergen-specific T cells. Eur J Immunol 1996;26:697–703.

64   Cho SS, Bacon CM, Sudarshan C, Rees RC, Finbloom D, Pine R, O'Shea JJ: Activation of STAT4 by IL-12 and IFN-α. Evidence for the involvement of ligand-induced tyrosine and serine phosphorylation. J Immunol 1996;157:4781–4789.

65   Pernis A, Gupta S, Gollob KJ, Garfein E, Coffman RL, Schindler C, Rothman P: Lack of interferon γ receptor β chain and the prevention of interferon γ signaling in T_H1 cells. Science 1995;269:245–247.

66   Bach EA, Szabo SJ, Dighe AS, Ashkenazi A, Aguet M, Murphy KM, Schreiber RD: Ligand-induced autoregulation of IFN-γ receptor β chain expression in T helper cell subsets. Science 1995; 270:1215–1218.

67   Paul WE, Seder RA: Lymphocyte responses and cytokines. Cell 1994;76:241–251.

68   Coffman RL, von der Weid T: Multiple pathways for the initiation of T helper 2 (Th2) responses. J Exp Med 1997;185:373–375.

69   Rincon M, Anguita J, Nakamura T, Fikrig E, Flavell RA: Interleukin (IL)-6 directs the differentiation of IL-4-producing CD4+ T cells. J Exp Med 1997;185:461–469.

70   Shaw J-P, Utz PJ, Durand DB, Toole JJ, Emmel EA, Crabtree GR: Identification of a putative regulator of early T cell activation genes. Science 1988;241:202–205.

71   Jain J, McCaffrey PG, Valge-Archer VE, Rao A: Nuclear factor of activated T cells contains Fos and Jun. Nature 1992;356:801–804.

72   Flanagan WM, Corthesy B, Bram RJ, Crabtree GR: Nuclear association of a T-cell transcription factor blocked by FK-506 and cyclosporin A. Nature 1991;352:803–807.

73   McCaffrey PG, Luo C, Kerppola TK, Jain J, Badalian TM, Ho AM, Burgeon E, Lane WS, Lambert JN, Curran T, Verdine GL, Rao A, Hogan PG: Isolation of the cyclosporin-sensitive T cell transcription factor NFATp. Science 1993;262:750–754.

74   Northrop JP, Ho SN, Chen L, Thomas DJ, Timmerman LA, Nolan GP, Admon A, Crabtree GR: NF-AT components define a family of transcription factors targeted in T-cell activation. Nature 1994;369:497–502.

75   Hoey T, Sun Y-L, Williamson K, Xu X: Isolation of two new members of the NF-AT gene family and functional characterization of NF-AT proteins. Immunity 1995;2:461–472.

76   Nolan GP: NF-AT-AP-1 and Rel-bZIP: Hybrid vigor and binding under the influence. Cell 1994; 77:795–798.

77   Szabo SJ, Gold JS, Murphy TL, Murphy KM: Identification of cis-acting elements controlling interleukin-4 expression in T cells: Roles for NF-Y and NF-ATc. Mol Cell Biol 1993;13:4793–4805.

78   Rooney JW, Hoey T, Glimcher LH: Coordinate and cooperative roles for NF-AT and AP-1 in the regulation of the murine IL-4 gene. Immunity 1995;2:473–483.

79   Cockerill PN, Shannon MF, Bert AG, Ryan GR, Vadas MA: The granulocyte-macrophage colony-stimulating factor/interleukin-3 locus is regulated by an inducible cyclosporin A-sensitive enhancer. Proc Natl Acad Sci USA 1993;90:2466–2470.

80   Goldfeld AE, McCaffrey PG, Strominger JL, Rao A: Identification of a novel cyclosporin-sensitive element in the human tumor necrosis factor α gene promoter. J Exp Med 1993;178:1365–1379.

81   Rao A: NF-ATp: A transcription factor required for co-ordinate induction of several cytokine genes. Immunol Today 1994;15:274–281.

82   Rooney JW, Hodge MR, McCaffrey PG, Rao A, Glimcher LH: A common factor regulates both Th1- and Th2-specific cytokine gene expression. EMBO J 1994;13:625–633.

83   Hodge MR, Ranger AM, Charles de la Brousse F, Hoey T, Grusby M, Glimcher LH: Hyperproliferation and dysregulation of IL-4 expression in NF-ATp-deficient mice. Immunity 1996;4:397–405.

84   Lederer JA, Liou JS, Kim S, Rice N, Lichtman A: Regulation of NF-κB activation in T helper 1 and T helper 2 cells. J Immunol 1996;156:56–63.

85   Lederer JA, Perez VL, DesRoches L, Kim SM, Abbas AK, Lichtman AH: Cytokine transcriptional events during helper T cell subset differentiation. J Exp Med 1996;184:397–406.

86   Ho I-C, Hodge MR, Rooney JW, Glimcher LH: The proto-oncogene c-maf is responsible for tissue-specific expression of interleukin-4. Cell 1996;85:973–983.

87   Hodge MR, Chun HJ, Rengarajan J, Alt A, Lieberson R, Glimcher LH: NF-AT-driven interleukin-4 transcription potentiated by NIP45. Science 1996;274:1903–1905.

88   Xu X, Sun Y-L, Hoey T: Cooperative DNA binding and sequence-selective recognition conferred by the STAT amino-terminal domain. Nature 1996;273:794–797.

Lars Rogge, Roche Milano Ricerche, Via Olgettina 58, I–20132 Milano (Italy)
Tel. (2) 2884 804, Fax (2) 2153 203, E-mail: roggel@dibit.hsr.it

Adorini L (ed): IL-12. Chem Immunol. Basel, Karger, 1997, vol 68, pp 54–69

....

Regulation of IL-12 Receptor Expression in Early T-Helper Responses Implies Two Phases of Th1 Differentiation: Capacitance and Development

Kenneth M. Murphy [a], *Theresa L. Murphy* [a], *Susanne J. Szabo* [a],
Nils G. Jacobson [a], *Mehmet L. Guler* [a], *James D. Gorham* [a] *and Ueli Gubler* [b]

[a] Department of Pathology, Washington University School of Medicine, St. Louis, Mo., and
[b] Department of Inflammation/Autoimmune Diseases, Hoffmann La-Roche Inc., Nutley, N.J. USA

Introduction

A great deal of effort by numerous investigators has gone into understanding the regulation of Th1 and Th2 development. Much of the effort has focused on trying to define the specific signals that determine which CD4 T cells may develop upon primary antigen activation. In the end, it appears that numerous parameters of T-cell activation can impact on the outcome of the overall balance of Th1/Th2 phenotype development. Clearly however, recent studies have defined a hierarchy among these parameters, with some acting directly at the level of the T cell to deliver the final signals inducing Th1 or Th2 differentiation, and others less proximal acting on APCs or other innate immune cells to modify levels of certain cytokines or costimulators. Among these various parameters are the APC used for T-cell priming [1], the dose of antigen used for T-cell activation [2–5], the structure of the antigen and particularly the affinity for the MHC and TCR [4, 6], the level of co-stimulation present during T-cell priming [7–9], the genetic background of the cells [10, 11], the presence or absence of certain pathogen-derived materials and the cytokines present in the priming milieu [12–28]. Changing any one of these parameters can alter the balance between Th1 and Th2 development. It is clear that IL-

12 and IL-4 act directly on T cells through STATs to deliver final and specific differentiation signals [29–31]. An unresolved issue concerns by what mechanisms these other non-cytokine parameters influence Th1/Th2 balance. We predict, based on early experiments, that many of the other parameters will be shown to act indirectly, by altering *initial* levels of IL-4, IL-12 or IFN-γ levels available to T cells during primary activation. These changes in primary levels of IL-4 or IL-12 will then mediate the observed changes in Th1/Th2 development.

This prediction is based on (1) our understanding of the antigen dose effect in the in vitro developmental system, and (2) on the lack of involvement of TCR signaling directly with the Jak/Stat pathway. First, it was clear that IL-4, through its activation of Stat6, acts to deliver specific and potent signals to induce Th2 pheonotype development [12, 13, 15, 18, 22, 29, 32–38], and that IL-12, through its activation of Stat4, acts to deliver equally specific and potent signals leading to Th1 development [30, 31, 39–43]. Second, while antigen dose changes can bring about a change in the apparent phenotype of the T cells in vitro [3], this effect was totally lost when cytokines (IL-4) were manipulated, indicating that cytokines are dominant in the hierarchy of these parameters. While the molecular downstream targets of Stat6 and Stat4 relevant to these differentiation pathways are still unknown, the cytokines, IL-4 and IL-12, which activate these two factors, appear to play the most dominant role in the hierarchy of phenotype-controlling parameters. Also, it is clear that altered strengths of signaling through the TCR can be achieved by alterations in the peptide antigen structure. However, TCR signaling does not activate any of the known STATs, and there is no direct evidence that a different quantity or quality of signals delivered through the TCR alone can direct the pathway of Th1/Th2 development. Rather, we feel that is very likely that altering the quantity of TCR signaling may produce changes in the initial level of IL-2 and IL-4 production by T cells, and these changes in cytokine levels feed back through the cytokine receptors to promote changes (via Stat6 in this case) to alter Th1/Th2 development. Nonetheless, this area currently represents one of the more active and interesting unsolved puzzles in Th1/Th2 developmental biology. Only time, and much more direct experimentation, will answer these issues for certain.

IFN-γ Modifies Early T-Cell Responses to IL-12

Along with several investigators, we identified IL-12 as a potent inducer of Th1 development in vitro [16, 19, 20, 44]. However, even in our earliest studies, we recognize that IFN-γ was a necessary but not sufficient factor for Th1 development in vitro induced by pathogen [45]. Thus, when we neutralized IFN-γ in cultures where Th1 development had been induced by the addition of *Listeria*, we noted a significant reduction in the overall level of Th1 development. Neutralizing IFN-γ could act at two levels: first, it could act on the APC to diminish the induction of IL-12 by *Listeria*, and second, it could somehow act on the T cell, perhaps by preventing a necesssary action on the T cell for Th1 development. In our study on the regulation of IL-12 p40 promoter [46], we noted that IFN-γ did indeed augment IL-12 production stimulated by heat-killed *Listeria*. These effects of IFN-γ could be mediated even at the level of a reporter construct, acting within the first 200 base pairs of the p40 promoter. While the most significant *cis* element residing within this region is the NF-κB site, induced by lipopolysaccharide (LPS) or lipoteichoic acid (LTA) [47], the specific and relevant site for mediating IFN-γ augmentation of p40 has not been identified. Within this region, there is no perfect consensus for Stat1 or for IRF1 that can be easily demonstrated to bind with high affinity to nuclear factors from activated macrophages [46, 48]. Interestingly, the phenotype of the ICSBP knockout includes diminished IL-12 production so that perhaps this IRF1 family member may participate in proximal promoter regulation [49]. The second potential target of IFN-γ for the above effects would be at the level of the T cell. Thus, under the conditions that were used in vitro, it might be necessary for IFN-γ to act on the T cell to enable that cell to respond appropriately to IL-12 for Th1 development [5]. This could be mediated by several different and nonexclusive types of mechanisms. In our study comparing the relative contributions of IFN-γ and IFN-α for murine Th1 development [50], we found that IFN-γ alone did not induce Th1 development in vitro, but appeared to promote the responsiveness of T cells to IL-12 during the first 7 days of development. Interestingly, this effect by IFN-γ was not provided by IFN-α. Thus, in the mouse system, we found that the IFN-α was unable to induce Th1 development, and was unable to prime T cells to respond to IL-12 as IFN-γ did. Here, it is important to note that these findings were done with T cells derived from the BALB/c background and analyzed in vitro using the DO11.10 TCR system. T cells from other backgrounds or analyzed in different ways might show differing requirements. However, our conclusion was that IFN-γ clearly acted also at the level of the T cell to enable naive CD4 cells to fully respond to IL-12. Since one potential mechanism of this action would be to induce expression of IL-12 receptors, we subsequently addressed the possibility (see below).

IL-12 Signaling

Our first initial approach several years ago to determine the molecular pathways for Th1 development were to identify the factors directly controlling IFN-γ production in a Th1 cell, and to work backwards towards the cell membrane. However, our studies of the IFN-γ promoter were stifled by the lack of an appropriate IL-12 responsive transfectable model cell line. Other studies of the IFN-γ have identified certain *cis* elements within the promoter and the intragenic regions [51, 52], but none of these have been identified as relevant for Th 1-specific expression of this gene. When the JAK/STAT pathway was identified as central to IFN-γ signaling [53–56], we turned our attention to test whether IL-12 could possibly signal via other members of this signaling family. We intentionally sought to identify IL-12-induced complexes using probes known to bind Stat1 [39]. Through this approach, we were able to identify Stat3 and Stat4 in addition to Stat1, as factors activated by murine IL-12. While several cytokines can activate either Stat1 or Stat3, Stat4 was apparently activated by no other cytokine than IL-12. Furthermore, at the time we did these studies, there had been no identification of any factor that activated Stat4. Stat4 had been identified solely through its homology to Stat1 [57, 58] and was therefore an orphan STAT. We showed that IL-12 treatment of Th1 cells led to the rapid phosphorylation of Stat4, and that there was a predominant complex apparently composed of a Stat4 homodimer, with the other complexes in the IL-12-treated extracts being Stat1 homodimer and Stat3/Stat4 heterodimers. Turning our attention back to the IFN-γ promoter, we are able to show that most of the proximal IFN-γ promoter failed to compete in gel shift assays for the IL-12-induced complexes [39]. This initially indicated that the IFN-γ promoter did not contain high affinity sites interacting with IL-12-induced complexes. Subsequently, a study by Hoey and co-workers [59] has shown that Stat4 has the unique ability to form higher order complexes, so that interactions between pairs of Stat4 dimers can take place, allowing greater interactions with low affinity sites. While this study showed the intragenic regions of IFN-γ contains several potential low affinity STAT sites, it did not test whether these sites actually participate functionally in IL-12-induced or Th1-selective-expression of IFN-γ.

Cytokine Signaling in Developing Th1 and Th2 Populations: What Goes Up ...

Knowing that IL-12 induces Stat4 in a specific manner, we next asked if this pathway was regulated during Th1/Th2 development. We compared the ability of Th2 cells and Th1 cells to activate complexes in response to several cytokines [43]. While IFN-α and IL-4 can activate STAT-containing complexes similarly in both Th1 and Th2 cells, we found that signaling for IL-12 and for IFN-γ differed between Th1 and Th2 cells. First, only Th1 cells appeared to induce complexes in response to IL-12. Th2 cells failed to induce complexes in response to IL-12, and this appeared to be a developmental process that occurred very rapidly following activation of primary cells. Even within 3 days following activation of FACS-sorted naive T cells, there was a substantial decrease in the ability of IL-12 to induce Stat4 phosphorylation. This capacity was completely lost by day 5 and continued to be absent thereafter. At that time, the molecular basis for this extinction of IL-12 signaling was unknown, so that it was only possible to demonstrate that high affinity binding sites were apparently equivalent for both Th1 and Th2 cells. Subsequently we have learned that there are two subunits comprising functional IL-12 receptors in both mouse and human [60–63]. The β subunit, cloned first by Gubler and co-workers [61] in the mouse system can confer substantial high affinity binding of the IL-12 heterodimer. This fact explains our observation that both Th1 and Th2 cells appeared to have high affinity binding sites. Gubler and co-workers subsequently cloned a second component of the IL-12 receptor, called the β2 subunit, that is responsible for STAT recruitment and signaling in response to IL-12 [62]. We examined Th1 and Th2 cells for expression of the signaling subunit of the IL-12 receptor. First, Th2 cells clearly lack expression of this signaling subunit. Second of all, this subunit is expressed in Th1 cells, and it appears to undergo specific regulation by the cytokines IL-4, IFN-γ, and IL-12 [64]. In the mouse system, it appears first that TCR activation is necessary to induce expression of the subunits of the IL-12 receptor, which are absent on naive T cells. Secondly, induction of the β2 subunit is inhibited by IL-4, leading to its extinction during Th2 development. However, and somewhat surprisingly, we found that IFN-γ can induce expression of the signaling subunit even when T cells are cultured with IL-4 and undergo development of an IL-4 producing phenotype. These effects were mediated at the level of transcription of the IL-12R β2 subunit. This observation explains our previous finding that IFN-γ appeared necessary for promoting IL-12 responsiveness. Since we had used T cells from the BALB/c background in our earlier studies, the IL-4 produced by these T cells was apparently sufficient to impose a repression of the β2 subunit, which IFN-γ appears necessary to overcome.

We have examined these issues in greater detail by crossing the DO11.10 TCR transgenic model onto Stat1- and Stat4-deficient backgrounds, and analyzing Th1/Th2 development in vitro under a variety of specific conditions. First, we confirm the finding that Stat4 is required for Th1 development. Stat4-

deficient T cells make extremely little IFN-γ under any circumstances. Whereas normal Th1 populations induced in the absence of IL-4 and in the presence of IL-12 can produce on day 7 IFN-γ in the range of >1,000 U/ml under our standard in vitro assay system. In contrast, identically treated Stat4-deficient T cells make between 10 and 20 U/ml. This level is above the threshold of detection and can be regulated by IL-4 and by IFN-γ exposure, so that we feel this very small level does represent a weak acquired developmental stage [Jacobson et al., in preparation]. It is perhaps a semantic issue whether these cells should be considered 'Th1' cells, since while they do not make IL-4, their IFN-γ production is clearly far less than normal Th1 cells. On the one hand, they produce no IL-4 (if IL-4 has been neutralized in the primary) and do produce some IFN-γ (although the amount is unlikely to be effective against *Leishmania*). Only further experiments, and discussion, will resolve this issue.

While Stat4 is required to allow IL-12 to augment IFN-γ production, it appears that Stat1 is required to provide for expression of the IL-12R β2 subunit. This conclusion stems from analysis of the pattern of responses of Stat1-deficient DO11.10 T cells to cytokines in vitro. In these cells, we found that Th1 development in response to IL-12 could occur as efficiently as in normal T cells, provided that the IL-12 receptors were present. In the absence of Stat1 however, IFN-γ is not able to induce receptor expression as in wild-type cells. IL-12R β2 expression in Stat1-deficient T cells requires IL-4 neutralization and IL-12 addition very early in development. Neutralizing IL-4 alone does not induce Th1 development. All of these finding are consistent with the previous findings in which IL-4 inhibited IL-12R β2 and IFN-γ induced IL-12R β2 expression. Thus we suggest that Th1 development can be considered at least a two-stage process (fig. 1). First, after initial TCR activation, the balance of IL-4 and IFN-γ can act to determine whether T cells will express sufficient IL-12 β2 subunit to allow for IL-12 responsiveness. Second, IL-12, although a process involving Stat4, acts to promote a process of development that provides for a significantly increased capacity for IFN-γ production.

IFN-α Signaling: A Mouse Is Not a Man

Dr. Francesco Sinigaglia (Roche Milano Ricerche, Milano, Italy) at the same time was carrying out parallel work on IL-12 receptor regulation in the human system, and we had the opportunity to compare and contrast our findings with the human system. In the mouse system, Th2 cells appear to completely extinguish IL-12 responsiveness through the complete loss of β2 expression. This may not be the case for human Th2 clones, since these cells

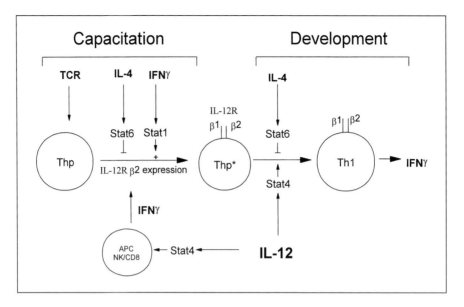

Fig. 1. Roles of cytokines in regulating early Th1 development: capacitance and development. In the very early response, CD4 cells activated by TCR/antigen will initiate expression of the IL-12 receptor subunits. Expression of the β2 subunit is inhibited in the presence of even quite low levels of IL-4 (in the BALB/c background). This inhibition is reversed in the presence of IFN-γ. While we find that addition of IL-12 also can induce β2 expression, our data with Stat1 and Stat4-deficient mice suggest that this effect is through induction of IFN-γ from APCs such as NK and CD8 T cells. Once IL-12R β1 and β2 subunits are expressed, IL-12 acts through Stat4, not Stat1, to promote Th1 development. The mechanisms of Stat4-induced Th1 development have yet to be worked out.

appear to maintain some low level of β2 expression, and therefore can respond to IL-12 treatment, activating Stat1, 3 and 4, which then can further induce the expression of this receptor. In contrast, in the mouse cells, sufficiently low levels of receptor are expressed by Th2 cells so that IL-12 treatment alone cannot achieve induction of the β2 receptor. A second difference between mouse and human was noted. IFN-γ treatment of developing murine Th2 cells appeared capable of inducing IL-12 receptor expression and functional IL-12 responsiveness. However, in the human system, IFN-γ does not act as an effective inducer of IL-12R β2 as it was in the mouse. IFN-α in contrast was effective at inducing expression of the β2 subunit in human T cells. Thus, whatever the basis of this difference turns out to be, it may imply that there are significant differences in the pattern of cytokine responses between human and mouse for control of the IL-12 receptor signaling chains.

Furthermore, there has recently been one report that might indicate a difference between IFN-α signaling between mouse and man for the pattern of STATs activated. This finding by O'Shea and co-workers [65] describes Stat4 activation to occur in human peripheral T-cell blasts in response to treatment with IFN-α. It was already known that IL-12 activated Stat4 in both mouse and human T cells [39, 40]. Because Stat4 appears to have a central role in inducing Th1 development in the mouse, based upon the knockout phenotype, this might predict that IFN-α might be able to induce Th1 development in human T cells. In fact there has been some uncertainty in the human system whether IL-12 is the only factor able to induce Th1 development, with some reports indicating an effect of IFN-α [66, 67]. In light of these findings, we have re-examined the actions of IFN-α in the mouse system. We have reconfirmed the fact that in the murine system IFN-α does not activate Stat4, nor does it induce Th1 development [50]. Our positive controls for the ability of IFN-α to act on mouse T cells was demonstrated by changes in class I MHC expression and the ability of IFN-α to activate Stat1 [50]. We have repeated the experiments of O'Shea's group and confirm their findings that IFN-α activates Stat4 in human T cells [Farrar and Murphy, in preparation]. Thus, there appears to be a real difference between human and mouse for which STATs become activated. The basis for this interesting and potentially important difference is unknown at present. This difference could reside either at the level of the receptor structure, for example in the cytoplasmic domains that recruit STAT factors within the IFN-α receptor, or could be based on potential heterogeneity of the specific type of IFN-α used for these studies. This will clearly be an active area for current and ongoing work since the relative actions of IFN-α and IL-12 have important implications for immunotherapy of infectious diseases in humans.

IFN-γ Signaling in Developing Th1 and Th2 Populations: What Goes Around

We also found a difference in IFN-γ signaling between Th1 and Th2 cells [43]. Namely, IFN-γ treatment of Th2 cells resulted in the formation of complexes in gel shift from extracts of Th2 cells, but not from extracts of Th1 cells. This finding, in our hands, appeared likely to be due to the high levels of exposure of Th1 cells to IFN-γ, rather than a difference between Th1 and Th2 cells based upon differentiation. We based this conclusion on an experiment where Th2 cells were activated in the presence of high levels of IFN-γ [43]. We noted that Th2 cells thus exposed to IFN-γ also became unresponsive to IFN-γ [43]. Therefore, we suspected that this phenomenon might be some form of ligand-induced down-regulation of IFN-γ signaling, and not a key signature of Th1 cells. To understand the molecular basis of this difference, we collaborated with Dr. Robert Schreiber, who has developed a number of important reagents to analyze IFN-γ signaling. The results of these studies indicated that the loss of IFN-γ signaling seen in Th1 cells is due to a down-regulation of the β chain of the IFN-γ receptor, which is essential for Stat1 recruitment and phosphorylation [68]. Thus, down-regulation of this subunit leads to the inability to signal for IFN-γ responses in either Th1 or Th2 cells. The significance of this down-regulation has not been tested in vivo. Several years ago, this phenomenon was first described by Fitch and Gajewski [69–71] who found that there was a significant antiproliferative response of IFN-γ exerted on Th2 cells, but not on Th1 cells. They speculated that this may indicate that IFN-γ would play an important role in skewing the phenotype of a population of emerging T cells based upon differential proliferative responses of distinct subpopulations. The magnitude of this effect is only approximately 2-fold [69–71]. Since that time, other factors have been found that direct phenotype development in quantitatively greater amounts, so that it is not necessary to invoke IFN-γ as a primary regulatory cytokine based upon its proliferative effects. Moreover, since we have shown that the mechanism of this difference relies upon exposure of T cells to IFN-γ, it is important to realize that in vivo, T cells of different antigen specificity reacting to different pathogens, may be exposed to common levels of extracellular IFN-γ, and therefore would fall under the same effects equally for down-regulation of the IFN-γ signaling pathway. Therefore, this pathway has yet to be verified as functionally operative in vivo.

Genetic Effects on Th1/Th2 Development

Another parameter regulating the balance between Th1 and Th2 development is genetic background. There are well-established genetic effects influencing Th1 or Th2 responses to specific pathogens and genetic linkages between certain loci and atopic conditions in humans. It is easy to understand how a genetic defect in any number of the structural genes for cytokines or receptors could lead to a defect in either Th1 or Th2 development. However, there have not been any naturally occurring defects such as those described in mice or humans as responsible for the strain–dependent susceptibilities dependent on Th1/Th2 balance. While such pathogen susceptibilities can be attributed to the inappropriate Th1 or Th2 phenotype response, the underlying genetic basis for the described strain differences appear to be multigenic and complex.

We have tried to begin analyzing these complex genetic aspects of T-helper development by using DO11.10 TCR transgene bred onto distinct H-2^d genetic backgrounds. This approach allows us to compare T cells of identical antigen specificity but on distinct genetic backgrounds. We are able to show that even though B10, BALB/c, and DBA2 genetic backgrounds responded similarly to the inducing stimuli of IL-4 or IL-12 for Th2 and Th1 development, there was a difference between these backgrounds when T cells were allowed to develop without direct manipulation of cytokines. We have operationally defined this condition of unmanipulated in vitro T cells development as the neutral condition or the 'default' pathway. These terms are not meant to imply that there is specific or unique 'default' mechanism programmed to operate differently from the known actions of other factors, but simply that the difference between genetic backgrounds is more apparent in vitro when T cells are activated with APCs and peptide but without other manipulations. We fully recognize that in vitro conditions of development, even without added antibodies or cytokines to manipulate phenotype, is itself a very artificial system, but have accepted that at present we have no more direct way to examine the genetic basis of differing T-cell responses. We have used comparisons of these neutral conditions to try to understand cellular and molecular mechanisms underlying genetic differences between these strains for phenotype development.

T cells from the B10.D2 genetic background appear to more strongly develop towards a Th1 phenotype when developing under neutral conditions compared to T cells from BALB/c background [24]. In our system, this difference is maintained independently of the genetic background of the APCs used to prime the T cells. Thus, in this system, we are identifying differences that reside within the T-cell compartment that tend to promote Th1 development in the B10 greater than in the BALB/c background. The basis for this difference appears to be complex. First, while IL-4 induced Th2 development in the B10 and the BALB/c T cells, we did observe residual IFN-γ produced by B10 T cells but not BALB/c T cells. In contrast, neutralization of IL-4 and addition of IL-12 led to nearly identical Th1 phenotypes developing from both backgrounds. The largest difference was in the neutral point, where B10 T cells were significantly higher in IFN-γ production and BALB/c's significantly higher in IL-4 production. To begin to unravel the disparate cellular mechanisms that might be involved in these differences, we carried out a series of mixing experiments [72]. The purpose of these experiments was to distinguish whether genetic effects acted by induction of distinct extracellular conditons in primary cultures, or through cell intrinsic differences (i.e., such as variations in an intracellular signaling pathway). For example, if BALB/c T cells simply were programmed to produce greater quantities of IL-4 on primary stimulation compared to B10, we would expect a mixing experiment to reveal this difference, since IL-4 produced by BALB/c T cells can act on both the BALB/c and B10.D2 T cells in a mixing experiment. The results from these mixing experiments indicated that both intrinsic and extrinsic differences exist between the B10 and BALB/c cells [72].

Another component we analyzed in these mixing experiments was the maintenance of IL-12 responsiveness, since we had recently found that this component of T-cell response determined by expression of the β2 subunit of the IL-12 receptor was expressed independently of strict Th1/Th2 phenotype definitions. Therefore, we carried out a series of mixing experiments in which phenotype and IL-12 responsiveness was measured. IL-12 responsiveness was measured in two ways: first, the induction of IFN-γ on secondary stimulation, and second, the induction of an IL-12-responsive cell surface marker, CD25. The results of these experiments indicated that both an intrinsic and extrinsic difference exist between BALB and B10 T cells. The intrinsic difference appears to allow B10 T cells to maintain IL-12 responsiveness, even when mixed in a population of BALB/c T cells where BALB/c cells predominate. In this setting, B10 remained more Th1-like producing higher IFN-γ, but more signifcantly remained IL-12-responsive whereas BALB/c lose IL-12 responsiveness under these conditions. In the reverse setting, where B10 are mixed at a majority, both B10 and BALB retain an IL-12-responsive phenotype, and BALB/c T cells show more of a Th1-type bulk phenotype pathway, producing higher IFN-γ than before.

We have measured the expression of the mRNA for the two IL-12 receptor subunits in this system. We find that the maintenance of IL-12 responsiveness at neutral conditions shown by B10 T cells correlates with expression of the IL-12R β2 subunit, while loss of IL-12 responsiveness in BALB/c correlates with its loss. Moreover, the maintenance of IL-12R β2 expression in the B10 appears regulated by cytokines generally as in the BALB/c, since it is induced by IFN-γ and inhibited by IL-4. At present we do not understand the underlying reasons for this difference. When we examined the pattern of inheritance of IL-12 responsiveness at neutral conditions, we found only one locus near the IL-4 gene on mouse chromosome 11 that was strongly linked to this phenotype [73]. That might imply that the IL-4 locus itself is different between these strains in a manner that preferentially skews BALB/c towards Th2 development more strongly than B10.D2. This could be due to, for example, an intrinsically more active IL-4 cytokine locus, so that IL-4 and the other Th2-specific cytokines genes located in this cluster are more easily induced or expressed at higher levels in BALB/c compared to B10.D2. On the other hand, it also could imply that some other gene resides in this region that is responsible for the observed phenotype, for example the presence of different alleles of IRF1, which is nearby IL-4. The results of the mixing experiments [72] seems to favor the second possibility, since the first mechanism would have predicted that mixing BALB/c and B10.D2 cells together would convert B10 cells toward IL-12 unresponsiveness, given that IL-4 can act extracellularly. However, that study only examined theF_1(B10.D2 × BALB/c) backcross to BALB/c, and not a full F_2 cohort of mice for genetic analysis, and this may have caused us to miss loci that could act in a recessive manner.

At present, it is clear only that there may be many differences between various strains., and individual humans, that potentially can generate differences in the character of Th1/Th2 development. These differences may be very important in understanding the causes of atopic diseases, such as the propensity to develop asthma, and may also extend to varying diseases related to Th1/Th2 balance, including autoimmunity. Because of the numerous feedback effects and the general complexity of Th1/Th2 regulation, it may be some time before any of these differences are identified with certainty. This situation is not at all unlike the current situations for certain other genetically-based, but extraordinarily complex disease models such as NOD, where numerous genetic linkages have seemed to defy their individual identification.

In summary: Our model of Th1/Th2 development in vitro has stressed the importance of IL-12 and IL-4 as final determinants of Th1 and Th2 development. Recently, much of our attention has been focused on analyzing the early regulation of IL-12 responsiveness of T-cell population. Because the extinction of IL-12 signaling in early Th2 development could potentially be important in imprinting a more permanent Th2 phenotype on a population of T cells, we sought to understand various parameters of regulation of IL-12 signaling. We place IFN-γ as a cofactor in Th1 development, because we find that it promotes expression of the signaling component of the IL-12 receptor, IL-12R β2. We propose that Th1 development can be considered in two stages, capacitance and development. We would define the first stage, capacitance, as that in which T cells decide whether to express sufficient IL-12R β2 subunit to become functionally IL-12-responsive. Expression of this receptor subunit is inhibited by IL-4, and this inhibition is overcome by IFN-γ. This balance also may be influenced by relatively weak parameters such as genetic background and by level of TCR activation. The second stage we propose is the true IL-12-induced developmental stage, likely involving expression of Stat4-inducible proteins. While it is formally possible that all of Stat4 actions on Th1 development may be exerted directly by Stat4 at the IFN-γ gene, we suggest that this model is unlikely to be correct. Rather, we are pursuing the hypothesis that Stat4 induces Th1 development by inducing one or several noncytokine genes, which act to define the transcriptional state of Th1 cell.

Acknowledgments

This work was supported by NIH grants AI34580, AI31238 and AI39676 and a grant from the American Cancer Society. S.J.S. was supported by training grant CA09547.

References

1   Chang T-L, Shea CM, Urioste S, Thompson RC, Boom WH, Abbas AK: Heterogeneity of helper/inducer T lymphocytes. III. Responses of IL-2 and IL-4-producing (Th1 and Th2) clones to antigens presented by different accessory cells. J Immunol 1990;145:2803–2808.
2   Parish CR, Liew FY:Immune response to chemically modified flagellin. 3. Enhanced cell-mediated immunity during high and low zone antibody tolerance to flagellin. J Exp Med 1972;135:298–311.
3   Hosken NA, Shibuya K, Heath AW, Murphy KM, O'Garra A: The effect of antigen dose on CD4+ T helper cell phenotype development in a T cell receptor-alpha beta-transgenic model. J Exp Med 1995;182:1579–1584.
4   Murray JS, Pfeiffer C, Madri J, Bottomly K: Major histocompatibility complex (MHC) control of CD4 T cell subset activation. II. A single peptide induces either humoral or cell-mediated responses in mice of distinct MHC genotype. Eur J Immunol 1992;22:559–565.
5   Constant S, Pfeiffer C, Woodward A, Pasqualini T, Bottomly K: Extent of T cell receptor ligation can determine the functional differentiation of naive CD4+ T cells. J Exp Med 1995;182:1591–1596.
6   Pfeiffer C, Murray J, Madri J, Bottomly K: Selective activation of Th1- and Th2-like cells in vivo – Response to human collagen IV. Immunol Rev 1991;123:65–84.
7   Freeman GJ, Boussiotis VA, Anumanthan A, Bernstein GM, Ke XY, Rennert, PD, Gray GS, Gribben JG, Nadler LM: B7-1 and B7-2 do not deliver identical constimulatory signals, since B7-2 but not B7-1 preferentially costimulates the initial production of IL-4. Immunity 1995;2:523–532.
8   Lenschow DJ, Ho SC, Sattar H, Rhee L, Gray G, Nabavi N, Herold KC, Bluestone JA: Differential effects of anti-B7-1 and anti-B7-2 monoclonal antibody treatment on the development of diabetes in the nonobese diabetic mouse. J Exp Med 1995;181:1145–1155.
9   Kuchroo VK, Das MP, Brown JA, Ranger AM, Zamvil SS, Sobel RA, Weiner HL, Nabavi N, Glimcher LH: B7-1 and B7-2 costimulatory molecules activate differentially the Th1/Th2 developmental pathways: Application to autoimmune disease therapy. Cell 1995;80:707–718.
10   Murphy EE, Terres G, Macatonia SE, Hsieh CS, Mattson J, Lanier L, Wysocka M, Trincheiri G, Murphy K, O'Garra A: B7 and interleukin-12 cooperate for proliferation and interferon-gamma production by mouse T helper clones that are unresponsive to B7 costimulation. J Exp Med 1994; 180:223–231.
11   Kubin M, Kamoun M, Trincheiri G: Interleukin-12 synergizes with B7/CD28 interaction in inducing efficient proliferation and cytokine production of human T cells. J Exp Med 1994;180:211–222.
12   Le Gros G, Ben-Sasson SZ, Seder RA, Finkelman FD, Paul WE: Generation of interleukin-4 (IL-4)-producing cells in vivo and in vitro: IL-2 and IL-4 are required for in vitro generation of IL-4-producing cells. J Exp Med 1990;172:921–929.
13   Swain SL, Weinberg AD, English M, Huston G: IL-4 directs the development of Th2-like helper effectors. J Immunol 1990;145:3796–3806.
14   Swain SL, Huston G, Tonkonogy S, Weinberg AD: Transforming growth factor-beta and IL-4 cause helper T cell percursors to develop into distinct effector helper cells that differ in lymphokine secretion pattern and cell surface phenotype. J Imunol 1991;147:2991–3000.
15   Hsieh C-S, Heimberger AB, Gold JS, O'Garra A, Murphy KM: Differential regulation of T helper phenotype development by interleukins 4 and 10 in alpha-beta-T-cell-receptor transgenic system. Proc Natl Acad Sci USA 1992;89:6065–6069.
16   Hsieh C-S, Macatonia SE, Tripp CS, O'Garra A, Murphy KM: Development of Th1 CD4+ T cells through IL-12 produced by Listeria-induced macrophages. Science 1993;260:547–549.

17   Sadick MD, Heinzel FP, Holaday BJ, Pu RT, Dawkins RS, Locksley RM: Cure of murine leishmaniasis with anti-interleukin-4 monoclonal antibody. J Exp Med 1990;171:115–127.

18   Maggi E, Parronchi P, Manetti R, Simonelli C, Piccinni M-P, Rugiu FS, de Carli M, Ricci M, Romagnani S: Reciprocal regulatory effects of IFN-gamma and IL-4 on the in vitro development of human Th1 and Th2 clones. J Immunol 1992;148:2142–2147.

19   Manetti R, Parronchi P, Giudizi MG, Piccinini M-P, Maggi E, Trincheiri G, Romagnani S: Natural killer cell stimulatory factor (interleukin-12 [IL-12]) induces T helper type 1 (Th1)-specific immune responses and inhibits the development of IL-4 producing Th cells. J Exp Med 1993;177:1199–1204.

20   Seder RA, Gazzinelli R, Sher A, Paul WE: Interleukin-12 acts directly on CD4 + T cells to enhance priming for interferon-gamma production and diminishes interleukin-4 inhibition of such priming. Proc Natl Acad Sci USA 1993;90:10188–10192.

21   Sypek JP, Chung CL, Mayor SEH, Subramanyam JM, Goldman SJ, Sieburth DS, Wolf SF, Schaub RG: Resolution of cutaneous leishmaniasis: Interleukin-12 initiates a protective T helper type 1 immune response. J Exp Med 1993;177:1797–1802.

22   Chatelain R, Varkila K, Coffman RL: IL-4 induces a Th2 response in *Leishmania major*-infected mice. J Immunol 1992;148:1182–1187.

23   Belosevic M, Finbloom DS, Van der Meide PH, Slayter MV, Nacy CA: Administration of monoclonal anti-IFN-gamma antibodies in vivo abrogates natural resistance of C3H/HeN mice to infection with *Leishmania major*. J Immunol 1989;143:266–274.

24   Hsieh CS, Macatonia SE, O'Garrra A, Murphy KM: T cell genetic background determines default T helper phenotype development in vitro. J Exp Med 1995;181:713–721.

25   Howard JG: Immunological regulation and control of experimental leishmaniasis. Int Rev exp Pathol 1986;28:79–116.

26   Heinzel FP, Sadick MD, Holaday BJ, Coffman RL, Locksley RM: Reciprocal expression of interferon-gamma or interleukin-4 during the resolution or progression of murine leishmaniasis. J Exp Med 1989;169:59–72.

27   Scott P, Natovitz P, Coffman RL, Pearce E, Sher A: Immunoregulation of cutaneous leishmaniasis. T cell lines that transfer protective immunity or exacerbation belong to different T helper subsets and respond to distinct parasite antigens. J Exp Med 1988;168:1675–1684.

28   Locksley RM, Scott P: Helper T-cell subsets in mouse leishmaniasis: Induction, expansion and effector function; in Ash C, Gallagher RB (eds): Immunoparasitology Today. London, Elsevier Trends Journals, 1991, pp a58–a61.

29   Kaplan MH, Schindler U, Smiley ST, Grusby MJ: Stat6 is required for mediating responses to IL-4 and for development of Th2 cells. Immunity 1996;4:313–319.

30   Kaplan MH, Sun YL, Hoey T, Grusby MJ: Impaired IL-12 responses and enhanced development of Th2 cells in Stat4-deficient mice. Nature 1996;382:174–177.

31   Thierfelder WE, van Deursen JM, Yamamoto K, Tripp RA, Sarwar SR, Carson RT, Sangster MY, Vignali DA, Doherty PC, Grosveld GC, Ihle JN: Requirement for Stat4 in interleukin-12-mediated reponses of natural killer and T cells. Nature 1996;382:171–174.

32   Kopf M, Le Gros G, Bachmann M, Lamers MC, Bleuthmann H, Kohler G: Disruption of the murine IL-4 gene blocks Th2 cytokine responses. Nature 1993;362:245–247.

33   Kuhn R, Rajewsky K, Muller W: Generation and analysis of interleukin-4 deficient mice. Science 1991;254:707–710.

34   Betz M, Fox BS: Regulation and development of cytochrome c-specific IL-4-producing T cells. J Immunol 1990;145:1046–1052.

35   Hou J, Schindler U, Henzel WJ, Ho TC, Brassuer M, McKnight SL: An interleukin-4-induced transcription factor: IL-4 Stat. Science 1994;265:1701–1706.

36   Quelle FW, Shimod K, Thierfelder W, Fischer C, Kim A, Ruben SM, Cleveland JL, Pierce JH, Keegan AD, Nelms K, et al: Cloning of murine Stat6 and human Stat6, Stat proteins that are tyrosine phosphorylated in responses to IL-4 and IL-3 but are not required for mitogenesis. Mol Cell Biol 1995;15:3336–3343.

37   Shimoda K, van Deursen J, Sangster MY, Sarawar SR, Carson RT, Tripp RA, Chu C, Quelle FW, Nosaka T, Vignali DA, Doherty PC, Grosveld G, Paul WE, Ihle JN: Lack of IL-4 induced Th2 response and IgE class switching in mice with disripted Stat6 gene. Nature 1996;380:630–633.

38 Takeda K, Tanaka T, Shi W, Matsumoto M, Minami M, Kashiwamura S, Nakanishi K, Yoshida N, Kishimoto T, Akira S: Essential role of Stat6 in IL-4 signalling. Nature 1996;380:627–630.

39 Jacobson NG, Szabo SJ, Weber-Nordt RM, Zhong Z, Schreiber RD, Darnell JE Jr. Murphy KM: Interleukin-12 signaling in T helper type 1 (Th1) cells involves tyrosine phosphorylation of signal transducer and activator of transcription (Stat)3 and Stat4. J Exp Med;1981:1755–1762.

40 Bacon CM, Petricoin EF III, Ortaldo JR, Rees RC, Larner AC, Johnston JA, O'Shea JJ: Interleukin-12 induces tyrosine phosphorylation and activation of STAT4 in human lymphocytes. Proc Nat Acad Sci USA 1995;92:7307–7311.

41 Mattner F, Magram J, Ferrante J, Launois P, Di Padova K, Behin R, Gately MK, Louis JA, Alber G: Genetically resistant mice lacking interleukin-12 are susceptible to infection with *Leishmania major* and mount a polarized Th2 cell response. Eur J Immunol 1996;26:1553–1559.

42 Magram J, Connaughton SE, Warrier RR, Carvajal DM, Wu CY, Ferrante J, Stewart C, Sarmiento U, Faherty DA, Gately MK: IL-12-deficient mice are defective in IFN-gamma production and type cytokine responses. Immunity 1996;4:471–481.

43 Szabo SJ, Jacobson NG, Dighe AS, Gubler U, Murphy KM: Developmental commitment to the Th2 lineage by extinction of IL-12 signaling. Immunity 1995;2:665–675.

44 Macatonia SE, Hsieh C-S, Murphy KM, O'Garra A: Dendritic cells and macrophages are required for Th1 development of CD4+ T cells from alpha beta TCR transgenic mice: IL-12 substitution for macrophages to stimulate IFN-gamma production is IFN-gamma-dependent. Int Immunol 1993;5:1119–1128.

45 Hsieh C-S, Macatonia SE, O'Garra A, Murphy KM: Pathogen-induced Th1 phenotype development in CD4+ alpha-beta-TCR transgenic T cells is macrophage dependent. Int Immunol 1993;5:371–382.

46 Murphy TL, Cleveleland MG, Kulesza P, Magram J, Murphy KM: Regulation of interleukin-12 p40 expression through an NF-kappa B half-site. Mol Cell Biol 1995;15:5258–5267.

47 Cleveland MG, Gorham JD, Murphy TL, Tuomanen E, Murphy KM: Lipoteichoic acid preparations of gram-positive bacteria induce interleukin-12 through a CD14-dependent pathway. Infect Immun 1996;64:1906–1912.

48 Ma X, Chow JM, Gri G, Carra G, Gerosa F, Wolf SF, Dzialo R, Trincheiri G: The interleukin-12 p40 gene promoter is primed by interferon-gamma in monocytic cells. J Exp Med 1996;183:147–157.

49 Holtschke T, Lohler J, Kanno Y, Fehr T, Giese N, Rosenbauer F, Lou J, Knobeloch KP, Gabriele L, Waring JF, Bachmann MF, Zinkernagel RM, Morse, Ozato K, Horak I: Immunodeficiency and chronic myelogenous leukemia-like syndrome in mice with a targeted mutation of the ICSBP gene. Cell 1996;87:307–317.

50 Wenner CA, Guler ML, Macatonia SE, O'Garra A, Murphy KM: Roles of IFN-gamma and IFN-alpha in IL-12 induced T helper cell-1 development. J Immunol 1996;156:1442–1447.

51 Sica A, Tan TH, Rice N, Kretzschmar M, Ghosh P, Young HA: The c-rel protooncogene product c-Rel but not NF-kappa B binds to the intronic region of the human interferon-gamma gene at a site related to an interferon-stimulable response element. Proc Nat Acad Sci USA 1992;89:1740–1744.

52 Penix L, Weaver WM, Pang Y, Young HA, Wilson HA, Wilson CB: Essential regulatory elements in the human interferon-gamma promoter confer activation-specific expression in T cells. J Exp Med 1993;178:1483–1496.

53 Shuai K, Schindler C, Prezioso VR, Darnell JE Jr: Activation of transcription by IFN-gamma: Tyrosine phosphorylation of a 91-kD †DNA binding protein. Science 1992;258:1808–1812.

54 Fu XY, Schindler C, Improta T, Aebersold R, Darnell JE Jr: The proteins of ISGF-3, the interferon-alpha-induced transcriptional activator, define a gene family involved in signal transduction. Proc Nat Acad Sci USA 1992;89:7840–7843.

55 Schindler C, Fu XY, Improta T, Aebersold R, Darnell Jr: Proteins of transcription factor ISGF-3: One gene encodes the 91- 84-kDa ISGF-3 proteins that are activated by interferon-alpha. Proc Nat Acad Sci USA 1992;89:7836–7839.

56 Darnell JE Jr, Kerr IM, Stark, GR: Jak-STAT pathways and transcriptional activation in response to IFNs and other extracellular signaling proteins (review). Science 1994;264:1415–1421.

57   Zhong Z, Wen Z, Darnell JE Jr: Stat3 and Stat4: Members of the family of signal transducers and activators of transcription. Proc Nat Acad Sci USA 1994;91:4806–4810.

58   Yamamoto K, Quelle FW, Thierfelder WE, Kreier BL, Gilbert DJ, Jenkins NA, Copeland NG, Silvennoinen O, Ihle JN: Stat4, a novel gamma interferon activation site-binding protein expressed in early myeloid differentiation. Mol Cell Biol 1994;14:4342–4349.

59   Xu X, Sun YL, Hoey T: Cooperative DNA binding and sequence-selective recognition conferred by the STAT amino-terminal domain (see comments). Science 1996;273:794–797.

60   Chau AO, Chizzonite R, Desai BB, Truitt TP, Nunes P, Minetti LJ, Warrier RR, Presky DH, Levine JF, Gately MK, et al: Expression cloning of a human IL-12 receptor component. A new member of the cytokine receptor superfamily with strong homology to gp130. J Immunol 1994;153:128–136.

61   Chau AO, Wilkinson VL, Presky DH, Gubler U: Cloning and characterization of a mouse IL-12 receptor-beta component. J Immunol 1995;155:4286–4294.

62   Presky DH, Yang H, Minetti LJ, Chua AO, Nabavi N, Wu CY, Gately MK, Gubler U: A functional interleukin-12 receptor complex is composed of two beta type cytokine receptor subunits. Proc Nat Acad Sci 1996;93:14002–14007.

63   Wy CY, Warrier RR, Carvajal DM, Chua AO, Minetti LJ, Chizzonite R, Mongini PKA, Stern AS, Gubler U, Presky DH, Gately MK: Interleukin-12, interluekin-12 receptor, interleukin-12 receptor beta chain. Biological function and distribution of human interleukin-12 receptor beta chain. Eur J Immunol 1996;26:345–350.

64   Szabo SJ, Dighe AS, Gubler U, Murphy KM: Regulation of the IL-12R beta2 subunit expression in developing Th1 and Th2 cells abstract. J Exp Med 1997; .

65   Cho SS, Bacon CM, Sudarshan C, Rees RC, Finbloom D, Pine R, O'Shea JJ: Activation of Stat4 by IL-12 and IFN-alpha – Evidence for the involvement of ligand-induced tyrosine and serine phosphorylation. J Immunol 1996;157:4781–4789.

66   Brinkmann V, Geiger T, Alkan S, Heusser CH: Interferon-alpha increases the frequency of interferon-gamma-producing human CD4+ T cells. J Exp Med 1993; 178:1655–1663.

67   Parronchi P, De Carli M, Manetti R, Simonelli C, Sampognaro S, Piccini MP, Macchia D, Maggi E, del Prete G, Romagnani S: IL-4 and IFN (alpha and gamma) exert opposite regulatory effects of the development of cytolytic potential by Th1 or Th2 human T cell clones. J Immunol 1992; 149:2977–2983.

68   Bach EA, Szabo SJ, Dighe AS, Ashkenazi A, Aguet M, Murphy KM, Schreiber RD: Ligand-induced autoregulation of IFN-gamma receptor beta chain expression in T helper cell subsets. Science 1995;270:1215–1218.

69   Gajewski TF, Fitch TW: Anti-proliferative effect of IFN-gamma in immune regulation. I. IFN-gamma inhibits the proliferation of Th2 but not Th1 murine helper T lymphocyte clones. J Immunol 1988;140:4245–4252.

70   Gajewski TF, Joyce J, Fitch FW: Antiproliferative effect of IFN-gamma in immune regulation. III. Differential selection of TH1 and TH2 murine helper T lymphocyte clones using recombinant IL-2 and recombinant IFN-gamma. J Immunol 1989;143:15–22.

71   Gajewski TF, Goldwasser E, Fitch FW: Anti-proliferative effect of IFN-gamma in immune regulation. II. IFN-gamma inhibits the proliferation of murine bone marrow cells stimulated with IL-3, IL-4, or granulocyte-macrophage colony-stimulating factor. J Immunol 1988;141:2635–2642.

72   Guler ML, Gorham JD, Hsieh CS, Mackey AJ, Steen RG, Dietrich WF, Murphy KM: Genetic susceptibility to Leishmania: IL-12 responsiveness in TH1 cell development. Science 1996;271: 984–987.

73   Gorham JD, Guler ML, Steen RG, Mackey AJ, Daly MJ, Frederick K, Dietrich WF, Murphy KM: Genetic mapping of murine locus controlling development of T helper 1 T helper 2 type responses. Proc Nat Acad Sci USA 1996;93:12467–12472.

Kenneth Murphy MD, PhD, Department of Pathology, Washington University School of Medicine, Campus Box 8118, 660 S. Euclid Avenue, St. Louis, MO 63110, (USA)

Adorini L (ed): IL-12. Chem Immunol. Basel, Karger, 1997, vol 68, pp 70–85

....

The Immunostimulatory Function of IL-12 in T-Helper Cell Development and Its Regulation by TGF-β, IFN-γ and IL-4

Edgar Schmitt, Erwin Rüde, Tieno Germann

Institute for Immunology, Johannes Gutenberg University, Mainz, Germany

IL-12 is a heterodimeric cytokine that is mainly produced by macrophages and dendritic cells preferentially in response to bacteria, bacterial products and parasites as well as in the interaction with activated T cells [1–3]. The biological activities of IL-12 on NK cells and CD4[+] and CD8[+] T cells comprise the stimulation of cytokine production, especially of IFN-γ, the proliferation and the enhancement of cytotoxic activity. IL-12 has profound antitumor activities that were at least partially mediated by CD8[+] T cells and by IFN-γ [4]. Using T cells from immunodeficient HIV patients, it was shown that IL-12 can restore the HIV-specific immune response in vitro and can block the programmed cell death of such T cells [5, 6]. Furthermore, the application of IL-12 in different infectious disease models clearly revealed a considerable protective effect that was obviously based on the strong Th-1-inducing activity of IL-12 in the initial phase of an infection. Thus, IL-12 is considered to be an 'initiation cytokine for cellular immunity' [7, 8]. Furthermore, IL-12 represents a decisive link between the nonspecific phagocytic system, that mediates natural resistance, and the highly specific Th1 cell-regulated cellular immune response. However, recent data suggested that IL-12, in the presence of IL-4, can also promote the development of Th2 cells and up-regulate via the production of antibodies a concomitant humoral response [9–13].

Optimal Th1 Development of Naive CD4$^+$ T Cells Depends on the Synergistic Actions of IL-12 and IFN-γ

Since the first studies on the role of IL-12-induced Th cell differentiation were done in vivo or using human PBMC [14–16] or CD4$^+$ T cells in the presence of spleen cells or B-cell hybridomas as accessory cells [17], it was not clear whether IL-12 acts directly on CD4$^+$ T cells or whether its effects on Th cell differentiation are indirect and mediated by other cell types as described for IL-10 [18]. Therefore, purified naive CD4$^+$ T cells from unimmunized mice were stimulated in the absence of accessory cells by immobilized anti-CD3 monoclonal antibodies (mAb) and the direct effect of IL-12 alone or in combination with additional cytokines on the development of naive CD4$^+$ T cells, was evaluated. Six days after primary activation, T cells of the different cultures were restimulated by immobilized anti-CD3 mAb solely to determine their cytokine profile as an indicator of their differentiation.

Using this experimental protocol, we found that IL-12 induces the development of naive murine CD4$^+$ T cells into Th1-type cells. IFN-γ was also reported to promote the development of Th1 cells [19]. Furthermore, it was shown that neutralizing anti-IFN-γ mAb abolished the development of Th1 cells in vivo [20]. Since IL-12 strongly promotes primary production of IFN-γ by freshly isolated CD4$^+$ T cells, these findings suggested that the IL-12-induced Th1 development might be a consequence of the enhanced endogenous primary IFN-γ production and it should be possible to replace IL-12 by exogenous IFN-γ. To test this assumption we activated CD4$^+$ T cells primarily by anti-CD3 mAb in combination either with IL-12 or mouse IFN-γ. After 4 days the IFN-γ concentration of the resulting supernatants was determined. Figure 1A shows that naive CD4$^+$ T cells produced a low but significant amount of IFN-γ which was substantially augmented in the presence of IL-12. Moreover, the amount of mouse IFN-γ (1,000 U/ml) initially added to the respective T-cell culture was only marginally reduced (809 U/ml) and exceeded the IFN-γ concentration in the culture supernatant which was originally supplemented with IL-12 (254 U/ml IFN-γ). Thus, in both cases (priming in the presence of IL-12 or mouse IFN-γ) a concentration of IFN-γ was present during the primary culture period that was saturating with respect to Th1 development. However, restimulation by plate-bound anti-CD3 mAb revealed that Th1 development as indicated by secondary IFN-γ production was not significantly promoted by the addition of mouse IFN-γ whereas the presence of IL-12 during primary culture resulted in a substantial increase of the secondary IFN-γ production. This indicates that IFN-γ by itself cannot support an optimal Th1 development of naive CD4$^+$ T cells in the absence of IL-12 (fig. 1B).

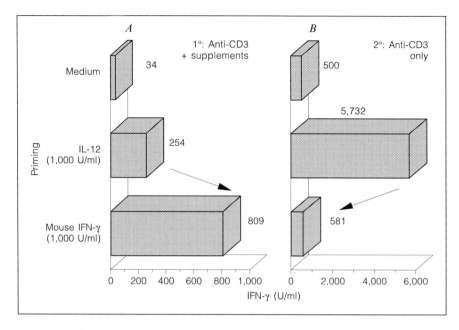

Fig. 1. The effect of exogenous IFN-γ and IL-12 on Th1 development of naive CD4+ T cells. Purified naive CD4+ T cells (1 × 10⁶/ml) from unimmunized mice were stimulated primarily with immobilized anti-CD3 mAb (5 μg/ml) in the presence of IL-12 or mouse IFN-γ. T cells were restimulated on day 6 for 18 h with immobilized anti-CD3 mAb (10 μg/ml) to test for secondary cytokine production. Supernatants from primary (*A*, 1°, harvested 4 days after primary activation) and secondary (*B*, 2°) cultures were tested for the presence of IFN-γ by ELISA to determine the Th phenotype.

To determine whether IL-12 stimulates Th1 development independently from endogenously produced IFN-γ, we chose the following approach: naive CD4+ T cells were stimulated in the presence of IL-12, neutralizing anti-mouse IFN-γ mAb (XMG 1.2), and rat IFN-γ. Because rat IFN-γ is active on murine cells but is not neutralized by the anti-mouse IFN-γ mAb, this experimental approach should allow to differentiate between the capacity of IL-12 to stimulate IFN-γ production and its role in inducing Th1 development. Figure 2A shows that IL-12 strongly enhanced the primary production of IFN-γ by CD3-activated naive CD4+ T cells. Application of anti-mouse IFN-γ mAb neutralized in each case the primarily secreted IFN-γ. Furthermore, priming naive CD4+ T cells in the presence of anti-mouse IFN-γ mAb alone, completely abrogated the relatively low secondary IFN-γ production observed when naive CD4+ T cells were stimulated with anti-CD3 mAb in medium

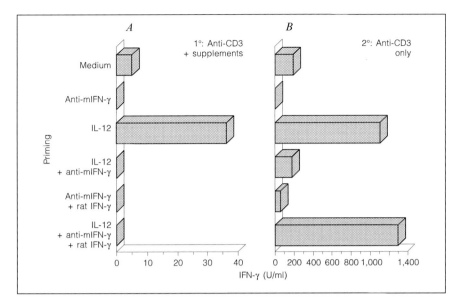

Fig. 2. Development of Th1 cells promoted by IL-12 is partially inhibited by anti-mouse IFN-γ mAb. Purified naive CD4$^+$ T cells were primed in the presence of IL-12 (1,000 U/ml), anti-mouse IFN-γ (XMG 1.2, 30 μg/ml) and rat IFN-γ (1,000 U/ml) in the indicated combinations. Primary (*A*, 1°) and secondary (*B*, 2°) production of IFN-γ were determined by ELISA.

(fig. 2B). IL-12, as expected, efficiently supported the development of Th1 cells. Priming with IL-12 in combination with anti-mouse IFN-γ mAb led to a substantial reduction of the secondary IFN-γ production indicating that the effect of IL-12 with regard to Th1 development is at least partially mediated by IFN-γ. This assumption was confirmed by addition of rat IFN-γ which completely compensated for the inhibition of Th1 differentiation caused by anti-mouse IFN-γ mAb when the T cells were primed in the presence of IL-12. In conclusion, this detailed analysis of the effect of IL-12 on Th1 differentiation of naive CD4$^+$ T cells revealed that (a) IFN-γ or IL-12 in the absence of IFN-γ induced only a weak Th1 development and (b) the IL-12-induced enhancement of Th1 differentiation depends on the coordinate action of IL-12 and IFN-γ [21]. These findings were supported in studies which demonstrate that the optimal Th1 development of naive antigen-specific CD4$^+$ T cells isolated from T-cell receptor transgenic mice depends on IL-12 and IFN-γ [22, 23]. However, Seder et al. [24] proposed a 'default' pathway of Th1 differentiation independent from primary IFN-γ production because these authors observed that Th1 development in vitro could be neither enhanced by exogenous IFN-γ nor inhibited by addition of neutralizing anti-mouse IFN-γ mAb. In accordance with these data, we found that Th1 development of naive CD4$^+$ T cells stimulated by plate-bound anti-CD3 mAb could not be enhanced by exogenous IFN-γ. On the contrary, in our experiments, addition of a neutralizing anti-mouse IFN-γ mAb to these cultures abolished secondary production of IFN-γ by the resulting T cells. This indicates that, in the absence of IL-12, IFN-γ is essential for the generation of Th1 cells. In agreement with our data, other groups reported that neutralization of IFN-γ during primary T-cell activation inhibited subsequent IFN-γ production of the developing Th cells [25, 26]. Moreover, it was shown in vivo that the induction of a Th1 response to the filarial helminth, *Brugia malayi,* was dependent on IFN-γ [27]. The apparently divergent results of Seder et al. [24] could be due to the stimulation of transgenic CD4$^+$ T cells in the presence of accessory cells which might serve as a source of cytokines like IL-12 and IFN-α, that was also reported to affect Th1 cell development of human T cells [28] and, in analogy to IL-12, to activate STAT4 [29]. Another cytokine, that was recently cloned as IFN-γ-inducing factor (IGIF), could also be a potential Th1 promoter [30, 31].

Recent studies with IFN-γ receptor 'knockout (KO)' mice revealed that Th1 differentiation can obviously occur when T cells cannot respond to endogenous IFN-γ, thus indicating that in vivo IL-12 alone or in combination with additional cytokines such as IGIF is sufficient for the development of Th1 cells [32]. In our experimental system, naive CD4$^+$ T cells isolated from such IFN-γ receptor KO mice also showed considerable Th1 development after priming with IL-12 [unpubl. results]. The role of IL-12 as a Th1-inducing factor is further substantiated by the work of Mattner et al. [33] who have shown that the Th1-mediated protection against an infection with *Leishmania major* in C57Bl/6 mice is completely abrogated in IL-12p40 KO mice of this strain. Detailed analysis of such mice revealed that they cannot mount a Th1 reaction in response to a *L. major* infection. Furthermore, it was shown with IL-12p40 KO mice that a KLH-specific Th1 response was strongly reduced and that the residual Th1 response depended on IFN-γ [34]. In addition, it was found that a KLH-specific Th1 response of the respective wild-type mice was considerably inhibited after treatment with neutralizing anti-mouse IFN-γ mAb. Thus, IL-12 and IFN-γ seem to be indispensable for an optimal Th1 development and obviously they serve as direct Th1 inducers. Moreover, they seem to be a part of a positive feedback mechanism with respect to the IL-12-promoted IFN-γ production by T cells and NK cells and the IFN-γ-enhanced competence of antigen-presenting cells to produce IL-12.

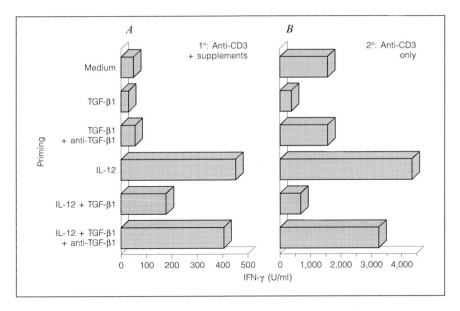

Fig. 3. TGF-β inhibits the Th1 development induced by IL-12 and IFN-γ. Purified naive CD4⁺ T cells were activated in the presence of IL-12 (1,000 U/ml), TGF-β1 (2 ng/ml), and anti-TGF-β1 Ab (3 μg/ml) in the indicated combinations. Primary (*A*, 1°) and secondary (*B*, 2°) production of IFN-γ were determined by ELISA.

Regulation of IL-12-Induced Th1 Development by TGF-β

It was suggested that TGF-β, like IL-12, strongly promotes the development of Th1 cells in vitro [35]. In contrast to these data, we found that the differentiation of CD3-activated naive CD4⁺ T cells to a Th1-like phenotype is substantially reduced by TGF-β even in the presence of the Th1-inducer IL-12 [21]. When naive CD4⁺ T cells were primed in the presence of TGF-β alone or in combination with IL-12, the primary as well as the secondary production of IFN-γ was strongly reduced. This indicates that Th1 differentiation of naive CD4⁺ T cells was rather inhibited than supported by TGF-β (fig. 3A, B). The specificity of this effect of TGF-β was confirmed by applying neutralizing anti-TGF-β Ab which restored the Th1 development that was diminished by TGF-β.

The reduction of primary IFN-γ production by TGF-β suggested that inhibition of Th1 differentiation caused by TGF-β might be due to the decreased IFN-γ production during the priming phase. In order to compensate for this inhibitory effect of TGF-β, rat IFN-γ was added during the priming

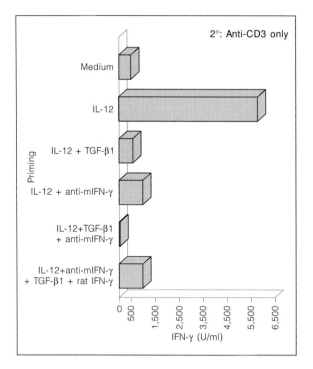

Fig. 4. Th1 development is promoted by IL-12 and abrogated by TGF-β and anti-mouse IFN-γ mAb. Purified naive CD4$^+$ T cells were primed in the presence of IL-12 (1,000 U/ml), TGF-β1 (2 ng/ml), anti-mouse IFN-γ mAb (XMG 1.2, 30 μg/ml) and rat IFN-γ (200 U/ml) in the indicated combinations. On day 6 after primary activation, secondary (2°) production of IFN-γ by the developing Th cells was determined by ELISA.

phase. As shown in figure 4, the secondary production of IFN-γ after priming with anti-CD3 mAb alone (medium) was strongly enhanced in the presence of IL-12. This Th1 development promoted by IL-12 was strongly reduced by priming naive CD4$^+$ T cells in the presence of either TGF-β or anti-mouse IFN-γ mAb. The limited Th1 differentiation that was induced by IL-12 in the presence of anti-mouse IFN-γ mAb, which is presumably due to a direct effect of IL-12 on naive CD4$^+$ T cells, could be completely abrogated by TGF-β, thus indicating that TGF-β can abolish IL-12-induced Th1 development in the absence of IFN-γ. A combination of IL-12, anti-mouse IFN-γ mAb, TGF-β and rat IFN-γ also led only to a limited secondary IFN-γ production. This is in agreement with the assumption that the effect of IL-12 on Th development is strongly inhibited in the presence of TGF-β because exogenous rat IFN-γ could not restore Th1 development abolished by a combination of anti-mouse IFN-γ mAb and TGF-β whereas in the absence of TGF-β the effect of anti-mouse IFN-γ mAb was compensated for by exogenous rat IFN-γ (see fig. 2B). These results suggest that Th1 development of naive CD4$^+$ T cells, which is promoted by a synergistic action of IL-12 and IFN-γ, is strongly reduced in the presence of TGF-β. TGF-β inhibits Th1 differentiation directly by interfering with the differentiation of T cells induced by IL-12 and indirectly by reducing the endogenous production of IFN-γ. In agreement with these findings, it was shown that the IL-12-induced IFN-γ production of neonatal human T cells was strongly suppressed by TGF-β [26]. Moreover, studies dealing with the phenomenon of oral tolerance also demonstrated that T cells which suppressed a myelin basic protein-specific Th1-dominated autoimmune response secreted IL-4 and/or TGF-β, implying that TGF-β inhibits the development of Th1 cells in vivo [36]. In IL-10-deficient mice, it was found that Th1 cells induce colitis [37]. In a second colitis model, it was shown recently that neutralizing IL-12 or blocking CD40-CD40L interaction can inhibit experimental colitis [38, 39] and that treatment with TGF-β has the same effect [40] thus implying that TGF-β is inhibitory by blocking the Th1-inducing capacity of IL-12. In agreement with these findings, preliminary data from our laboratory show that Th1 development in vivo, which was induced by immunizing CBA/J mice with KLH in combination with IL-12, was inhibited when TGF-β was applied simultaneously [unpubl. data]. Interestingly, the splenomegaly which occurred in the course of the IL-12 treatment was also reduced by TGF-β.

Additional studies that were performed to clarify the discrepant results with respect to the effect of TGF-β on Th1 differentiation revealed that TGF-β promotes or inhibits Th1 development depending on the mouse strain used [41]. Detailed analyses revealed that this puzzling property of TGF-β is mainly due to the different ability of the respective T cells to produce IL-2 upon primary activation, and to the different sensitivity of the T cells to the TGF-β-mediated suppression of this primary IL-2 production. TGF-β inhibits Th1 differentiation in the presence of low amounts of IL-2 (<50–100 ng/ml) and stimulates it in the presence of relatively high amounts of IL-2 (>100–200 ng/ml). The TGF-β-mediated inhibition of Th1 development could not be compensated by the addition of IL-12.

The Th2 Promoter IL-4 Dominates the Th1-Inducing Capacity of IL-12

When naive CD4$^+$ T cells were stimulated in the presence of both IL-12 and IL-4 in comparable concentrations, the effect of IL-12 on Th1 differenti-

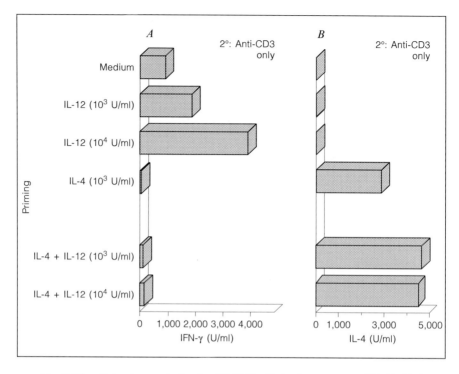

Fig. 5. Th cell development of naive CD4+ T cells in the presence of IL-12, IL-4 or a combination of both cytokines. Purified naive CD4+ T cells (1×10^6/ml) were primed with immobilized anti-CD3 mAb (5 µg/ml) in the presence of IL-4 or IL-12 or a combination of both cytokines. T cells were restimulated on day 6 only with immobilized anti-CD3 mAb (10 µg/ml) without the addition of cytokines. Supernatants were harvested after 18 h and tested for the presence of IFN-γ (*A*) and IL-4 (*B*) by ELISA to determine the Th phenotype.

ation was largely inhibited by IL-4 (fig. 5A). This dominance of IL-4 might be based on a rapid extinction of IL-12 signaling in the developing Th2 cells within 3 days after primary activation [42]. This corresponds to the lack of IL-12 responsiveness by Th2 cells as described by our group [43] which was also recently demonstrated for human allergen-specific Th2 cells [44]. These Th2 cells do not respond to IL-12 because of a total lack of IL-12-induced phosphorylation of STAT4, a transcription factor that is typically involved in IL-12 signalling.

When naive CD4+ T cells were stimulated in the presence of IL-4, addition of IL-12 exerted no inhibitory effect on IL-4-induced Th2 differentiation but rather enhanced the secondary production of IL-4 after restimulation of the T cells (fig. 5B) [12]. This finding was confirmed by recently published data

[9, 10, 17, 45–47]. In addition, it was shown that IL-12 increases the production of IL-4 and IL-10 of human Th0- and Th2-type T-cell clones and freshly isolated peripheral blood T cells [48–50]. Thus, in contrast to the above mentioned allergen-specific Th2 cell clones, other clones remain responsive to IL-12. One could speculate whether the heterogeneity of human Th cells regarding their IL-12 responsiveness is a consequence of different concentrations of IL-4 present during priming. High concentrations of IL-4 might result in a loss of IL-2 responsiveness, whereas low concentrations of IL-4 might lead only to a Th2-like population which still responds to IL-12. Presumably, the differential capacity of human Th2 cells to respond to IL-12 depends also on the different genetic background of the distinct T-cell clones as was shown for the development of murine Th2 cells [51, 52].

Codevelopment of Th1 and Th2 Cells in the Presence of IL-12 and Low Concentrations of IL-4 and Potent Adjuvant Effect of IL-12 for Humoral Immune Reponses

Priming with low amounts of IL-4 (10^2 U/ml) in combination with a high level of IL-12 (10^4 U/ml) led to a Th cell population that simultaneously produced relatively high amounts of IL-4 and IFN-γ after secondary activation by anti-CD3 mAb (fig. 6) [53]. This could be due to the coexistence of Th1 and Th2 cells or to the development of Th0 cells which produce a mixed pattern of lymphokines. Immunofluorescence double staining of intracellular IL-4 and IFN-γ in combination with flow cytometry (FACS) revealed that most of the emerging Th cells produced either IL-4 or IFN-γ and only very few double producers could be detected (fig. 7). This indicates that individual naive CD4$^+$ T cells can differentiate under the same conditions either into Th1 or Th2 cells and implicates that the development of Th1 and Th2 cells in this experimental model is a stochastic process depending on the concentration of IL-4 and IL-12.

These in vitro findings probably reflect observations made in vivo where IL-12, although promoting Th1 development, failed to interfere with the development either of Th2 cells or Th2 cell-dependent antibody production. In susceptible mice infected with *Candida albicans,* which mount a Th2-type response, treatment with IL-12 failed to inhibit the progression of systemic disease and did not alter the course of the mucosal infection. Although IFN-γ production was up-regulated in IL-12-treated mice, IL-12 failed to suppress the production of Th2-type cytokines such as IL-4 and IL-10 [9].

Certain strains of mice develop very strong Th2/IgE responses upon immunization with low concentrations of protein antigens adsorbed to aluminum

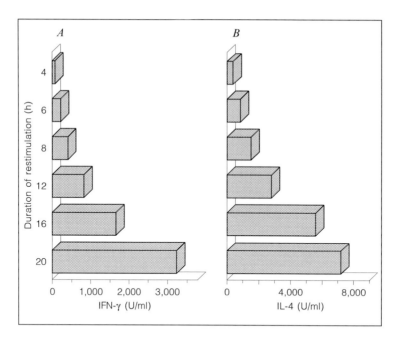

Fig. 6. Priming of naive CD4[+] T cells in the presence of low IL-4 and high IL-12 leads to a Th cell population producing IFN-γ (*A*) and IL-4 (*B*). Purified naive CD4[+] T cells (1 × 10^6/ml) were primarily stimulated with plate-bound anti-CD3 mAb (5 µg/ml) in the presence of IL-4 (100 U/ml) together with IL-12 (10,000 U/ml). Th cells were restimulated on day 6 with immobilized anti-CD3 mAb (5 µg/ml) without the addition of cytokines. Supernatants were collected after the indicated time periods and the content of IFN-γ and IL-4 was determined by ELISA.

hydroxide [54]. Administration of IL-12 promoted the development of Th1 cells and resulted in enormously increased serum levels of antibodies of the Th1-type such as IgG2a and IgG2b [55]. However, under most conditions the synthesis of IgE was not down-regulated by IL-12 in these mice [11]. The slight inhibition of IgE synthesis achieved by treatment with high concentrations of IL-12 was mediated by IFN-γ since neutralization of IFN-γ or similar experiments performed in IFN-γ receptor-deficient mice demonstrated that, in the absence of functional IFN-γ, IL-12 promoted the development of Th1 cells and Th2 cells. Furthermore, the serum levels of Th2-type antibodies (IgG1, IgE) were highest in such mice [unpubl. observations]. Our results are in agreement with recent reports [10, 56] which showed that IL-12 stimulated IL-4 and IgE synthesis after neutralization of endogenous IFN-γ or in IFN-γ receptor-deficient mice injected with eggs from *Schistosoma mansoni*, whereas

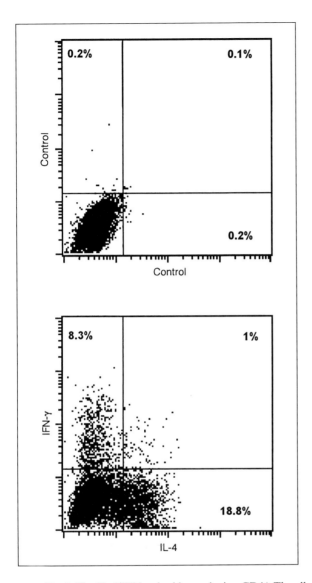

Fig. 7. The IL-4/IFN-γ double-producing CD4$^+$ Th cell population consists mainly of a mixture of IFN-γ-producing Th1 and IL-4-producing Th2 cells. CD4$^+$ T cells were primarily stimulated with plate-bound anti-CD3 mAb (5 µg/ml) in the presence of IL-4 (100 U/ml) in combination with IL-12 (10,000 U/ml). Th cells were restimulated at day 6 with immobilized anti-CD3, harvested after 20 h and stained for intracellular IL-4 and IFN-γ. Quadrants were set on the basis of the corresponding cytokine-blocked negative controls.

it inhibited IL-4 and IgE in wild-type mice. Thus, IL-12 by itself and in the absence of functional IFN-γ appears to promote Th1 and Th2 development. Moreover, these results document the potent adjuvant effect of IL-12 for humoral immune responses as well.

Conclusion

During the early response of the phagocytic cell system in the course of a microbial infection, IL-12 is produced by antigen-presenting cells and subsequently induces a cell-mediated Th1-regulated immune response. Thus, IL-12 functions as an early switch toward cell-mediated immunity. We and others have shown that IL-12 directly stimulates the Th1 development of naive CD4$^+$ T cells, especially in combination with IFN-γ. TGF-β was found to strongly inhibit this effect of IL-12. In addition, IL-4 which is the essential Th2 promoter was also shown to efficiently inhibit the Th1-inducing capacity of IL-12, whereas IL-12 could not prevent the ability of IL-4 to prime Th cells for IL-4 production. Therefore, these data imply that the development either of a Th1- or a Th2-dominated immune response depends on the presence and the concentrations on the one hand of IL-12 and IFN-γ and on the other hand of IL-4 and TGF-β early in the immune response.

References

1   Shu U, Kiniwa M, Wu CY, Maliszewski C, Vezzio N, Hakimi J, Gately M, Delespesse G: Activated T cells induce interleukin-12 production by monocytes via CD40-CD40 ligand interaction. Eur J Immunol 1995;25:1125–1128.
2   Macatonia SE, Hosken NA, Litton M, Vieira P, Hsieh CS, Culpepper JA, Wysocka M, Trinchieri G, Murphy KM, O'Garra A: Dendritic cells produce IL-12 and direct the development of Th1 cells from naive CD4+ T cells. J Immunol 1995;154:5071–5079.
3   Skeen MJ, Miller MA, Shinnick TM, Ziegler HK: Regulation of murine macrophage IL-12 production. Activation of macrophages in vivo, restimulation in vitro, and modulation by other cytokines. J Immunol 1996;156:1196–1206.
4   Nastala CL, Edington HD, McKinney TG, Tahara H, Nalesnik MA, Brunda MJ, Gately MK, Wolf SF, Schreiber RD, Storkus WJ, Lotze MT: Recombinant IL-12 administration induces tumor regression in association with IFN-gamma production. J Immunol 1994;153:1697–1706.
5   Clerici M, Sarin A, Coffman RL, Wynn TA, Blatt SP, Hendrix CW, Wolf SF, Shearer GM, Henkart PA: Type 1/type 2 cytokine modulation of T-cell programmed cell death as a model for human immunodeficiency virus pathogenesis. Proc Natl Acad Sci USA 1994;91:11811–11815.
6   Clerici M, Lucey DR, Berzofsky JA, Pinto LA, Wynn TA, Blatt SP, Dolan MJ, Hendrix CW, Wolf SF, Shearer GM: Restoration of HIV-specific cell-mediated immune responses by interleukin-12 in vitro. Science 1993;262:1721–1724.
7   Scott P: IL-12: initiation cytokine for cell-mediated immunity (comment). Science 1993;260:496–497.
8   Wang Z, Zheng S, Corry DB, Dalton DK, Seder RA, Reiner SL, Locksley RM: Interferon-gamma-independent effects of interleukin-12 administered during acute or established infection with *Leishmania major*. Proc Natl Acad Sci USA 1994;91:12932–12936.

9   Romani L, Mencacci A, Tonnetti L, Spaccapelo R, Cenci E, Puccetti P, Wolf SF, Bistoni F: IL-12
      is both required and prognostic in vivo for T helper type 1 differentiation in murine candidiasis.
      J Immunol 1994;153:5167–5175.
10   Wynn TA, Jankovic D, Hieny S, Zioncheck K, Jardieu P, Cheever AW, Sher A: IL-12 exacerbates
      rather than suppresses T-helper 2-dependent pathology in the absence of endogenous IFN-γ. J Im-
      munol 1995;154:3999–4009.
11   Germann T, Guckes S, Bongartz M, Dlugonska H, Schmitt E, Kolbe L, Kölsch E, Podlaski FJ,
      Gately MK, Rüde E: Administration of interleukin-12 during ongoing immune responses fails to
      permanently suppress and can even enhance the synthesis of antigen-specific IgE. Int Immunol
      1995;7:1649–1657.
12   Schmitt E, Hoehn P, Germann T, Ruede E: Differential effects of IL-12 on the development of
      naive mouse CD4$^+$ T cells. Eur J Immunol 1994;24:343–347.
13   Wynn TA, Reynolds A, James S, Cheever AW, Caspar P, Hieny S, Jankovic D, Sher A: IL-12
      enhances vaccine-induced immunity to schistosomes by augmenting both humoral and cell-mediated
      immune responses against the parasite. J Immunol 1996;157:4068–4078.
14   Manetti R, Parronchi P, Giudizi MG, Piccinni MP, Maggi E, Trinchieri G, Romagnani S: Natural
      killer cell stimulatory factor (interleukin-12 [IL-12]) induces T helper type 1 (Th1)-specific immune
      responses and inhibits the development of IL-4-producing Th cells. J Exp Med 1993;177:1199–
      1204.
15   Heinzel FP, Schoenhaut DS, Rerki RM, Rosser LE, Gately MK: Recombinant interleukin-12 cures
      mice infected with *Leishmania major.* J Exp Med 1993;177:1505–1509.
16   Sypek JP, Chung CL, Mayor SE, Subramanyam JM, Goldman SJ, Sieburth DS, Wolf SF, Schaub
      RG: Resolution of cutaneous leishmaniasis: Interleukin-12 initiates a protective T helper type 1
      immune response. J Exp Med 1993;177:1797–1802.
17   Hsieh CS, Macatonia SE, Tripp CS, Wolf SF, O'Garra A, Murphy KM: Development of TH1
      CD4 + T cells through IL-12 produced by Listeria-induced macrophages (see comments). Science
      1993;260:547–549.
18   Fiorentino DF, Zlotnik A, Vieira P, Mosmann TR, Howard M, Moore KW, O'Garra A: IL-10
      acts on the antigen-presenting cell to inhibit cytokine production by Th1 cells. J Immunol 1991;
      146:3444–3451.
19   Gajewski TF, Fitch FW: Anti-proliferative effect of IFN-gamma in immune regulation. I. IFN-
      gamma inhibits the proliferation of Th2 but not Th1 murine helper T lymphocyte clones. J Immunol
      1988;140:4245–4252.
20   Belosevic M, Finbloom DS, Van Der Meide PH, Slayter MV, Nacy CA: Administration of mono-
      clonal anti-IFN-gamma antibodies in vivo abrogates natural resistance of C3H/HeN mice to infection
      with *Leishmania major.* J Immunol 1989;143:266–274.
21   Schmitt E, Hoehn P, Huels C, Goedert S, Palm N, Rüde E, Germann T: T helper type 1 development
      of naive CD4 + T cells requires the coordinate action of interleukin-12 and interferon-gamma and
      is inhibited by transforming growth factor-β. Eur J Immunol 1994;24:793–798.
22   Bradley LM, Dalton DK, Croft M: A direct role for IFN-gamma in regulation of Th1 cell develop-
      ment. J Immunol 1996;157:1350–1358.
23   Wenner CA, Guler ML, Macatonia SE, O'Garra A, Murphy KM: Roles of IFN-gamma and IFN-
      alpha in IL-12-induced T helper cell-1 development. J Immunol 1996;156:1442–1447.
24   Seder RA, Paul WE, Davis MM, Fazekas de St Groth B: The presence of interleukin-4 during in
      vitro priming determines the lymphokine-producing potential of CD4 + T cells from T cell receptor
      transgenic mice. J Exp Med 1992;176:1091–1098.
25   Macatonia SE, Hsieh CS, Murphy KM, O'Garra A: Dendritic cells and macrophages are required
      for Th1 development of CD4$^+$ T cells from αβ TCR transgenic mice: IL-12 substitution for macro-
      phages to stimulate IFN-gamma production is IFN-gamma-dependent. Int Immunol 1993;5:1119–
      1128.
26   Wu CY, Demeure C, Kiniwa M, Gately M, Delespesse G: IL-12 induces the production of IFN-
      gamma by neonatal human CD4 T cells. J Immunol 1993;151:1938–1949.
27   Pearlman E, Heinzel FP, Hazlett FE Jr, Kazura JW: IL-12 modulation of T helper responses to
      the filarial helminth, *Brugia malayi.* J Immunol 1995;154:4658–4664.

28 Brinkmann V, Geiger T, Alkan S, Heusser CH: Interferon-α increases the frequency of interferon-τ-producing human CD4$^+$ T cells. J Exp Med 1993;178:1655–1663.

29 Cho SS, Bacon CM, Sudarshan C, Rees RC, Finbloom D, Pine R, O'Shea JJ: Activation of STAT4 by IL-12 and IFN-alpha: Evidence for the involvement of ligand-induced tyrosine and serine phosphorylation. J Immunol 1996;157:4781–4789.

30 Micallef MJ, Ohtsuki T, Kohno K, Tanabe F, Ushio S, Namba M, Tanimoto T, Torigoe K, Fujii M, Ikeda M, Fukuda S, Kurimoto M: Interferon-gamma-inducing factor enhances T helper 1 cytokine production by stimulated human T cells: Synergism with interleukin-12 for interferon-gamma production. Eur J Immunol 1996;26:1647–1651.

31 Okamura H, Tsutsi H, Komatsu T, Yutsudo M, Hakura A, Tanimoto T, Torigoe K, Okura T, Nukada Y, Hattori K, Akita K, Namba M, Tanabe F, Konishi K, Fukuda S, Kurimoto M: Cloning of a new cytokine that induces IFN-gamma production by T cells. Nature 1995;378:88–91.

32 Swihart K, Fruth U, Messmer N, Hug K, Behin R, Huang S, Del Giudice G, Aguet M, Louis JA: Mice from a genetically resistant background lacking the interferon-gamma receptor are susceptible to infection with *Leishmania major* but mount a polarized T helper cell 1-type CD4 + T cell response. J Exp Med 1995;181:961–971.

33 Mattner F, Magram J, Ferrante J, Launois P, Di Padova K, Behin R, Gately MK, Louis JA, Albert G: Genetically resistant mice lacking interleukin-12 are susceptible to infection with *Leishmania major* and mount a polarized Th2 cell response. Eur J Immunol 1996;26:1553–1559.

34 Magram J, Connaughton SE, Warrier RR, Carvajal DM, Wu CY, Ferrante J, Stewart C, Sarmiento U, Faherty DA, Gately MK: IL-12-deficient mice are defective in IFN-gamma production and type 1 cytokine responses. Immunity 1996;4:471–481.

35 Negelkerken L, Gollob KJ, Tielemans M, Coffman RL: Role of transforming growth factor-β in the preferential induction of T helper cells of type 1 by staphylococcal enteroxin. Eur J Immunol 1993;23:2306–2310.

36 Chen Y, Kuchroo VK, Inobe J, Hafler DA, Weiner HL: Regulatory T cell clones induced by oral tolerance: Suppression of autoimmune encephalomyelitis. Science 1994;265:1237–1240.

37 Davidson NJ, Leach MW, Fort MM, Thompson Snipes L, Kuhn R, Muller W, Berg DJ, Rennick DM: T helper cell 1-type CD4 + T cells, but not B cells, mediate colitis in interleukin-10-deficient mice. J Exp Med 1996;184:241–251.

38 Neurath MF, Fuss I, Kelsall BL, Stuber E, Strober W: Antibodies to interleukin-12 abrogate established experimental colitis in mice. J Exp Med 1995;182:1281–1290.

39 Stuber E, Strober W, Neurath M: Blocking the CD40L-CD40 interaction in vivo specifically prevents the priming of T helper 1 cells through the inhibition of interleukin-12 secretion. J Exp Med 1996; 183:693–698.

40 Neurath MF, Fuss I, Kelsall BL, Presky DH, Waegell W, Strober W: Experimental granulomatous colitis in mice is abrogated by induction of TGF-beta-mediated oral tolerance. J Exp Med 1996; 183:2605–2616.

41 Hoehn P, Goedert S, Germann T, Koelsch S, Jin S, Palm N, Ruede E, Schmitt E: Opposing effects of TGF-β2 on the Th1 cell development of naive CD4 + T cells isolated from different mouse strains. J Immunol 1995;155:3788–3793.

42 Szabo SJ, Jacobson NG, Dighe AS, Gubler U, Murphy KM: Development commitment to the Th2 lineage by extinction of IL-12 signaling. Immunity 1995;2:665–675.

43 Germann T, Gately MK, Schoenhaut DS, Lohoff M, Mattner F, Fischer S, Jin SC, Schmitt E, Rüde E: Interleukin-12/T cell stimulating factor, a cytokine with multiple effects on T helper type 1 (Th1) but not on Th2 cells. Eur J Immunol 1993;23:1762–1770.

44 Hilkens CMU, Messer G, Tesselaar K, van Rietschoten AGI, Kapsenberg ML, Wierenga EA: Lack of IL-12 signaling in human allergen-specific Th2 cells. J Immunol 1996;157:4316–4321.

45 Seder RA, Gazzinelli R, Sher A, Paul WE: Interleukin-12 acts directly on CD4 + T cells to enhance priming for interferon-gamma production and diminishes interleukin-4 inhibition of such priming. Proc Natl Acad Sci USA 1993;90:10188–10192.

46 Finkelman FD, Madden KB, Cheever AW, Katona IM, Morris SC, Gately MK, Hubbard BR, Gause WC, Urban JFJ: Effects of interleukin-12 on immune responses and host protection in mice infected with intestinal nematode parasites (see comments). J Exp Med 1994;179:1563–1572.

47   Gerosa F, Paganin C, Peritt D, Paiola F, Scupoli MT, Aste Amezaga M, Frank I, Trinchieri G: Interleukin-12 primes human CD4 and CD8 T cell clones for high production of both interferon-gamma and interleukin-10. J Exp Med 1996;183:2559–2569.

48   Meyaard L, Hovenkamp E, Otto SA, Miedema F: IL-12-induced IL-10 production by human T cells as a negative feedback for IL-12-induced immune responses. J Immunol 1996;156:2776–2782.

49   Jeannin P, Delneste Y, Seveso M, Life P, Bonnefoy JY: IL-12 synergizes with IL-2 and other stimuli in inducing IL-10 production by human T cells. J Immunol 1996;156:3159–3165.

50   Jeannin P, Delneste Y, Life P, Gauchat JF, Kaiserlian D, Bonnefoy JY: Interleukin-12 increases interleukin-4 production by established human Th0- and Th2-like T cell clones. Eur J Immunol 1995;25:2247–2252.

51   Guler ML, Gorham JD, Hsieh CS, Mackey AJ, Steen RG, Dietrich WF, Murphy KM: Genetic susceptibility to Leishmania: IL-12 responsiveness in TH1 cell development (see comments). Science 1996;271:984–987.

52   Gorham JD, Güler ML, Steen RG, Mackey AJ, Daly MJ, Frederick K, Dietrich WF, Murphy KM: Genetic mapping of a murine locus controlling development of T helper 1/T helper 2 type responses. Proc Natl Acad Sci USA 1996;93:12467–12472.

53   Palm N, Germann T, Goedert S, Hoehn P, Koelsch S, Rüde E, Schmitt E: Co-development of naive CD4+ cells toward T helper type 1 or T helper type 2 cells induced by a combination of IL-12 and IL-4. Immunobiology 1997;196:475–484.

54   Kolbe L, Heusser C, Kolsch E: Antigen dose-dependent regulation of B epsilon-memory cell expression. Int Arch Allergy Appl Immunol 1991;95:202–206.

55   Germann T, Bongartz M, Dlugonska H, Hess H, Schmitt E, Kolbe L, Kölsch E, Podlaski FJ, Gately MK, Rüde E: IL-12 profoundly upregulates the synthesis of antigen-specific, complement-fixing IgG2a, IgG2b and IgG3 antibody subclasses in vivo. Eur J Immunol 1995;25:823–829.

56   Wynn TA, Oswald IP, Eltoum IA, Caspar P, Lowenstein CJ, Lewis FA, James SL, Sher A: Elevated expression of Th1 cytokines and nitric oxide synthase in the lungs of vaccinated mice after challenge infection with *Schistosoma mansoni.* J Immunol 1994;153:5200–5209.

Edgar Schmitt, Institute for Immunology, Johannes Gutenberg University,
D–55101 Mainz (Germany)

Adorini L (ed): IL-12. Chem Immunol. Basel, Karger, 1997, vol 68, pp 86–109

....

The Role of IL-12 and IL-4 in
Leishmania major Infection

Frank Mattner[a], *Gottfried Alber*[a], *Jeanne Magram*[b], *Manfred Kopf*[c]

[a] Department of Infectious Diseases, Hoffmann-La Roche AG, Basel, Switzerland;
[b] Department of Biotechnology, Hoffmann-La Roche, Nutley, N.J., USA and
[c] Basel Institute for Immunology, Basel, Switzerland

Introduction

It is well established in both mouse and human systems that CD4[+] T cells can be divided into two subsets, designated Th1 and Th2 [for reviews, see 1–3]. These subsets are defined by the profile of lymphokines they secrete. Typically, Th1 cells produce primarily IFN-γ, whereas Th2 cells produce characteristically a panel of cytokines including IL-4, IL-5, IL-6, IL-9, IL-10 and IL-13. Functionally, Th1 responses mediate predominantly cellular immunity, whereas Th2 cells are responsible for allergic and humoral responses characterized by high IgG1 and IgE levels, eosinophilia, and mastocytosis. IL-12 and IL-4 have been shown to be key factors, which mediate the in vivo development of Th1 and Th2 cells, respectively [4–9]. Both in vitro and in vivo experiments have demonstrated the crucial importance of IL-12 in mice in initiating and establishing both innate immunity- and cell-mediated resistance to intracellular pathogens, including *Listeria monocytogenes, Toxoplasma gondii,* and *Mycobacterium tuberculosis* in mice [10–13].

Cutaneous infection of mice with *Leishmania major* is a well-established experimental model of chronic human disease caused by an intracellular parasite [for review, see 14]. The infection of mice of different genetic backgrounds with *L. major* results in one of two contrasting patterns of disease. In BALB/c and a few other mouse strains, local infection is not effectively controlled by the immune response and the disease disseminates to involve visceral organs, eventually resulting in a fatal outcome. Infection of most other inbred strains (e.g. C57Bl/6, C3H/HeN, 129Sv) causes a localized lesion that heals spontaneously after a few weeks. The resolution of lesions is accompanied by the development of complete resistance to reinfection. MHC class II-restricted CD4$^+$ T cells are of critical importance for the development of clinical disease [15–18], whereas MHC class I-restricted CD8$^+$ T cells are of minor importance during the primary infection [19]. Cure or exacerbation of infection with *L. major* has become a paradigm for the role of different T-helper subsets during the infection. Resistant strains develop predominantly Th1 responses, whereas susceptible strains develop predominantly Th2 responses [17–20]. Consistent with this paradigm, depletion of IL-4 by neutralization with an mAb makes susceptible mice resistant [21–23] and depletion of IFN-γ by either mAb neutralization or gene disruption renders resistant mice susceptible to infection [24–26]. Furthermore, neutralization of IL-12, a cytokine promoting Th1 and suppressing Th2 development, abrogates resistance, whereas the supplementation of rIL-12 to susceptible mice allows them to resolve the infection [27–29].

In this review, we summarize the latest results that contribute to further the understanding of the role of IL-4 and IL-12 during *L. major* infection. We emphasize on studies of IL-12- and IL-4-deficient mice on both a genetically resistant and susceptible genetic background [30, 31].

Early Events of *L. major*-Infected Macrophages: Suppression of IL-12 as a Parasite Evasion Mechanism

In contrast to a variety of intracellular pathogens (e.g. Listeria, Toxoplasma), *L. major* promastigotes enter into macrophages in a relatively 'silent' way. In vitro, it has been demonstrated that promastigotes avoid the initiation of activation signals for proinflammatory cytokines, chemokines and host defense factors (e.g. IL-12, IL-1α, IL-1β, TNF, MCP-1, and iNOS). IL-12 mRNA and protein production, in particular, were actively inhibited by promastigotes [32, 33]. Identical outcomes were observed comparing infected macrophages from resistant C57Bl/6 and susceptible BALB/c mice, suggesting that the preferential development of Th2 cells during infection of BALB/c mice cannot be explained by differences in the ability to produce IL-12 [32]. Indeed, a delayed induction of IL-12p40 mRNA was found for both resistant and susceptible mice in vivo [33]. In another study, however, BALB/c mice produced elevated levels of IL-12p40 transcripts 1 day after infection [29]. Our own studies support the observations in this report, as expression of IL-12p40 in BALB/c mice started at day 1 after infection and became increased at day 6 and 8, a time-point where IL-12p40 transcripts in C57Bl/6 mice have just begun to be expressed [M. Kopf, unpubl. data]. Induction of Th1 cells in

BALB/c mice may be antagonized by a stronger early IL-4 response in BALB/c mice early during the course of infection (see below) [34], or by delayed expression of the high affinity IL-12 receptor on Th1 cells, as suggested by Murphy's group [35, 36].

In vitro, IL-12 inhibition was independent of the presence or absence of IFN-γ costimulation, but dependent on intact promastigotes. Both heat-killed *L. major* and a recombinant Leishmania antigen, which is expressed on promastigotes and amastigotes, were able to stimulate IL-12 production from macrophages [32, 37]. Additionally, IL-12 inhibition was also not mediated by the *L. major* cell surface protein lipophosphoglycan (LPG) [32]. IL-10, a potent inhibitor of macrophage-dependent cytokine synthesis including IL-12 after infection with *T. gondii* and *L. monocytogenes* [38, 39], seems not to down-regulate IL-12 synthesis by *L. major*-infected macrophages [32]. This is consistent with the finding that mice treated with anti-IL-10 mAb remain resistant to infection with *L. major* [14].

The Role of Costimulatory Interactions for Cytokine Secretion Patterns and T-Helper Cell Polarization

For an adaptive immune response to occur after infection, specific T cells must receive a minimum of two signals. This requirement is believed to provide a safeguard mechanism to avoid inappropriate activation and autoimmunity [40, 41]. Upon cognate interaction of antigen-presenting cell (APC) and CD4$^+$ T cell, signal 1 is provided by the ternary complex MHC class II, antigenic peptide and T-cell receptor (TCR). Signal 2 is a hierarchy of nonantigen-driven additional stimuli provided by costimulatory receptor-ligand interaction, the most important being CD40-CD40L, CD28-B7 and/or CTLA4-B7 [42, 43].

CD40 is expressed by APCs (e.g. B cells, macrophages, dendritic cells) and a variety of other cell types, such as microglia, vascular endothelial cells, fibroblasts and thymic epithelial cells [for review, see 44]. Its cognate ligand (CD40L) is expressed transiently by CD4$^+$ T cells during activation. Disruption of CD40-CD40L interaction abrogates humoral responses and critically effects cell-mediated immune response [45–49]. Individuals with a mutant CD40L display the X-linked hyper-IgM syndrome, an immunodeficient disease characterized by the absence of IgG and IgA antibodies, and they are highly susceptible to infections (e.g. Cryptococcus, Pneumocystis and Histoplasma). Similarly, mice carrying disrupted alleles of CD40 or CD40L lack germinal centers and the ability to switch antibody classes. Further, these knockouts have been used to establish the importance of CD40-CD40L interaction for protective cell-mediated immunity to Leishmania. Both CD40L- and CD40-

deficient mice on a genetically resistant background became susceptible to infection with *L. major* [50, 51]. Inflammatory macrophages (peritoneal exudate cells, PEC) of mutant mice could not be induced to produce IL-12, which was not an intrinsic defect, but due to the inability of T cells to activate macrophages. As a consequence, T cells failed to develop a protective Th1 response. Furthermore, CD40L-deficient mice infected with *Leishmania amazonensis*, a species to which most inbred strains of mice are susceptible, showed a greatly increased parasite burden and a decreased Th1 response [52]. IL-4-dependent IgE responses were also reduced. Cocultures of PEC and draining lymph node cells from CD40L-deficient mice stimulated with parasite failed to induce nitrite production, whereas IL-12 levels were comparable to controls. It should be noted, however, that promastigotes of the species *L. amazonensis* seem to poorly stimulate IL-12 production and that levels measured in cultures may have resulted from unspecific stimulation. Together, these reports demonstrate that CD40-CD40L interaction is important for both Th1 development and proper activation of macrophages. Whether the absence of Th1 induction by disruption of CD40-CD40L interaction allows default Th2 development remains controversial. In *L. major*-infected CD40-deficient but not the CD40L-deficient mice, elevated levels of IL-4 were observed. Interestingly, in this context, signaling exclusively through CD40 with an agonistic anti-CD40 mAb was sufficient to confer protection to *L. major* to the normally susceptible BALB/c mice [W. Ferlin, DNAX, pers. commun.].

Work over the last years has demonstrated that CD28 is one of the major costimulatory receptors on the surface of resting T cells [for review, see 43]. CD28 ligation acts synergistically with TCR ligation to maximize T-cell activation, promote T-cell differentiation and expansion, and to regulate survival of T cells. CD28 interacts with at least two natural ligands, CD80 (B7-1) and CD86 (B7-2), which are expressed upon stimulation of professional APCs. CD80 and CD86 have been reported to differentially regulate lymphokine production [53]. The system appears extremely complex, considering that activated T cells also express a CD28 homologue, CTLA-4, which is a high affinity binder for both CD80 and CD86. Engagement of CTLA-4 seems to transmit a negative signal for T-cell activation [54, 55]. During infection with *L. major*, CD28 seems to play a limited role. CD28-deficient C57Bl/6 mice are fully capable of controlling infection and mounting a normal IFN-γ response, whereas CD28-deficient BALB/c mice remain susceptible to infection unless treated with anti-IL-4 mAb [56]. This indicates that in vivo IL-4 responses are not critically affected in the absence of CD28 costimulation. In contrast, in vitro restimulation cultures of draining lymph node cells of CD28-deficient BALB/c mice show a strongly diminished capacity to produce IL-4. Physical disruption of the cognate architecture may limit compensatory interactions and/or the supply of appropriate soluble factors. A similar discrepancy has been described for lymphocyte proliferation in the absence of IL-2, which is inhibited in vitro, but still functional when assessed in vivo after viral infection [57, 58].

Both IL-12p35$^{-/-}$ and IL-12p40$^{-/-}$ Mice Develop High Susceptibility to Infection with *L. major*

Mice with a homozygous disruption of either the IL-12p35 or IL-12p40 gene on a normally resistant genetic background (129Sv/Ev) fail to control infection with *L. major* and develop progressive disease, as determined by footpad swelling, ulceration of lesion, and parasite titer, (fig. 1A, 2A) [30]. Accordingly, IL-12p35/p40 doubly deficient mice are highly susceptible to *L. major* infection and develop disease comparable to IL-12p35 or IL-12p40 singly deficient mice (fig. 1A). This indicates that a functional IL-12(p35/p40) heterodimer is required for containment of *L. major* and that a monomer or homodimer of either of the individual subunits has no agonistic activity in this infection. Interestingly, the footpad swelling reaction started sooner after infection in susceptible BALB/c mice compared to normally resistant 129Sv mice rendered susceptible by disruption of either IL-12 or IFN-γR1 (fig. 1A, 8). This may be related to strain-specific (129Sv versus BALB/c) genetic factor(s) other than IL-12 and IFN-γ, which regulate extravasation and/or chemoattraction of inflammatory cells. Alternatively, cell trafficking itself is regulated by IL-12 and/or IFN-γ. The observation of a delayed footpad swelling in IL-12-deficient mice on the BALB/c background (fig. 1B), similar to IL-12-deficient mice on the 129Sv background, may argue for the latter hypothesis.

Enumeration of the number of parasites in draining lymph nodes 11 weeks after infection showed a 10-fold and 80- to 400-fold increase in BALB/c and IL-12-deficient 129Sv/Ev mice, respectively, indicating that the disease is worse in IL-12-deficient 129Sv mice compared to susceptible BALB/c mice (fig. 2A). Differences in number of parasites in IL-12p35- and IL-12p40-deficient mice were statistically insignificant. It is interesting that IL-12-deficient mice on a resistant background develop significantly higher parasite burdens than genetically susceptible BALB/c mice do. A similar situation was observed in IFN-γR1-deficient mice (129Sv). These mice succumbed to infection between weeks 6 and 9 displaying fatal visceral leishmaniasis and severe liver histopathology, whereas BALB/c mice were found without obvious liver histopathology, when euthanized due to necrotic lesions [31]. This indicated that the type 1 pathway in *L. major*-infected BALB/c mice is partially intact and contributes to the limiting of parasite visceralization. Indeed, it has become evident from other studies that susceptible and resistant mice do not considerably differ in

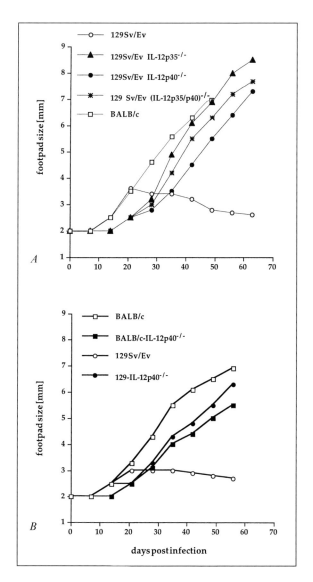

Fig. 1. Disease phenotype in response to infection of IL-12-deficient mice. Groups of 5 mice were infected in the left hind footpad with 3×10^6 *L. major* promastigotes (MRHO/SU/59/P). The course of disease was monitored weekly using a metric caliper to quantitate the swelling at the site of inoculation. Designated infection groups included mice on a normally genetically resistant background (129Sv/Ev) disrupted of IL-12p35 (129Sv/Ev-IL-12p35$^{-/-}$), IL-12p40 (129Sv/Ev-IL-12p40$^{-/-}$), both IL-12p35 and IL-12p40 (129Sv/Ev-IL-12p35/p40)$^{-/-}$, and wild-type 129Sv/Ev and BALB/c mice (*A*); mice disrupted of IL-12p40 on both a genetically susceptible (BALB/c) and a resistant (129Sv/Ev) background (*B*), and congenic wild-type controls. Values represent the mean of each group.

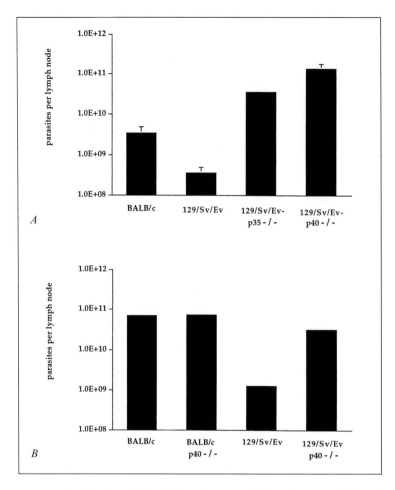

Fig. 2. A, B Parasite load in lymph nodes of infected IL-12-deficient mice. Groups of infected mice as represented in legend to figure 1 were sacrificed at day 75 and the number of viable parasites was determined by limiting dilution. Values represent the mean of each group.

IFN-γ levels and IFN-γ-producing cells within the first 3 weeks of infection [25, 33, 59]. However, a consistent feature of BALB/c mice is a reduced ratio of IFN-γ to IL-4 during the entire course of infection [60].

To test the role of IL-12 in susceptible BALB/c mice, both the IL-12p40 and IL-12p35 mutant genes were backcrossed for 5 generations from 129Sv/Ev to the BALB/c background. Following intercross, mice homozygous for these mutations were obtained and were infected with *L. major* promastigotes

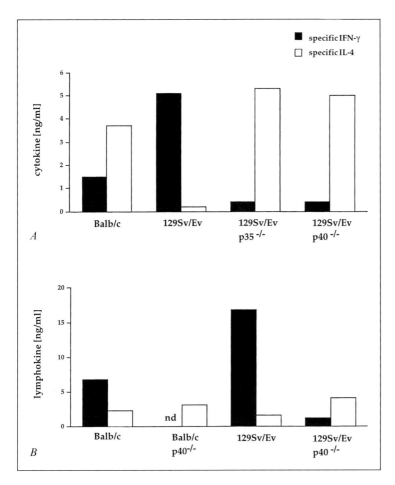

Fig. 3. A, B In vitro cytokine production from IL-12-deficient mice. Draining lymph node cells of groups of infected mice as presented in legend to figure 1 were stimulated for 72 h in the presence of specific antigen (freeze-thawed promastigotes) equivalent to 10^6 promastigotes/ml. Supernatants were assayed for IL-4 and IFN-γ by ELISA. Values represent the mean of triplicate cultures; nd = not detectable.

(strain LV 39). Expectedly, similar to IL-12-deficient mice on the 129Sv/EV background, IL-12p40-deficient BALB/c mice were susceptible to infection, as measured by footpad swelling (fig. 1B) and parasite titer (fig. 2B). However, it should be noted that in 3 out of 4 experiments the parasite load in IL-12-deficient BALB/c mice was not higher compared to wild-type BALB/c mice, although the IFN-γ levels went down to baseline. Again, no differences were observed between IL-12p35 and IL-12p40 mutants mice (not shown).

CD4$^+$ T-Cell Development in the Absence of IL-12

Protection and exacerbation of infection with *L. major* has been clearly related to the development of Th1 and Th2 cells, respectively, which presumably arise from a common naive precursor (Thp) [61]. A number of factors have been suggested to influence Thp commitment to either Th1 or Th2 subsets including cytokines, hormones, type of APC, dose of antigen, epitope specificity, and costimulatory receptors [for a detailed review, see 2]. As to the influence of cytokines, there has been substantial evidence that IL-12 and IL-4 are the major factors determining the capacity of primed CD4$^+$ T cells to develop into Th1 and Th2 cells, respectively. Moreover, IL-4 and IL-12 have been suggested to act in a cross-regulatory manner and to mutually inhibit Th subset development directly or indirectly by IL-10 and IFN-γ [10, 62, 63]. Analysis of draining lymph node cells of late stage ($>$ 10 weeks) infected IL-12-deficient mice (both IL-12p35 and IL-12p40) on the 129Sv/Ev background demonstrated dramatically impaired Th1 (IFN-γ) responses (fig. 3A). In vivo IFN-γ-specific transcripts and ex vivo Leishmania antigen-stimulated IFN-γ protein production were 50- to 100-fold reduced in IL-12-deficient mice. By contrast, IL-4 transcript and protein levels were 50- to 100-fold elevated indicating the up-regulation of Th2 responses in the absence of IL-12. Interestingly, IFN-γ production in infected BALB/c mice was increased 10-fold compared to IL-12-deficient 129Sv/Ev. BALB/c IFN-γ production was dependent on IL-12, for it was completely inhibited in IL-12-deficient BALB/c mice concomitant with a further increase of IL-4 production (fig. 3B). To the extent that delayed-type hypersensitivity (DTH) responses are mediated by Th1 cells, their absence in IL-12-deficient mice further indicates the absence of functionally intact Th1 cells [30]. Taken together, these results clearly demonstrate that: (i) IL-12 is crucial for Th1 development; (ii) IL-12 inhibits Th2 development, and (iii) Th1 development is not defective in susceptible BALB/c mice but it is antagonized by IL-4. Whether the inhibition of Th2 development in resistant mice is mediated by IFN-γ still remains unclear. Infected IFN-γ-deficient mice on the C57Bl/6 background undergo default Th2 development [25], whereas IFN-γR1-deficient mice on the 129Sv background maintain Th1 development [26]. Independent of Th development, however, the outcome of infection in both deficient strains is fatal. The discrepancy between IFN-γR1- and IFN-γ-deficient mice may reflect a genetic difference (129Sv versus C57Bl/6 strains) in Th development. Alternatively, the conflict may be resolved by assuming that the IFN-γ receptor β chain (IFN-γR2), which is intact in IFN-γ receptor α chain (IFN-γR1)-deficient mice, can bind IFN-γ and transduce a negative signal for Th2 development. Interestingly, it has been shown that the IFN-γ receptor β chain is present and signals in Th2 but not in Th1 clones [64].

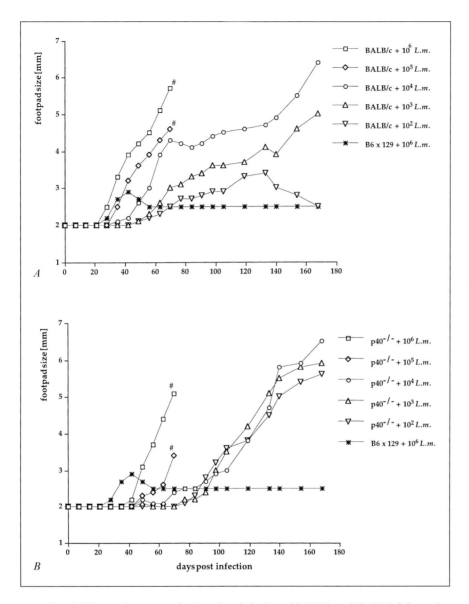

Fig. 4. Disease phenotype after low dose infection of BALB/c and IL-12-deficient mice. Groups of 5 mice were infected in the left hind footpad with the indicated numbers of promastigotes of *L. major* (*L.m.*), strain LV 39. The course of disease was monitored weekly. Infected mice evaluated in the same experiment included wild-type BALB/c (*A*), IL-12p40-deficient (B6 × 129 IL-12p40$^{-/-}$) (*B*), and control wild-type C57Bl/6 × 129Sv/Ev mice (B6 × 129). Mice were sacrificed because of necrosis of lesions at days indicated (#).

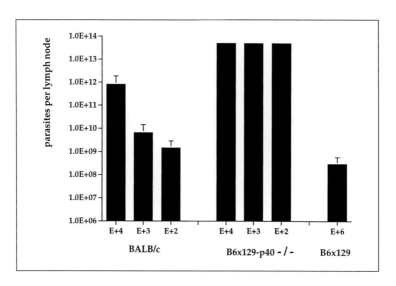

Fig. 5. Parasite load after low dose infection of BALB/c and IL-12-deficient mice. Number of viable parasites recovered from lymph nodes of groups of mice described in legend to figure 4 were determined by limiting dilution at day 168 after infection. Values represent the mean of each group.

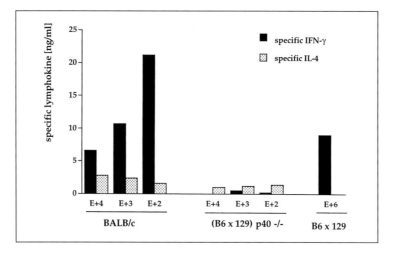

Fig. 6. In vitro cytokine production from low dose infected BALB/c and IL-12-deficient mice. Lymph node cells of groups of mice described in legend to figure 4 were harvested at day 168 after infection, stimulated with specific antigen and cytokines determined as described in legend to figure 3.

Inhibition of Th1 development by IL-4 in BALB/c mice becomes quantitatively measurable only at later stages of infection, as suggested by the observation that IL-4-deficient BALB/c mice have increased IFN-γ production 9 weeks but not 3 weeks after infection [31], and that the number of IFN-γ-producing cells does not considerably differ comparing susceptible and resistant mice within the first 3–4 weeks of infection [25]. This is surprising considering that immune interventions, such as treatment with anti-IL-4 or recombinant IL-12, allow BALB/c mice to resolve infection only when administered within the first week [14].

The Early IL-4 Response

It has been shown recently that, in contrast to resistant mice, susceptible BALB/c mice exhibit a peak of IL-4 mRNA expression extremely rapidly after infection with *L. major* [34]. Interestingly, NK1.1$^-$ CD4$^+$ T cells were responsible for this rapid IL-4 response that could be down-regulated by IL-12 administered prior to injection of parasites. Although the role of this rapid IL-4 response in driving the subsequent differentiation of Th2 cells in BALB/c mice has not yet been directly ascertained, indirect evidence suggest that these two events are related. In this context, it is of great interest that, in contrast to wild-type (C57Bl/6 × 129Sv/Ev)F$_2$ mice, IL-12-deficient mice exhibited an early peak of IL-4 mRNA either in the spleens 90 min after intravenous injection of parasites or in lymph nodes 16 h after subcutaneous injection [30]. This demonstrates that (i) in resistant mice, IL-12 down-regulates the early IL-4 response observed in BALB/c mice, and that (ii) early induction of IL-4 in IL-12-deficient mice correlates with subsequent Th2 development. Thus, the rapid IL-4 response indeed may be decisive for Th2 development and the fatal outcome of infection.

The Role of Antigen Dose on T-Helper Subset Development: Comparison of IL-12-Deficient Mice and BALB/c Mice Exposed to Low Number of Parasites

It has been shown earlier that susceptible BALB/c mice resist an infection consisting of a relatively small number of parasites, and that this resistance is associated with the development of stable cell-mediated immunity. Furthermore, these mice aquired resistance to a larger, normally pathogenic rechallenge [65]. Thus *L. major* infection of BALB/c mice can serve as an important in vivo model for vaccination regimens.

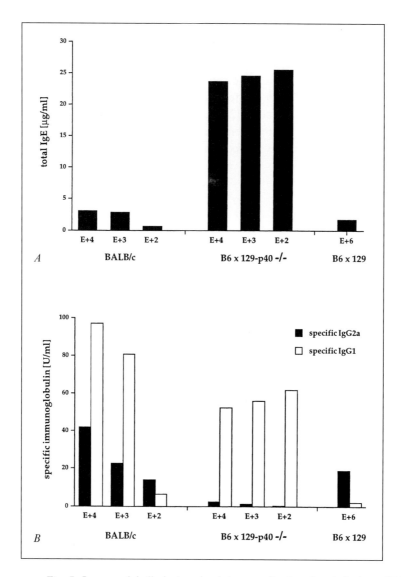

Fig. 7. Immunoglobulin isotype levels in sera after low dose infection of BALB/c and IL-12-deficient mice. Groups of mice as presented in figure 4 were bled at sacrifice and *L. major*-specific immunoglobulin levels of isotype IgE (*A*), IgG1 and IgG2a (*B*) were determined by ELISA.

To compare low dose parasite exposure in susceptible BALB/c mice and genetically resistant mice rendered susceptible by disruption of the IL-12 subunit gene(s), groups of mice were infected with a serial decrease in number of promastigotes (strain LV 39). In keeping with results of Bretscher et al. [65], BALB/c mice infected with a high dose ($>10^5$) of parasites developed large lesions with high parasite load, whereas low dose (10^2) inocula resulted in late appearance of small lesions, which could be resolved (fig. 4A). More than 5 months after infection, the number of viable parasites derived from lymph nodes of these low dose infected BALB/c mice was comparable to resistant mice (F_2: C57Bl/6 × 129) injected with a high dose (fig. 5). Infection of BALB/c mice with intermediate parasite doses (10^3–10^4) showed a 'milder' disease pattern based on parasite burden and a delay of lesion development, which eventually could not be resolved. Concomitant with the decrease of parasite inocula was a gradual reduction of IL-4 and a mutual increase of IFN-γ responses in BALB/c mice. This shift of T-helper subset responses was associated with a shift from a humoral to a cell-mediated immune response, demonstrated by the loss of specific IgG1 and IgE isotypes in low dose infected BALB/c mice (fig. 7). In contrast, IL-12-deficient 129Sv/Ev mice were highly susceptible independent of the number of injected promastigotes. Comparing low dose (100 parasites) infected BALB/c and IL-12-deficient mice, only the latter were found to develop ulcerating lesions (fig. 4B), a 10^5-fold increase in parasite load (fig. 5), and to maintain IL-4 and humoral responses (e.g. IgG1, IgE) at the expense of IFN-γ and associated cellular responses (e.g. IgG2a) (fig. 6, 7).

These results confirmed previously published results by Bretscher et al. [65], which demonstrate that susceptibility and Th2 development can be reversed in BALB/c mice infected with a low dose of *L. major* promastigotes [65]. In a secondary response, low dose pre-exposed mice acquire resistance to a high dose exposure. Resistance is not restricted to either a particular site of infection or to a particular parasite strain [60]. However, to achieve resistance requires severalfold fewer parasites of a high compared to a low virulent strain [60]. This may become important in the discussion of whether IL-4-deficient BALB/c mice are resistant or susceptible to infection. In the case of IL-12-deficient mice, default Th2 development and susceptibility cannot be reversed by low dose exposure to *L. major*. Development of a protective type 1 response is crucially dependent on IL-12.

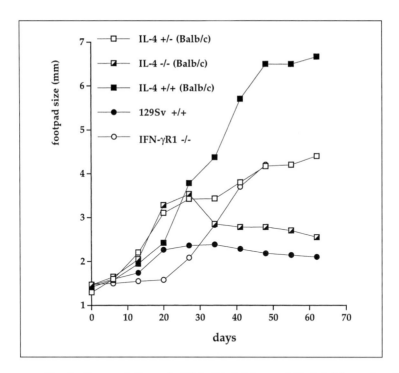

Fig. 8. Course of disease in IFN-γR1-deficient and IL-4-deficient mice. Groups of 5 mice were infected in the left hind footpad with *L. major* promastigotes (MHOM/IL/81/FEBNI). The course of disease was monitored weekly. Infected mice included IL-4$^{-/-}$ (BALB/c), IL-4$^{+/-}$ (BALB/c), IFN-γR1$^{-/-}$ (129Sv), wild-type BALB/c, and wild-type 129Sv mice. IFN-γR1$^{-/-}$ succumbed to infection at weeks 6–8.

The Role of IL-4: Paradigm Lost?

During the last decade, the murine model of cutaneous leishmaniasis has become a paradigm, mainly because of the observation that susceptible BALB/c mice can be cured by distinct immune interventions including sublethal irradiation, low dose infection, depletion of CD4$^+$ T cells, treatment with cyclophosphamide, anti-IL-4, anti-IL-2, CTLA4-Ig, or recombinant IL-12, which all had one immunological effect in common: the attenuation of the IL-4 response [14]. Paradoxically, mice disrupted of the IL-4 gene appear to confront this dogma. Noben-Trauth et al. [66] reported that IL-4-deficient BALB/c mice remain every bit as susceptible as control BALB/c mice. However, by using the same strain of IL-4-deficient mice to study the outcome of infection with *L. major*, we arrived at opposite conclusions. The IL-4-deficient mice contained the infection and did not develop progressive disease [31].

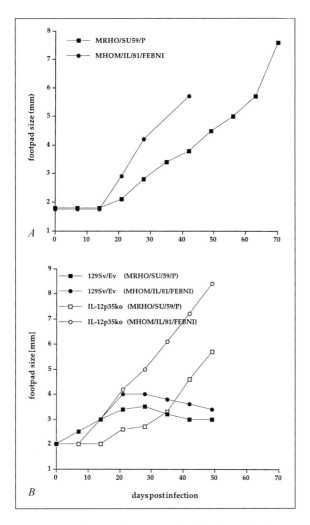

Fig. 9. Disease phenotype after infection with different strains of L. major. Groups of 5 mice were infected in the left hind footpad with 2×10^6 L. major promastigotes of either strain MHOM/IL/81/FEBNI or strain MRHO/SU/59/P (LV 39) as indicated. The course of disease was monitored weekly. Infected mice included wild-type BALB/c (A), IL-12p35$^{-/-}$ (129Sv/Ev), and wild-type 129Sv/Ev mice (B).

Furthermore, as compared to homozygous IL-4 wild-type mice, heterozygous IL-4$^{+/-}$ animals consistently developed smaller lesions with less ulceration and necrosis, indicating the likelihood of gene-dosage effects (fig. 8). This result suggests that the magnitude of the IL-4 response correlates directly with the severity of disease, as suggested earlier by studies comparing different inbred strains covering the range of susceptibility to disease [67]. The conflicting results obtained with IL-4-deficient mice are not easy to reconcile, but might lie in the different parasite strains used. For a direct comparison, BALB/c wild-type, IL-12-deficient 129Sv and IL-4-deficient BALB/c mice were infected with 2×10^6 *L. major* promastigotes derived of strain MRHO/SU/59/P (LV 39) and of strain MHOM/IL/81/FEBNI, which had been used in the published reports of Noben-Trauth et al. [66] and Kopf et al. [31], respectively. Infection of both susceptible BALB/c and IL-12-deficient mice with promastigotes of strain MRHO/SU/59/P compared to MHOM/IL/81/FEBNI showed a delayed kinetic of footpad swelling and ulceration of the lesion suggesting that the latter strain is more virulent (fig. 9A). Infection of IL-4-deficient BALB/c mice with MRHO/SU/59/P promastigotes resulted in a massive swelling reaction, as reported by Noben-Trauth et al. [66] (fig. 10A). However, compared to BALB/c wild-type mice, the IL-4-deficient mice were able to eventually restrict progression. The lesions were not necrotic, although they remained relatively big in size (4–5 mm) and did not resolve during the time observed (5 months). Furthermore, 12 weeks after infection, the enumeration of parasites in draining lymph nodes showed a 1,000-fold reduction in IL-4-deficient BALB/c mice compared to BALB/c wild-type controls (fig. 11A). However, parasite elimination in IL-4-deficient mice was not as efficient as in genetically resistant C57Bl/6 mice with a 10^6-fold reduction compared to BALB/c mice. Infection with a very high dose (2×10^7) of promastigotes resulted in a similar result. Wild-type BALB/c mice had to be euthanized with completely necrotic lesions 7 weeks after infection, while in IL-4-deficient mice, lesions remained in a 'steady state' for several months without necrosis. Moreover, parasite spread appeared to be under control, since the higher dose (2×10^7- versus 2×10^6-fold) did not result in concomitant increase in numbers of parasites recovered from draining lymph nodes of IL-4-deficient mice. In addition to infection of IL-4-deficient BALB/c mice, we infected anti-IL-4 mAb (11B11)-treated wild-type BALB/c mice with promastigotes of strain MRHO/SU/59/P. According to the literature, we expected this treatment to heal infected mice. Surprisingly, in our hands, IL-4 neutralization failed to restrict growth of *L. major* (MRHO/SU/59/P strain). However, lesion development was delayed and slightly impaired as compared to BALB/c mice treated with control mAb. The efficacy of mAb treatment was demonstrated by the finding that Th2 responses including IL-4 and specific IgE production were inhibited (data not shown). While we do not understand why IL-4 neutralization had no effect at all on parasite growth, despite the inhibition of Th2 responses, lesion development was similar to IL-4-deficient mice infected with strain MRHO/SU/59/P. Thus, mice treated with neutralizing antibody do not behave much differently compared to mice disrupted of the IL-4 gene, which

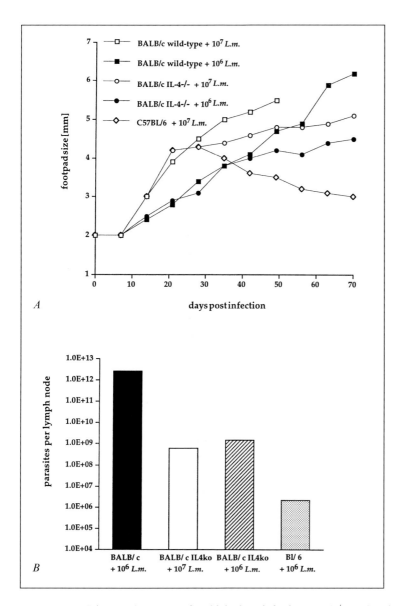

Fig. 10. Disease phenotype after high dose infection. IL-4$^{-/-}$ (BALB/c), wild-type BALB/c, and C57Bl/6 mice were infected with the indicated numbers of *L. major* promastigotes (strain MRHO/SU/59/P). Disease progression is depicted as mean lesion size for each group (*A*). The parasite load in draining lymph nodes was determined 10 weeks after infection (*B*) and is given as a mean value for each group.

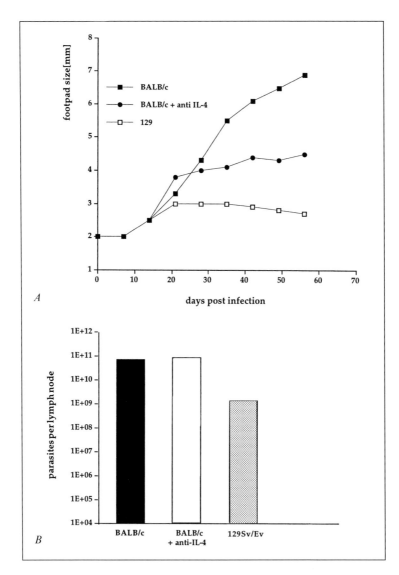

Fig. 11. Disease phenotype in BALB/c mice after treatment with anti-IL-4 mAb. BALB/c and 129Sv/Ev mice were infected with 10^6 *L. major* promastigotes (strain MRHO/SU/59/P). Designated group of BALB/c mice was treated with 5 mg anti-IL-4 mAb (11B11) at day 0. Disease progression is depicted as mean lesion size for each group (*A*). The parasite load in draining lymph nodes was determined 8 weeks after infection (*B*) and is given as a mean value for each group.

have been suggested to display an IL-4 redundant activity not seen in wild-type mice [66]. Our results obtained with IL-4-deficient mice infected with strain MRHO/SU/59/P are almost identical with results published by Noben-Trauth et al. [66]. However, we do disagree with their suggestion that IL-4-deficient mice remain susceptible. The absence of IL-4 eventually limits fatal cutaneous leishmaniasis independent of the parasite strain used for infection. IL-4-deficient mice can be kept for more than 6 months without visible necrosis of the lesion. Indeed, the other investigators show that both parasitemia and lesion size were already declining in IL-4-deficient BALB/c mice, while they were still progressing in BALB/c wild-type controls at a later time-point (7 weeks) after infection, when the experiment was terminated [66]. It remains to be determined by what mechanism particular parasite strains can regulate lesion development independent of an IL-4 response.

Together, our results strongly indicate that *L. major*-infected IL-4-deficient mice: (i) can control disease exacerbation independent of the parasite strain; (ii) may develop quite massive lesions dependent on the parasite strain, and (iii) are not as efficient in parasite control as a 'resistant' strain. Indeed, this implies that IL-4 is not the only factor determining susceptibility in BALB/c mice. However, the presence of IL-4 clearly tips the balance toward being worse. Previous studies by others already suggested that genetic traits which allow cure of an *L. major* infection can direct disease outcome from both T-cell and non-T-cell compartments, and that the presence of the curing genotype in only one compartment is sufficient to confer cure [68]. The detrimental trait in the T-cell compartment of BALB/c mice is an overwhelming IL-4 response.

Acknowledgement

We thank our colleagues M. Gately, F. Brombacher, W. Solbach for instrumental support and K. Di Padova, K. Lefrang, K.H. Widmann for excellent technical assistance.

References

1   Abbas AK, Murphy KM, Sher A: Functional diversity of helper T lymphocytes. Nature 1997;383: 787–793.
2   Seder RA, Paul WE: Acquisition of lymphokine-producing phenotype by CD4+ T cells. Annu Rev Immunol 1994;12:635–673.
3   Mosmann TR, Schumacher JH, Street NF, Budd R, O'Garra A, Fong TA, Bond MW, Moore KW, Sher A, Fiorentino DF: Diversity of cytokine synthesis and function of mouse CD4+ T cells. Immunol Rev 1991;123:209–229.
4   Kaplan MH, Sun YL, Hoey T, Grusby MJ: Impaired IL-12 responses and enhanced development of Th2 cells in Stat4-deficient mice. Nature 1996;382:174–177.

5   Thierfelder WE, van Deursen JM, Yamamoto K, Tripp RA, Sarawar SR, Carson RT, Sangster MY, Vignali DA, Doherty PC, Grosveld GC, Ihle JN: Requirement for Stat4 in interleukin-12-mediated responses of natural killer and T cells. Nature 1996;382:171–174.

6   Kopf M, Le Gros G, Bachmann M, Lamers MC, Bluethmann H, Köhler G: Disruption of the murine IL-4 gene blocks Th2 cytokine responses. Nature 1993;362:245–248.

7   Kaplan MH, Schindler U, Smiley ST, Grusby MJ: Stat6 is required for mediating responses to IL-4 and for development of Th2 cells. Immunity 1996;4:313–319.

8   Shimoda K, van Deursen J, Sangster MY, Sarawar SR, Carson RT, Tripp RA, Chu C, Quelle FW, Nosaka T, Vignali DA, Doherty PC, Grosveld G: Lack of IL-4-induced Th2 response and IgE class switching in mice with disrupted Stat6 gene. Nature 1996;380:630–633.

9   Takeda K, Tanaka T, Shi W, Matsumoto M, Minami M, Kashiwamura S, Nakanishi K, Yoshida N, Kishimoto T, Akira S: Essential role of Stat6 in IL-4 signalling. Nature 1996;380:627–630.

10 Hsieh CS, Macatonia SE, Tripp CS, Wolf SF, O'Garra A, Murphy KM: Development of TH1 CD4+ T cells through IL-12 produced by Listeria-induced macrophages (see comments). Science 1993;260:547–549.

11 Tripp CS, Wolf SF, Unanue ER: Interleukin-12 and tumor necrosis factor alpha are costimulators of interferon gamma production by natural killer cells in severe combined immunodeficiency mice with listeriosis, and interleukin-10 is a physiologic antagonist. Proc Natl Acad Sci USA 1993;90: 3725–3729.

12 Gazzinelli RT, Wysocka M, Hayashi S, Denkers EY, Hieny S, Caspar P, Trinchieri G, Sher A: Parasite-induced IL-12 stimulates early IFN-gamma synthesis and resistance during acute infection with *Toxoplasma gondii*. J Immunol 1994;153:2533–2543.

13 Cooper AM, Roberts AD, Rhoades ER, Callahan JE, Getzy DM, Orme IM: The role of interleukin-12 in acquired immunity to *Mycobacterium tuberculosis* infection. Immunology 1995;84:423–432.

14 Reiner SL, Locksley RM: The regulation of immunity to *Leishmania major*. Annu Rev Immunol 1995;13:151–177.

15 Titus RG, Ceredig R, Cerottini JC, Louis JA: Therapeutic effect of anti-L3T4 monoclonal antibody GK1.5 on cutaneous leishmaniasis in genetically-susceptible BALB/c mice. J Immunol 1985;135: 2108–2114

16 Sadick MD, Heinzel FP, Shigekane VM, Fisher WL, Locksley RM: Cellular and humoral immunity to *Leishmania major* in genetically susceptible mice after in vivo depletion of L3T4+ cells. J Immunol 1987;139:1303–1309.

17 Heinzel FP, Sadick MD, Holaday BJ, Coffman RL, Locksley RM: Reciprocal expression of interferon gamma or interleukin-4 during the resolution or progression of murine leishmaniasis. Evidence for expansion of distinct helper T cell subsets. J Exp Med 1989;169:59–72.

18 Locksley RM, Reiner SL, Hatam F, Littman DR, Killeen N: Helper T cells without CD4: Control of leishmaniasis in CD4-deficient mice. Science 1993;261:1448–1451.

19 Wang ZE, Reiner SL, Hatam F, Heinzel FP, Bouvier J, Turck CW, Locksley RM: Targeted activation of CD8 cells and infection of beta-2-microglobulin-deficient mice fail to confirm a primary protective role for CD8 cells in experimental leishmaniasis. J Immunol 1993;151:2077–2086.

20 Heinzel FP, Sadick MD, Mutha SS, Locksley RM: Production of interferon gamma, interleukin-2, interleukin-4, and interleukin-10 by CD4+ lymphocytes in vivo during healing and progressive murine leishmaniasis. Proc Natl Acad Sci USA 1991;88:7011–7015.

21 Sadick MD, Heinzel FP, Holaday BJ, Pu RT, Dawkins RS, Locksley RM: Cure of murine leishmaniasis with anti-interleukin-4 monoclonal antibody. Evidence for a T cell-dependent, interferon gamma-independent mechanism. J Exp Med 1990;171:115–127.

22 Sadick MD, Street N, Mosmann TR, Locksley RM: Cytokine regulation of murine leishmaniasis: Interleukin-4 is not sufficient to mediate progressive disease in resistant C57BL/6 mice. Infect Immun 1991;59:4710–4714.

23 Chatelain R, Varkila K, Coffman RL: IL-4 induces a Th2 response in *Leishmania major*-infected mice. J Immunol 1992;148:1182–1187.

24 Belosevic M, Finbloom DS, Van Der Meide PH, Slayter MV, Nacy CA: Administration of mono-clonal anti-IFN-gamma antibodies in vivo abrogates natural resistance of C3H/HeN mice to infection with *Leishmania major*. J Immunol 1989;143:266–274.

25   Wang ZE, Reiner SL, Zheng S, Dalton DK, Locksley RM: CD4+ effector cells default to the Th2 pathway in interferon gamma-deficient mice infected with *Leishmania major*. J Exp Med 1994;179: 1367–1371.

26   Swihart K, Fruth U, Messmer N, Hug K, Behin R, Huang S, Del-Giudice G, Aguet M, Louis JA: Mice from a genetically resistant background lacking the interferon gamma receptor are susceptible to infection with *Leishmania major* but mount a polarized T helper cell 1-type CD4+ T cell response. J Exp Med 1995;181:961–971.

27   Sypek JP, Chung CL, Mayor SE, Subramanyam JM, Goldman SJ, Sieburth DS, Wolf SF, Schaub RG: Resolution of cutaneous leishmaniasis: Interleukin-12 initiates a protective T helper type 1 immune response. J Exp Med 1993;177:1797–1802.

28   Heinzel FP, Schoenhaut DS, Rerko RM, Rosser LE, Gately MK: Recombinant interleukin-12 cures mice infected with *Leishmania major*. J Exp Med 1993;177:1505–1509.

29   Scharton Kersten T, Afonso LC, Wysocka M, Trinchieri G, Scott P: IL-12 is required for natural killer cell activation and subsequent T helper 1 cell development in experimental leishmaniasis. J Immunol 1995;154:5320–5330.

30   Mattner F, Magram J, Ferrante J, Launois P, Di Padova K, Behin R, Gately MK, Louis JA, Alber G: Genetically resistant mice lacking interleukin-12 are susceptible to infection with *Leishmania major* and mount a polarized Th2 cell response. Eur J Immunol 1996;26:1553–1559.

31   Kopf M, Brombacher F, Kohler G, Kienzle G, Widmann KH, Lefrang K, Humborg C, Ledermann B, Solbach W: IL-4-deficient Balb/c mice resist infection with *Leishmania major*. J Exp Med 1996; 184:1127–1136.

32   Carrera L, Gazinelli RT, Badolato R, Hieny S, Muller W, Kuhn R, Sacks DL: *Leishmania* promastigotes selectively inhibit interleukin-12 induction in bone marrow-derived macrophages from susceptible and resistant mice. J Exp Med 1996;183:515–526.

33   Reiner SL, Zheng S, Wang ZE, Stowring L, Locksley RM: Leishmania promastigotes evade interleukin-12 induction by macrophages and stimulate a broad range of cytokines from CD4+ cells during initiation of infection. J Exp Med 1994;179:447–456.

34   Launois P, Ohteki T, Swihart K, MacDonald HR, Louis JA: In susceptible mice, *Leishmania major* induce very rapid interleukin-4 production by CD4+ T cells which are NK1.1-. Eur J Immunol 1995;25:3298–3307.

35   Szabo SJ, Dighe AS, Gubler U, Murphy KM: Regulation of the interleukin-12R β2 subunit expression in developing T helper 1 (Th1) and Th2 cells. J Exp Med 1997;185:817–824.

36   Guler ML, Gorham JD, Hsieh C-S, Mackey AJ, Steen RG, Dietrich WF, Murphy KM: Genetic susceptibility to Leishmania: IL-12 responsiveness in Th1 cell development. Science 1996;271:984–987.

37   Skeiky YA, Guderian JA, Benson DR, Bacelar O, Carvalho EM, Kubin M, Badaro R, Trinchieri G, Reed SG: A recombinant Leishmania antigen that stimulates human peripheral blood mononuclear cells to express a Th1-type cytokine profile and to produce interleukin-12. J Exp Med 1995; 181:1527–1537.

38   Gazzinelli RT, Wysocka M, Hieny S, Scharton Kersten T, Cheever A, Kuhn R, Muller W, Trinchieri G, Sher A: In the absence of endogenous IL-10, mice acutely infected with *Toxoplasma gondii* succumb to a lethal immune response dependent on CD4+ T cells and accompanied by overproduction of IL-12, IFN-gamma and TNF-alpha. J Immunol 1996;157:798–805.

39   Dai WJ, Kohler G, Brombacher F: Both innate and acquired immunity to *Listeria monocytogenes* infection are increased in IL-10-deficient mice. J Immunol 1997;158:2259–2267.

40   Bretscher P, Cohn-M: A theory of self-nonself discrimination. Science 1970;169:1042.

41   Lafferty KJ, Prowse SJ, Simeonovic CJ: Immunobiology of tissue transplantation: A return to the passenger leukocyte concept. Annu Rev Immunol 1983;1:143–173.

42   Jenkins MK: The ups and downs of T cell costimulation. Immunity 1994;1:443–446.

43   Bluestone J: New perspectives of CD28-B7 mediated T cell costimulation. Immunity 1995;2:555–559.

44   Banchereau J, Bazan F, Blanchard D, Briere F, Galizzi JP, van-Kooten C, Liu YJ, Rousset F, Saeland S: The CD40 antigen and its ligand. Annu Rev Immunol 1994;12:881–922.

45   Kawabe T, Naka T, Yoshida K, Tanaka T, Fujiwara H, Suematsu S, Yoshida N, Kishimoto T, Kikutani H: The immune responses in CD40-deficient mice: Impaired immunoglobulin class switching and germinal center formation. Immunity 1994;1:167–178.

46   Castigli E, Alt FW, Davidson L, Bottaro A, Mizoguchi E, Bhan AK, Geha RS: CD40-deficient mice generated by recombination-activating gene-2-deficient blastocyst complementation. Proc Natl Acad Sci USA 1994;91:12135–12139.
47   Renshaw BR, Fanslow WR, Armitage RJ, Campbell KA, Liggitt D, Wright B, Davison BL, Maliszewski CR: Humoral immune responses in CD40 ligand-deficient mice. J Exp Med 1994;180: 1889–1900.
48   Xu J, Foy TM, Laman JD, Elliott EA, Dunn JJ, Waldschmidt TJ, Elsemore J, Noelle RJ, Flavell RA: Mice deficient for the CD40 ligand. Immunity 1994;1:423–431.
49   Grewal IS, Flavell RA: A central role of CD40 ligand in the regulation of CD4+ T cell responses. Immunol Today 1996;17:410–414.
50   Campbell KA, Ovendale PJ, Kennedy MK, Fanslow WC, Reed SG, Maliszewski CR: CD40 ligand is required for protective cell-mediated immunity to Leishmania major. Immunity 1996;4: 283–289.
51   Kamanaka M, Yu P, Yasui T, Yoshida K, Kawabe T, Horii T, Kishimoto T, Kikutani H: Protective role of CD40 in Leishmania major infection at two distinct phases of cell-mediated immunity. Immunity 1996;4:275–281.
52   Soong L, Xu JC, Grewal IS, Kima P, Sun J, Longley B Jr, Ruddle NH, McMahon-Pratt D, Flavell RA: Disruption of CD40-CD40 ligand interactions results in an enhanced susceptibility to Leishmania amazonensis infection. Immunity 1996;4:263–273.
53   Kuchroo VK, Das MP, Brown JA, Ranger AM, Zamvil SS, Sobel RA, Weiner HL, Nabavi N, Glimcher LH: B7-1 and B7-2 costimulatory molecules activate differentially the Th1/Th2 developmental pathways: Application to autoimmune disease therapy. Cell 1995;80:707–718.
54   Tivol EA, Borriello F, Schweitzer AN, Lynch WP, Bluestone JA, Sharpe AH: Loss of CTLA-4 leads to massive lymphoproliferation and fatal multiorgan tissue destruction revealing a critical negative regulatory role of CTLA-4. Immunity 1995;3:541–547.
55   Waterhouse P, Penninger JM, Timms E, Wakeham A, Shahinian A, Lee KP, Thompson CB, Griesser H, Mak TW: Lymphoproliferative disorders with early lethality in mice deficient in Ctla-4. Science 1995;270:985–988.
56   Brown DR, Green JM, Moskowitz NH, Davis M, Thompson CB, Reiner SL: Limited role of CD28-mediated signals in T helper subset differentiation. J Exp Med 1996;184:803–810.
57   Schorle H, Holtschke T, Hunig T, Schimpl A, Horak I: Development and function of T cells in mice rendered interleukin-2 deficient by gene targeting. Nature 1991;352:621–624.
58   Kundig TM, Schorle H, Bachmann MF, Hengartner H, Zinkernagel RM, Horak I: Immune responses in interleukin-2-deficient mice. Science 1993;262:1059–1061.
59   Morris L, Troutt AB, Handman E, Kelso A: Changes in the precursor frequencies of IL-4 and IFN-gamma secreting CD4+ cells correlate with resolution of lesions in murine cutaneous leishmaniasis. J Immunol 1992;149:2715–2721.
60   Menon JN, Bretscher PA: Characterization of the immunological memory state generated in mice susceptible to Leishmania major following exposure to low doses of L. major and resulting in resistance to a normally pathogenic challenge. Eur J Immunol 1996;26:243–249.
61   Kamogawa Y, Minasi LA, Carding SR, Bottomly K, Flavell RA: The relationship of IL-4- and IFN gamma-producing T cells studied by lineage ablation of IL-4-producing cells. Cell 1993;75: 985–995.
62   Seder RA, Paul WE, Davis MM, Fazekas de St Groth B: The presence of interleukin-4 during in vitro priming determines the lymphokine-producing potential of CD4+ T cells from T cell receptor transgenic mice. J Exp Med 1992;176:1091–1098.
63   Hsieh CS, Heimberger AB, Gold JS, O'Garra A, Murphy KM: Differential regulation of T helper phenotype development by interleukins 4 and 10 in an alpha beta T-cell-receptor transgenic system. Proc Natl Acad Sci USA 1992;89:6065–6069.
64   Pernis A, Gupta S, Gollob KJ, Garfein E, Coffman RL, Schindler C, Rothman P: Lack of interferon-γ receptor β chain and the prevention of interferon-γ signaling in Th1 cells. Science 1995;269: 245–247.
65   Bretscher PA, Wei G, Menon JN, Bielefeldt-Ohmann H: Establishment of stable, cell-mediated immunity that makes 'susceptible' mice resistant to Leishmania major. Science 1992;257:539–542.

66   Noben-Trauth N, Kropf P, Muller I: Susceptibility to *Leishmania major* infection in interleukin-4-deficient mice. Science 1996;271:987-990.
67   Morris L, Troutt AB, McLeod KS, Kelso A, Handman E, Aebischer T: Interleukin-4 but not gamma interferon production correlates with the severity of murine cutaneous leishmaniasis. Infect Immun 1993;61:3459-3465.
68   Shankar AH, Titus RG: T cell and non-T cell compartments can independently determine resistance to *Leishmania major*. J Exp Med 1995;181:845-855.

Manfred Kopf, Basel Institute for Immunology, Grenzacherstrasse 487, Postfach,
CH-4005 Basel (Switzerland)
E-mail: KOPF@BII.CH

Adorini L (ed): IL-12. Chem Immunol. Basel, Karger, 1997, vol 68, pp 110–135

....

Initiation of T-Helper Cell Immunity to *Candida albicans* by IL-12: The Role of Neutrophils

Luigina Romani [a], *Francesco Bistoni* [a], *Paolo Puccetti* [b]

Departments of Experimental Medicine and Biochemical Sciences,
[a] University of Perugia and
[b] University of Rome 'Tor Vergata', Italy

Fungal infections in humans can range in severity from easily treated superficial infections of the skin and mucosa to asymptomatic pulmonary infections to difficult-to-treat life-threatening disseminated infections, which involve multiple organ systems. Opportunistic mycoses, such as those typically caused by fungal species that are normally harmless to the immunocompetent host (i.e. *Candida, Aspergillus, Fusarium* and *Trichosporon* species, also Zygomycetes and *Cryptococcus neoformans*), occur in highly immunosuppressed cancer patients or immunologically debilitated individuals, such as transplant recipients and patients with AIDS. In this latter group of patients, *Histoplasma capsulatum* and *Coccidioides immitis* have also emerged as major opportunistic fungal pathogens.

Although much progress has been made toward developing effective yet nontoxic antifungal therapies, the goal of finding an ideal agent for systemic fungal infections is far from being achieved, and the morbidity and mortality rates associated with infections by opportunistic fungi remain high. An increased understanding of the immune defense to fungal infections may be instrumental in the development of rational approaches to immunotherapy of opportunistic mycoses, particularly in neutropenic and AIDS patients. These two types of immunocompromised individuals epitomize the two major conditions that predispose to systemic and superficial infections, respectively, the defect in antifungal effector function and the defect in T-cell directive immunity [1, 2].

Within a conceptual framework provided by the Th1/Th2 paradigm of acquired immunity in *Candida albicans* infection in mice, we have previously proposed a unifying view of phagocyte-dependent immunity to *Candida*. In this model, Th1 and Th2 cells are thought to provide critical cytokine-mediated activation and deactivation signals to fungicidal phagocytes, i.e. neutrophils and tissue macrophages [3, 4]. The relative importance of directive Th1/Th2 cells and of effector granulocytes/macrophages to the outcome of experimental challenge depends on numerous factors, including localization [5, 6] and virulence [7–10] of the primary infection, early cytokine response of the host to the yeast [11–16], and predominant type of Th cells activated by challenge, namely host-protective Th1 or disease-promoting Th2 cells [17–19]. The qualitative pattern of cytokines secreted by T cells will ultimately determine the efficacy of the effector response mediated by phagocytes [20–25].

As we expand on this hypothesis, we now review recent evidence supporting reciprocal influences between T cells and phagocytes in candidal infections, with a major focus on the role of IL-12 and IL-10 production by polymorphonuclear phagocytes for development of directive Th cell immunity. IL-12/IFN-γ on one side and IL-4/IL-10 on the other appear, in fact, to be the major cytokines governing Th cell development to *Candida* [26–28]. The possible therapeutic implications of these findings for immunotherapy of fungal infections are discussed.

Biological Significance of Th Cell Dichotomy to *Candida*

As the complex nature of the cytokine response to *Candida* has recently been reviewed in detail [29], we will consider here only those cytokines that may serve immunoregulatory or effector roles in Th cell-dependent immunity to the yeast. In attempting to accommodate the complexity of the spectrum of *Candida* diseases in humans with the deterministic and apparently reductionist approach provided by the Th1/Th2 paradigm in experimental animals, several points need to be considered. First, the highly polarized cytokine responses that are induced by injection of large yeast inocula into inbred mice with widely different degrees of susceptibility undoubtedly reflect the extreme conditions of testing. Yet, they may provide a unitary basis for explaining the yeast commensualistic relationship with humans and its ability to dynamically modulate the host's response so as to favor its own persistence, and may also clarify several aspects of the mechanisms of fungal pathogenicity and immunopathology. When environmental conditions are favorable, and/or within the context of a particular genetic background, the saprophytic carriage of the yeast can lead to symptomatic local infection, but may also trigger local or systemic immunopathology in the absence of overt infection. A pathogenic role of *Candida*-specific Th2-type responses may be operative in asthma [30], recurrent vaginitis [31, 32], atopic dermatitis [33, 34], and immunopathology associated with several disease states [35], including some of the unusual skin disorders that are by contrast common in AIDS [3]. Evidence in vitro for a possible association between predominance of Th2 rather than Th1 responses to *Candida* has recently been obtained in patients with chronic mucocutaneous candidiasis, suggesting that the manifestations seen in these patients (i.e. impairment of cell-mediated immunity, high levels of *Candida*-specific antibodies, and susceptibility to certain types of bacterial infections) could be the consequence of imbalanced cytokine production and regulation [36, 37].

Second, human studies have identified several effector mechanisms that result in *Candida* killing. Yet, no convincing link has been established so far between a particular clinical condition and any specific effector mechanism [29], despite the long-recognized associations between systemic candidiasis and neutrophil deficiency and between chronic mucosal infections and abnormalities in the cell-mediated response [38]. The concept of a reciprocal regulation between the phagocyte system and the T-cell compartment may provide a unifying thread between the systemic immune response and events occurring at the mucosal surface. As observed previously [4, 29], this notion emphasizes that the anticandidal responses that have been characterized in systemic and mucosal infections are not unique to either condition.

Finally, as in other experimental models of parasitic and retroviral infections [39–41], whatever is learned about the consequences of *Candida* infection for anti-infectious resistance, immunopathology, or coinfection can be used as a useful theoretical framework in the analysis of the general pathways of immunoregulation.

Th Cell Control Over Phagocyte Function: Induction of Antifungal Activity

Underlying immunity to *C. albicans* is usually present in adult immunocompetent individuals as a result of lifelong commensalism initiated at birth by yeast colonization of the host gastrointestinal mucosa [38]. This commensualistic relationship with humans, and a variety of virulence factors [42, 43], enable the yeast to multiply and replace much of the normal flora when environmental conditions are favorable. Localized disease, such as oral candidiasis [44] and vaginitis [45], may develop. Decreased neutrophil function, combined with the breakdown of anatomic defenses, may permit an endogenous focus of superficial colonization/infection to initiate a systemic disease [46, 47]. Due to their action on circulating leukocytes, the cytokines produced by *Candida*-specific T cells may be instrumental in mobilizing and activating anticandidal effectors. Interfacial and hence continuously critical in the mucosal association between the yeast and its host, the role of T cells will become operative in systemic infections when recruitment of antigen-specific lymphocytes and locally high cytokine concentrations are required for full expression of the anticandidal potential of phagocytes [4, 29].

Early studies in vitro indicating IFN-γ as a major activating factor for fungicidal phagocytes [48–51] have been confirmed by recent in vivo data [52]. In mice with protective Th1 responses induced by systemic inoculation of a *C. albicans* live vaccine strain (LVS), IFN-γ is the major effector cytokine released by specific CD4[+] and CD8[+] cells [18–22]. Analysis of cytokine gene expression in peripheral blood mononuclear cells from healthy humans stimulated in vitro with *Candida* antigens has revealed appreciable levels of IFN-γ mRNA [53]. The heightened candidacidal activity induced by IFN-γ in phagocytes involves both oxidative and nonoxidative pathways, the former relying on production of oxygen [50, 51] and nitrogen [24, 25] intermediates. Besides this effector function, the role of IFN-γ in experimental candidiasis encompasses early regulatory effects on Th cell differentiation leading to onset of protective immunity [10, 11], as will be discussed later. Overproduction of IFN-γ, however, may be involved in the acute pathology of fungal septic shock [4, 28].

Th Cell Control Over Phagocyte Function: Suppression of Antifungal Activity

The down-regulation of a strong, potentially immunopathological Th1 response could be beneficial to the host [55, 56], and this may have a role in limiting the gastrointestinal damage caused by *Candida* colonization and subsequent inflammatory stimuli in mice with intragastric challenge [6, 28]. However, it is likely as a result of an evasive strategy that the yeast has evolved mechanisms to down-modulate effector Th1 responses that can resolve an acute infection. Depending on environmental conditions, the immunomodulatory properties of the yeast may permit the maintenance of a commensualistic relationship with its host, but may also result in chronicity or exacerbation of infection.

Candida antigens can inhibit cell-mediated (or phagocyte-dependent) immunity [57, 58], and Th2 responses predominate in mice with ultimately fatal infections (i.e. genetically susceptible animals with LVS infection or mice with virulent yeast challenge) [3, 4]. As in leishmaniasis and other parasitic infections where Th2 cells serve a disease-promoting role [59–61], IL-4 and IL-10 are the major effector cytokines that oppose IFN-γ-mediated responses at the macrophage level, by suppressing cytotoxic mechanisms [13, 24, 25]. In addition, uptake of *Candida* yeast forms by macrophages is mediated by the mannose receptor, an event that can lead to phagocyte abuse if not accompanied by the coordinate activation of the cell cytotoxic machinery [62]. Increased expression of the receptor with no induced cytotoxicity could be a primary effect of macrophage exposure to IL-4 [63]. In contrast, IFN-γ down-regulates the expression of macrophage mannose receptors, yet results in effective killing, presumably via increased coupling of the receptor to the production of candidacidal molecules [49]. Both IL-4 and IL-10 are strong inhibitors of the induction of nitric oxide synthase in macrophages [64], and their activity may be potentiated by TGF-β in mice with lethal candidiasis [16].

Regulation of Phagocyte-Dependent Immunity to *Candida* in Humans

Therefore, in mixed Th1/Th2 such as those typically occurring in mucosal colonization of mice [6, 65–67] and presumably humans [53, 68], phagocyte-dependent resistance to *Candida* is regulated, at the effector level, by two sets of opposing cytokines, IFN-γ and IL-4/IL-10. In systemic infection of mice with virulent challenge ('nonhealer' mice), IL-4 responses clearly outweigh Th1 reactivity, whereas in genetically resistant mice with LVS infection ('healer' mice) the Th2 cytokines, IL-4 and IL-10, are not detected. While it is clear that these healer and nonhealer combinations display the appropriate Th1 and Th2 cytokine profiles [for review, see 4], a pivotal question is how these responses become established in primary colonization/infection, whether they are stable, and how these findings relate to the human conditon.

The basic models with healer and nonhealer yeast/host combinations may not be sufficiently informative per se for a general understanding of the complex regulation of Th cell-dependent immunity to *Candida* in human health and disease. As mentioned above, a true 'primary' infection in humans occurs only in the early neonate and, in adult life, *Candida* diseases will develop in the face of initial/underlying specific Th1-type reactivity [53]. Apart from the obvious increase in *Candida* infectivity caused by immunsuppressive or antibacterial therapy, neutropenia, or breakdown of anatomic defenses, it is possible that several factors related to the host (e.g. altered cytokine balance in disease states, coinfection, immunomodulatory therapy, etc.) or to the yeast (e.g. antigens, fungal load, localization of infection, etc.) may alter with time the stability or predominance of the Th1 cell response under specific conditions

Table 1. Manipulations known to modify the biologic response to *Candida* in healing and nonhealing infection models

Type of infection	Superimposed condition[1]
Primary systemic LVS infection (healing)	Serologic ablation of CD4, CD8, NK cells Granulocyte depletion ± exogenous IL-12 Neutralization of endogenous IFN-γ, IL-12, TGF-β Genetic deficiency of IL-6 production ± exogenous IL-6 or anti-IL-10 Administration of exogenous IL-4, IL-10, IL-12, TGF-β Administration of inhibitors of nitric oxide production Streptozotocin-induced diabetes
Primary systemic challenge with virulent yeast (nonhealing)	Serologic ablation of granulocytes Administration of exogenous CSF-1, IL-4, IL-10, IL-12, TGF-β Neutralization of endogenous IL-4 or TGF-β Superantigen-induced anergy in Vβ8 cells
Primary systemic LVS infection in genetically susceptible mice (nonhealing)	Neutralization of endogenous IL-10 Administration of exogenous IL-4, IL-10, IL-12
Primary intragastric challenge (healing)	Neutralization of endogenous IL-4 Administration of exogenous IL-4, IL-10, IL-12 Administration of cholera toxin
Secondary virulent challenge after LVS immunization (healing)	Serologic ablation of CD4/CD8 cells, IFN-γ, neutrophils Administration of exogenous IL-4 or IL-10

[1] Work referenced in text. Also reviewed in 3, 4, 28.

(e.g. immune abnormalities, AIDS). Such an effect would be reciprocal to that outlined above of a possible impact of *Candida* carriage/infection on concomitant pathology, and would support the occurrence of bidirectional influences between reactivity to the yeast and different disease states.

The following discussion will deal with the issue of selective Th cell differentiation to *Candida* in naive (healer or nonhealer) hosts and with the effect of superimposed conditions (table 1), such as an imbalanced production of endogenous cytokines, $CD4^+$ cell depletion, neutropenia, or exogenous cytokine administration, that might either modulate the expression or change the qualitative nature of the T-cell response to the yeast.

Selective Th1 Differentiation to *Candida*: Role of Endogenous IL-12

The mechanisms responsible in mice for the preferential expansion of *Candida*-reactive Th1 cells are now beginning to be clarified. In terms of cytokine regulatory activity and contribution to a systemic response, Th1 differentiation in vivo requires that two conditions at least be satisfied: (i) the relative absence of IL-4/IL-10 production, which is per se necessary [12, 13] and sufficient [25] to drive the Th2 polarization, and (ii) the combined effects of different cytokines acting on several cell types, including IFN-γ [10, 11], IL-12 [69, 70], TGF-β [16], and IL-6 [71]. Although deficient IFN-γ [69], TGF-β [16], and IL-6 [71] responses may each block the induction of protective immunity, none of these cytokine is as correlative of Th1 development as is IL-12 [70]. This puts a major focus on IL-12 in studies of CD4$^+$ subset differentiation to *Candida*.

We have monitored message levels of IL-12 in splenic macrophages and of IFN-γ, IL-4, and IL-10 in CD4$^+$ and CD8$^+$ cells using healer and nonhealer yeast/host combinations [69]. Two major qualitative differences in cytokine gene expression between healer and nonhealer mice were that IL-4 mRNA was uniquely expressed by CD4$^+$ cells from nonhealer animals and that IL-12 transcripts were persistently expressed by macrophages from healer but not nonhealer mice. Cytokine levels were measured in sera, and antigen-driven cytokine production by CD4$^+$ and CD8$^+$ cells was assessed in vitro, while IFN-γ-producing cells were enumerated in CD4$^-$ and CD8$^-$ cell fractions. These results showed that: (i) antigen-specific secretion of IFN-γ protein in vitro by CD4$^+$ cells occurred only in the healing infection; (ii) IL-4- and IL-10-producing CD4$^+$ cells expanded in nonhealer mice in the face of high levels of circulating IFN-γ, likely released by CD4$^-$ CD8$^-$ lymphocytes, including γδ T cells [3]: high endogenous levels of IFN-γ are not sufficient per se to inhibit Th2 development in candidiasis; (iii) a finely regulated IFN-γ production correlated in the healer mice with IL-12 mRNA detection, and IL-12 was required in vitro for yeast-induced development of IFN-γ-producing CD4$^+$ cells.

Combined with the finding that IL-12 also serves an obligatory role in *Candida*-driven Th1 differentiation in vivo [70], these observations allow a number of points to be made regarding the relationship between IFN-γ and IL-12 in the induction of a Th1 response to *Candida*. The occurrence of early and sustained levels of IFN-γ in *Candida*-driven Th2 development makes it unlikely that IL-12 plays only an indirect role in Th1 differentiation, by providing, soon after infection, the IFN-γ acting as an essential requirement for CD4$^+$ cell priming for IFN-γ production. This is consistent with the finding that serologic ablation of NK cells does not impair Th1 development [72] and with the detection of higher IFN-γ levels in early sera from nonhealer than healer mice [69].

The relative roles of IL-12 and autocrine IFN-γ in enhancing CD4$^+$ cell priming are not fully understood [73–76], and there is also considerable debate as to whether IFN-γ is required for the initial production of IL-12 [77]. Our in vivo data based on serologic ablation of either cytokine suggest that, irrespective of whether high or low levels of IFN-γ are present early in infection, it is the availability of IL-12 at the level of the antigen recognition triad (accessory cells, antigen, CD4$^+$ cells) that allows the latter cells to utilize IFN-γ, initiate their own production of IFN-γ, and differentiate into Th1 cells.

Altogether, it would appear that IL-12 is necessary for the development of a Th1 response in vivo to *Candida*, yet many questions remain to be answered. These include: (i) What cytokines negatively regulate the response? (ii) Can they revert an established and predominant Th1 phenotype in vivo? (iii) What is the major cellular source of endogenous IL-12 in systemic infection with a *C. albicans* LVS that results in protective immunity? (iv) Is exogenous IL-12 sufficient for initiating a Th1 response? These questions will be addressed in the following sections.

What Cytokines Negatively Regulate the Response?

To ascertain whether susceptibility to candidal infection may be linked to a dominant and suppressive Th2 response, IL-4 antagonists (i.e. neutralizing antibody or the soluble IL-4 receptor) or antibody to IL-10 were administered to genetically resistant or susceptible mice challenged with wild-type or LVSs of *C. albicans*, respectively. Mice infected with virulent yeast and receiving anti-IL-4 therapy at the time of infection were cured [12, 14], as were susceptible mice treated with anti-IL-10 at the time of LVS challenge [13]. In both yeast/host combinations, cure was associated with the onset of durable anticandidal protection, and higher frequencies of IFN-γ-secreting cells were found in splenic CD4$^+$ cells, that expressed lower levels of Th2 cytokine transcripts. Cure was also associated with histologic evidence of disease resolution, effective clearance of yeast cells from infected organs, onset of *Candida*-specific delayed-type hypersensitivity, suppression of the IgE response, and increased Th1-dependent B-cell isotype expression. In both yeast/host combinations, the cured mice displayed early macrophage expression of IL-12 transcripts [70].

These data provide strong support to the notion that IL-4 and IL-10 suppress protective anticandidal Th1 responses at both the macrophage and T-cell levels, and that anti-IL-4 or anti-IL-10 therapy in their respective infection models causes a marked shift from a predominant Th2 to a Th1 pattern of reactivity. Of particular interest, and apparently characteristic of the infection of genetically susceptible mice with a yeast LVS, may be the observation of an early and important regulatory role of IL-10 in the qualitative development of the Th cell response to *Candida*. Although the underlying mechanisms are unclear, the ability of anti-IL-10 to operate a phenotypic switch in the reponse of susceptible mice may be related to up-regulation of an intrisically deficient innate response, which exerts a major influence over subsequent Th subset selection, as will be discussed later. This may allow the susceptible mice to initiate Th1 development in response to LVS infection in a way similar to that of the genetically resistant mice [13].

Although a basal production of TGF-β [16] and IL-6 [71] appears to be required for optimal development of systemic Th1 reactivity in response to LVS challenge, overproduction of IL-6 in transgenic mice [15], and high levels of TGF-β [16] in nonhealer mice, are associated with Th2 development. This reinforces the notion that several cytokines, in the early stages of infection, contribute to cell recruitment and to the creation of a specific microenvironment that is highly favorable to development of Th1 cells [55]. In addition to the subtraction of cytokines with direct effects on CD4$^+$ cells, critical perturbations in the cytokine milieu may also result in an impaired Th1 cell response.

Can Th2 Cytokines Revert an Established Th1 Phenotype?

Among the different conditions that predispose to superficial or deep-seated fungal infections, the most striking association undoubtedly occurs between infection with the human immunodeficiency virus (HIV) and mucosal candidiasis. The latter often represents the first clinical sign or symptom of HIV disease [78], typically follows a hierarchical pattern of mucosal (i.e. oropharyngeal, esophageal, and vulvovaginal) involvement [79], and is associated with specific, yet unclarified pathologic processes rather than presence of the virus in mucosal tissue [80]. Neither a reduction in CD4$^+$ cells [78, 79] nor a deficient mucosal immune response [81] may be the only explanations for the impressive association of mucosal candidiasis with HIV infection [82], and oral (often asymptomatic) infection may develop before circulating CD4$^+$ lymphocytes decline to the levels typically associated with opportunistic infections [83].

Although *C. albicans* is frequently isolated from the human mouth, few healthy carriers develop clinical signs of disease, and it is the host's immune competence that ultimately determines whether clearance, colonization, or candidiasis occurs [84]. We have already hypothesized that the changes in cytokine secretion patterns which may occur early in HIV infection, involving IL-4 [85–87], IL-10 [88] and IL-12 [89], could contribute to *Candida* infectivity in AIDS [3, 4, 26]. This would imply that the balance between a Th1 and Th2 response to *Candida* in humans is labile, and is capable of being influenced not only by the virulence of the yeast strain and the genetic context in which infection takes place (as demonstrated by the healer and nonhealer combinations in mice), but also by environmental conditions perturbing the local or systemic cytokine balance.

In a recent study [25], we have examined the effect of IL-4 and IL-10 administration on the course of self-limiting (Th1-associated) gastrointestinal candidiasis and of healing and nonhealing systemic infections in mice. Under all conditions of testing, treatment with IL-4 and/or IL-10 greatly exacerbated the course of primary disease, and rendered healer mice, inoculated with a yeast LVS, susceptible to infection. However, neither cytokine, given alone or in combination, was able to modify the expression of estabished and predominant Th1 cell reactivity in immunized mice challenged systematically with the yeast. Thus, immune dysregulation resulting in overproduction, or administration of Th2 cytokines might exacerbate disseminated candidiasis only in the absence of strong established protective immunity.

These results may offer an explanation for the relative rarity of disseminated candidiasis in AIDS patients, in spite of the high frequency of a mucosal disease. If HIV induces a moderate bias toward Th0/Th2 responses and takes advantage of such responses to replicate more effectively [85–87], this might increase infectivity of the yeast in foci of mucosal colonization by interfering with the efficiency of candidacidal mechanisms (e.g. via IL-10 suppression of nitric oxide production). Any cytokine-induced modulation of Th1 cell effector function would have an immediate impact on the balance between the status of *Candida* as a commensal or pathogen, resulting in asymptomatic or symptomatic infection and perhaps in the selection of more virulent strains or biotypes of the yeast [90]. Yet, the overall expression of systemic acquired immunity would not be significantly impaired. Unless a marked drop in $CD4^+$ effector cell counts occurs, the host can be expected to effectively oppose candidemia [91] and onset of a systemic disease.

Later in HIV disease, however, it is likely that the reduction in $CD4^+$ cell counts contributes significantly to *Candida* disease. Although the effect of T-cell deficiency on anticandidal resistance may be dependent on the respective predominance of Th1- or Th2-type responses [4], the absence of $CD4^+$ cells has been found to be highly detrimental in most experimental models of mucosal infection, which typically results in the prevailing activation of local and systemic Th1 cells [5, 65–67, 92].

Table 2. Indirect evidence for a role of neutrophils in candidiasis that goes beyond their effector function

Observation	Possible implications
Early and sustained neutrophilia occurs in LVS infection [7]	Neutrophils provide the immediate and critical handling of blood-borne yeasts
LVS injection into IL-6-deficient mice results in impaired neutrophil response and Th1 development [71]	Failure to recruit neutrophils to the early response adversely affects Th1 development
Initial, albeit transient, neutropenia triggers a Th2-biased response [4]	Neutrophil role is critical in early Th1 development
Lymphomononuclear more than polymorphonuclear infiltrate predicts healing in late disseminated infection [10, 12-14, 18]	Neutrophils may be more important early in infection than for later resolution of local disease
Chronic systemic candidiasis in humans may persist in spite of normal neutrophil counts and adequate antifungal therapy [98]	Neutrophil effector function may not be adequately assisted by a T-cell response initiated by neutropenia

What Is the Major Cellular Source of Endogenous IL-12 in Systemic Candidiasis?

Although IL-12 was originally discovered as a product of B-cell lines, B cells do not represent the most important physiological producers of IL-12. The cytokine appears to be released mainly by phagocytes [93, 94], and the biological significance of IL-12 production by other cell types remains doubtful [95]. In addition to monocytes, human neutrophils respond in vitro to mitogen stimulation with the production of IL-12 p40 protein and, to a lesser extent, of the biologically active p70 heterodimer [96]. On a per cell basis, neutrophils produce less IL-12 p40 or p70 than monocytes. However, because of the large number of the former cells in the blood or inflammatory tissues, it has been suggested that neutrophil-derived IL-12 plays an important role in the inflammatory response to bacterial or parasitic infection [95, 97].

Several lines of indirect evidence led us to consider the possibility that neutrophil production of cytokines may influence the early development of the T-cell response in mice infected with *C. albicans* (table 2). Sustained neutrophilia accompanies the development of durable anticandidal protection in LVS-infected resistant mice [7]. Chronic systemic candidiasis initiated in humans by neutropenia may persist in spite of normal neutrophil counts and adequate antifungal therapy [98]. Antibody-mediated granulocyte depletion concurrent with LVS infection triggers a Th2-dominated progressive disease, despite the substantial recovery of granulocyte function within a few days of infection [4]. LVS injection into IL-6-deficient mice results in impaired neutrophil response and Th1 development, and both functions are restored by exogenous IL-6 [71]. Finally, despite the adverse effect of early neutropenia in healer mice, resolution of visceral foci of *Candida* infection is associated with a change from a predominantly polymorphonuclear to a lymphomononuclear infiltrate, suggesting that neutrophils may be more important early in systemic infection than for later resolution of local disease [10, 12–14, 18].

Recent studies in our laboratory have begun to address the issue of the possible different roles of neutrophils at different stages of infection and of the possible biological relevance of neutrophil-derived cytokines to the development of Th responses to *Candida*.

Differential Effects of Neutrophil Ablation According to Experimental Conditions

We have examined the effect of specific antibody-mediated depletion of neutrophils on the induction and expression of mucosal and systemic anticandidal protection and the course of Th2-associated, progressive systemic infection [99]. Consistent with a major role of granulocytes in providing a first line of defense against *Candida*, we found that early neutropenia increased infectivity of the yeast in all models of primary candidiasis (table 3). In particular, in self-limiting systemic infection caused by LVS challenge, granulocyte depletion at the time of infection increased the initial candidemia, favored dissemination to visceral organs, and initiated a progressive, ultimately fatal disease. A similar treatment led to accelerated mortality in nonhealer mice with virulent yeast challenge. However, neutrophil depletion performed on day 3 (or later) of LVS infection did not change the outcome of a healing infection. Even more striking was the observation of a protective effect of neutrophil ablation when performed late (on day 7) in the course of an otherwise lethal disease.

On the one hand, these observations reinforce that notion that neutrophils may be most important in the early stages of a self-limiting, Th1-associated infection. On the other, they suggest that neutrophils may even contribute to pathology late in the course of an overwhelming infection. This is not altogether unexpected, as we have already observed that granulocyte dysregulation in mice bearing a large fungal burden may lead to the uncontrolled release of proinflammatory cytokines and thus activate mechanisms of fungal septic shock [28].

Table 3. Differential effects of neutrophil serologic ablation depending on time of treatment and type of *Candida* challenge

Type of infection	Effect of neutrophil depletion
Primary systemic LVS infection	Early treatment (up to 24 h postinfection) operates a switch from a Th1- to a Th2-type response
Primary systemic challenge with virulent yeast	Early treatment accelerates mortality
Primary intragastric challenge	Early treatment enhances infectivity in esophagus and stomach, and hematogenous dissemination as well
Secondary virulent challenge after LVS immunization	Treatment concurrent with reinfection ablates vaccine-induced protection
Primary systemic challenge with virulent yeast	Treatment on day 7 postinfection improves outcome

Most relevant, however, to the present discussion may be the observation that the anticandidal effector function of granulocytes can be compensated effectively by other cell types (e.g. monocytes/macrophages) in the presence of an appropriate and sufficient T-cell response, as demonstrated by the lack of effect of late (day 3) neutrophil ablation on the outcome of LVS challenge. Therefore, the deleterious impact of early neutropenia is unlikely to be due only to defective granulocyte effector function in the face of an appropriate/ sufficient T-cell response, but rather suggests an ititial requirement for neutrophils in Th1 development. Although the underlying mechanisms may be multiple, the early production of directive cytokines by neutrophils in response to *Candida* makes an attractive possibility. This would be consistent with the observed conversion of the Th phenotype operated by neutropenia at the time of LVS infection [4, 99].

Production of IL-12 and IL-10 by Neutrophils in Response to *Candida*

By examining IL-12 and IL-10 production by neutrophils in vitro in response to *Candida*, we have recently obtained direct evidence that neutrophils can produce both cytokines. Most importantly, IL-12 appeared to be released only in response to the LVS strain (which initiates Th1 development in vivo), whereas IL-10 in response to the virulent strain [100]. The quantitative production of IL-12 (p40 and p70) was similar to that observed in vitro with established cellular sources of biologically relevant cytokine, such as activated macrophages, dendritic cells, keratinocytes, and Langerhans' cells [101]. The cytokine gene expression patterns of early neutrophils from healer and non-healer mice were consistent with a selective association of IL-12 detection with the healing response, and of IL-10 with the progressive disease. In line with our previous data [4, 99], early neutropenia in LVS infection, which leads to mortality, would also change the cytokine gene expression and secretion patterns of CD4$^+$ cells. More importantly, administration of recombinant IL-12 to the neutropenic, LVS-infected mice altered both the disease outcome and phenotype of the T-cell response, with a reversion from a Th2 to a Th1 type of reactivity [100]. Thus, neutrophil production of IL-12 and IL-10 to *Candida* is associated with the respective development of Th1 and Th2 responses. Replacement therapy with IL-12 will restore protective Th1 reactivity in otherwise susceptible neutropenic mice infected with a LVS of the yeast.

Besides identifying a potentially critical source of endogenous IL-12 in Th1 development to *Candida*, these studies may provide some insight into the mechanisms governing Th2 differentiation in nonhealer mice. We have already mentioned that IL-10, produced within the context of the innate response of genetically susceptible mice, may adversely affect the early handling of the yeast by phagocytes, leading to suppressed IL-12/IFN-γ responses [102]. If neutrophil-derived IL-12 has a role in Th1-associated anticandidal protection, it is also possible that production of IL-10 by neutrophils contributes to the Th2 development. While IL-10 neutralization will improve outcome in neutropenic mice with LVS infection [99], thus suggesting that neutrophils are not an exclusive source of IL-10, the most convincing example of neutrophil production of biologically relevant IL-10 may be provided by nongranulocytopenic mice treated with exogenous IL-12. This will be discussed in detail in the following section.

Is Exogenous IL-12 Sufficient for Initiating a Th1 Response?

IL-12 has been shown to protect susceptible mice from *Leishmania* infection [103, 104] and to exert an adjuvant effect in a vaccine against the parasite [105]. Marked activity against *Toxoplasma gondii* has also been reported [106], and the cytokine is likewise protective in a variety of infectious disease models [107–110], including mice with cryptococcosis [111] or retrovirus-induced immunodeficiency [112]. Although not all of these models are characterized by a dichotomy of Th responses and NK cell-dependent IFN-γ release may be the critical event in the IL-12-induced protection, the ability of IL-12 to oppose Th2 cytokines [113] could, in principle, be beneficial in a generality of Th2-dominated responses to *C. albicans.*

Earlier studies, involving IL-12 administration to nongranulocytopenic mice with systemic or mucosal yeast infection, did not support this contention [28, 70]. In systemically infected nonhealer mice (either genetically resistant or susceptible), IL-12 did not exert beneficial activity, and cytokine treatment did not result in any change in the qualitative development of the Th cell response. Remarkably, early in infection and as a result of IL-12 exposure, an increase was found in circulating levels of not only IFN-γ but also IL-10 and IL-4. Even more striking, however, was the observation of an exacerbating effect of IL-12 in the mucosal infection model, where the spontaneous development of Th1-associated acquired resistance was somewhat impaired to the benefit of an emerging Th2-biased reactivity [70]. Based on the observation of similar IL-10 induction by exogenous IL-12 in other models [114] including experimental infection [115, 116], and considering the dominant role of IL-10 in candidiasis [13], we have hypothesized that the Th1-promoting role of exogenous IL-12 may be blunted in this latter infection by the coordinate induction of IL-10 [28].

Our recent data of therapeutic efficacy of IL-12 treatment in neutropenic mice with candidal infection not only strengthen the previous suggestion that the induction of IL-10 may serve as a regulatory response to challenge with IL-12 [28, 114], but also suggest that neutrophils may represent a major source of IL-10 induced by IL-12 in nongranulocytopenic hosts (fig. 1). On the other hand, IL-12 induction of IL-10 production by neutrophils may be only one of several mechanisms whereby exogenous IL-12 exerts detrimental or immunotoxic activity in experimental candidiasis (fig. 1, table 4). For example, IFN-γ-dependent priming of mucosal tissue to local damage by inflammatory stimuli might contribute to the exacerbating effects of IL-12 in gastrointestinal infection [28]. Also, in otherwise healer mice with LVS challenge relatively high dosages of IL-12 result in acute pathology and mortality, suggesting the onset of septic shock associated with neutrophil dysregulation [28]. While precautions appear to be warranted by these findings in designing possible therapeutic interventions with exogenous IL-12 in humans, preliminary evidence suggests the utility of IL-12 therapy in experimental fungal infections other than candidiasis.

IL-12 Therapy in Other Fungal Infections

C. neoformans is also an opportunistic fungal pathogen that causes serious life-threatening disease in both healthy and immunocompromised individuals

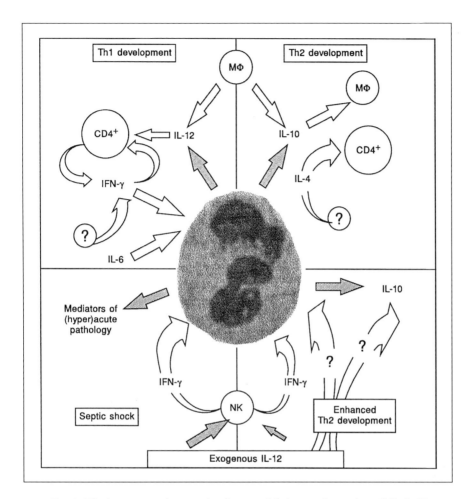

Fig. 1. The immunoregulatory role of neutrophils in experimental candidiasis. Neutrophils, in addition to macrophages, may represent an important source of biologically relevant IL-12 in the initiation of systemic Th1-type responses upon vaccination with a *C. albicans* attenuated strain, which requires IL-6 to effectively recruit neutrophils to the early response. However, neutrophils also appear to release IL-10 in response to virulent yeast challenge, possibly contributing to Th2 development. This effect may be most pronounced following administration of recombinant IL-12, when IL-10 release by neutrophils acts as a regulatory response to challenge with the exogenous cytokine. In acute candidemia associated with a large fungal burden, or as a result of relatively high dosages of exogenous IL-12 concomitant with yeast challenge, neutrophil dysregulation may occur, resulting in the production of several mediators of fungal septic shock.

Table 4. Complexity of the effects of exogenous IL-12 in candidiasis

Observation	Proposed mechanism(s)
Fails to alter disease outcome and Th phenotype in nonhealer mice [70]	Lack of IL-4/IL-10 suppressing activity; induction of IL-10
Worsens disease course in Th1-associated mucosal infection [28, 70]	Induction of IL-10; IFN-γ-dependent priming to local damage by inflammatory stimuli
High dosages trigger acute mortality in LVS-infected mice [28]	IFN-γ-mediated induction of fungal septic shock, resulting in neutrophil dysregulation
Cures neutropenic mice with LVS infection [100]	Th1-promoting role unopposed by IL-10 induction

[1, 2]. A recent study has examined the potential of immunomodulation of the host immune response by IL-12 as a treatment regimen in a murine model of systemic cryptococcosis. In addition, because conventional antifungal chemotherapy may not be curative in the treatment of the human infection, IL-12 was also given in conjunction with a suboptimal (noncurative) dosage of an antifungal agent to assess its possible utility as an adjunctive therapy [111]. The results showed that IL-12, given alone or in combination with chemotherapy, is an effective therapy in systemic, and particularly brain, cryptococcosis. The mechanims underlying the therapeutic activity of the exogenous cytokine were interpreted as involving primarily IFN-γ-mediated stimulation of the phagocytic/cytotoxic potential of antifungal effectors, including microglial cells in the brain [111]. A subsequent study supported the contention that IL-12 is effective when administered in the early stages of pulmonary cryptococcal infection [117].

Invasive aspergillosis is often observed as a secondary infection, and is associated with high mortality. The prolonged survival of profoundly immuno-compromised patients with AIDS has contributed to the increasing recognition of *Aspergillus* infections as an emerging problem [118]. Although in murine allergic aspergillosis exposure to particulate fungal infections elicits a strong Th2 response [119], little is known concerning immunoregulation in invasive aspergillosis [2]. It is therefore of interest that in a murine model of the disease, exogenous IL-12 has been found to protect animals from invasive *Aspergillus* infection via IFN-γ-dependent effects [120].

Histoplasmosis has become an important mycosis in regions of endemicity in North and Central America [121]. In the immunocompetent host, specific T-cell-mediated immunity develops in a few weeks and controls infection, but in individuals with immune deficiency, histoplasmosis is a severe and potentially fatal disease. Resistance to disease is due primarily to T cells and macrophages, IFN-γ being the critical cytokine in activating macrophages to kill the organism [2]. A recent study has examined the regulation of cytokine induction of mice infected with *H. capsulatum* and the effect of IL-12 administration on the course of disease [122]. Mice treated with IL-12 early in infection showed a substantial decrease in fungal burden, and improved clinical course and survival were also observed. Again, these effects were dependent on the production of endogenous IFN-γ.

Coccidioidomycosis is also a mycotic disease that, endemic to the southwestern United States and parts of Central and South America, may develop as a severe, progressive, and often fatal condition in immunocompromised individuals [2]. According to a pattern that appears to be similar, yet inverse to that of experimental candidiasis, DBA/2 mice are genetically resistant to infection and develop Th1-associated protective immunity, whereas BALB/c mice exhibit Th2-associated susceptibility to systemic challenge with *C. immitis* [123]. A recent study showed that administration of IL-12 to the susceptible mouse strain before and after challenge significantly ameliorated the course of the experimental infection [124].

Summary and Overall Conclusions

The Th1/Th2 paradigm of acquired immunity is proving essential for a better understanding of immunoregulation in candidiasis and perhaps other fungal infections, conditions that may be life-threatening in humans and difficult to control by chemotherapy alone, especially in neutropenic and severely immunocompromised patients [26]. In its basic conception applied to *Candida* infection in mice, this paradigm calls for: (i) an association between Th1 responses and the onset/maintenance of phagoctye-dependent immunity, critical for opposing infectivity of the commensal, focusing an infection, and clearing the yeast from infected tissue; (ii) the ability of the yeast to activate Th2 response as an evasive strategy; (iii) the reciprocal regulation of Th1 and Th2 responses, resulting in a dynamic balance between these two types of reactivity [6]. This balance, in concert with a variety of environmental factors, may regulate the status of the yeast as a commensal or pathogen in the mucosal tissue of colonized humans, but may also determine the outcome of deep-seated systemic infections once hematogenous dissemination of the yeast has occurred.

An important corollary of this hypothesis may be the possible combined effects on Th immunity of *Candida* carriage/infection and various disease states. While immune deficiency or dysregulation, resulting in an altered cytokine balance as may occur in AIDS, can reasonably be expected to increase local infectivity of the yeast [25], it is even more intriguing that antifungal chemotherapy will resolve some of the unusual skin (atopic dermatitis-like) disorders frequently observed in this clinical setting, patients with AIDS [125, 126]. Besides, an immunopathologic role for *Candida* has been suggested for atopic dermatitis [33, 34], atopy [30], and other conditions, overtly associated [31, 32, 36, 37] or not [35] with *Candida*. Thus, the Th cell dichotomy to *Candida* may have important implications not only for regulation of the balance between commensalism and infection, but may also contribute to the onset or dominance of Th2 responses in other disease states. A similar example, although with different effects, may be provided by the temporary improvement seen in atopic dermatitis patients in concomitance with acute severe infections, an effect that has been proposed to result from transient down-regulation of the predominant Th2 cell reactivity [127].

With a view to either controlling *Candida* infections or opposing *Candida*-related immunopathology, the promotion of yeast-specific Th1 responses appears to be a promising immunotherapeutic approach. This, in principle, could be achieved by subtraction of Th2 cytokines or by administration of Th1-promoting cytokines [26]. However, our initial studies with exogenous IL-12 were unsuccessful, suggesting that the recombinant cytokine: (i) is unable to oppose Th2 differentiation driven in vivo by IL-4/IL-10; (ii) may induce endogenous IL-10 production as a regulatory response, and (iii) may potentiate local inflammatory responses in gastrointestinal infection or even trigger IFN-γ-dependent mechanisms of fungal septic shock [28]. More recent studies seem to provide encouraging results, at least under specific conditions of testing. In acute candidemia, neutrophils appear to be a major source of the directive cytokines, IL-12 and IL-10, thus contributing to the selection of Th1 and Th2 cell responses to LVS or virulent infection, respectively. Neutrophils may also be an important source of IL-10 released in response to challenge with exogenous IL-12. As a result, the Th1-promoting role of IL-12 may be largely unopposed (by IL-10 induction) in neutropenic mice, which would otherwise succumb to LVS challenge. These animals are, in fact, cured by replacement therapy with IL-12 and acquire durable, Th1-associated anticandidal protection [100]. These findings may be very important for immunotherapy of fungal infections in humans. Neutropenic patients are those at the highest risk for developing systemic candidal infections. Although such patients may have different risk factors for the development of disseminated fungal infections [128], the present data suggest that IL-12 therapy could benefit neutropenic individuals with a responsive T-cell compartment, and extend the potential applications of IL-12 therapy to treatment or prophylaxis of severe fungal infections.

As outlined earlier, the significance of our current studies in experimental candidiasis could be manifold. Besides suggesting novel strategies for immunotherapy of candidal and other infections, they may provide important insights into the general mechanisms of immunoregulation. The ability of murine granulocytes to secrete cytokines that affect, either directly or indirectly, their own function supports a general function of IL-12 in regulating the neutrophil compartment in inflammation and infection, thus adding to the crucial role of this cytokine in bridging innate and adaptive immunity.

Acknowledgments

Many thanks are due to numerous collaborators over the years in different sections of the work described: in particular, to Antonella Mencacci, Elio Cenci, and Roberta Spaccapelo for carrying out most of the experiments, and to Eileen Zannetti for constant and invaluable secretarial support. This work was supported by a series of grants from the AIDS Project and the National Research Council (CNR) Project 'Cytokines', Italy.

References

1   Murphy JW, Friedman H, Bendinelli M: Fungal Infections and Immune Responses. New York, Plenum Press, 1993.
2   Romani L, Howard DH: Mechanisms of resistance to fungal infections. Curr Opin Immunol 1995; 7:517–523.
3   Romani L, Cenci E, Mencacci A, Bistoni F, Puccetti P: T helper cell dichotomy to *Candida albicans*: Implications for pathology, therapy, and vaccine design. Immunol Res 1995;14:148–162.
4   Romani L, Puccetti P, Bistoni F: Biological role of Th cell subsets in candidiasis. Chem Immunol 1996;63:115–137.
5   Bistoni F, Cenci E, Mencacci A, Schiaffella E, Mosci P, Puccetti P, Romani L: Mucosal and systemic T helper cell function after intragastric colonization of adult mice with *Candida albicans*. J Infect Dis 1993;168:1449–1457.
6   Cenci E, Mencacci A, Spaccapelo R, Tonnetti L, Mosci P, Enssle K-H, Puccetti P, Romani L, Bistoni F: T helper cell type 1 (Th1)- and Th2-like responses are present in mice with gastric candidiasis but protective immunity is associated with Th1 development. J Infect Dis 1995;171: 1279–1288.
7   Bistoni F, Verducci G, Perito S, Vecchiarelli A, Puccetti P, Marconi P, Cassone A: Immunomodulation by a low-virulence, agerminative variant of *Candida albicans*. Further evidence for macrophage activation as one of the effector mechanisms of nonspecific anti-infectious protection. J Med Vet Mycol 1988;26:285–299.
8   Vecchiarelli A, Cenci E, Puliti M, Blasi E, Puccetti P, Cassone A, Bistoni F: Protective immunity induced by low-virulence *Candida albicans*: Cytokine production in the development of the anti-infectious state. Cell Immunol 1989;124:334–344.
9   Cenci E, Bartocci A, Puccetti P, Mocci S, Stanley ER, Bistoni F: Macrophage colony-stimulating factor in murine candidiasis: Serum and tissue levels during infection and protective effect of exogenous administration. Infect Immun 1991;59:868–872.
10   Romani L, Mencacci A, Cenci E, Mosci P, Vitellozzi G, Grohmann U, Puccetti P, Bistoni F: Course of primary candidiasis in T-cell depleted mice infected with attenuated variant cells. J Infect Dis 1992;166:1384–1392.

11   Romani L, Cenci E, Mencacci E, Spaccapelo R, Grohmann U, Puccetti P, Bistoni F: Gamma interferon modifies CD4$^+$ subset expression in murine candidiasis. Infect Immun 1992;60:4950–4952.

12   Romani L, Mencacci A, Grohmann U, Mocci S, Mosci P, Puccetti P, Bistoni F: Neutralizing antibody to interleukin-4 induces systemic protection and T helper type 1-associated immunity in murine candidiasis. J Exp Med 1992;176:19–25.

13   Romani L, Puccetti P, Mencacci A, Cenci E, Spaccapelo R, Tonnetti L, Grohmann U, Bistoni F: Neutralization of IL-10 up-regulates nitric oxide production and protects susceptible mice from challenge with Candida albicans. J Immunol 1994;152:3514–3521.

14   Puccetti P, Mencacci A, Cenci E, Spaccapelo R, Mosci P, Enssle K-H, Romani L, Bistoni F: Cure of murine candidiasis by recombinant soluble interleukin-4 receptor. J Infect Dis 1994;169: 1325–1331.

15   Screpanti I, Romani L, Musiani P, Modesti A, Fattori E, Lazzaro D, Sellitto C, Scarpa S, Bellavia D, Lattanzio G, Bistoni F, Frati L, Cortese R, Gulino A, Ciliberto G, Costantini F, Poli V: Lymphoproliferative disorder and imbalanced T-helper response in C/EBPβ deficient mice. EMBO J 1995;14:1932–1941.

16   Spaccapelo R, Romani L, Tonnetti L, Cenci E, Mencacci A, Del Sero G, Tognellini R, Reed SG, Puccetti P, Bistoni F: TGF-β is important in determining the in vivo patterns of susceptibility or resistance in mice infected with Candida albicans. J Immunol 1995;155:1349–1360.

17   Romani L, Mocci S, Bietta C, Lanfaloni L, Puccetti P, Bistoni F: Th1 and Th2 cytokine secretion patterns in murine candidiasis. Association of Th1 responses with acquired resistance. Infect Immun 1991;59:4647–4654.

18   Romani L, Mencacci A, Cenci E, Spaccapelo R, Mosci P, Puccetti P, Bistoni F: CD4$^+$ subset expression in murine candidiasis. Th responses correlate directly with genetically determined susceptibility or vaccine-induced resistance. J Immunol 1993;150:925–931.

19   Romani L, Puccetti P, Mencacci A, Spaccapelo R, Cenci E, Tonnetti L, Bistoni F: Tolerance to staphylococcal enterotoxin B initiates Th1 cell differentiation in mice infected with Candida albicans. Infect Immun 1994;62:4047–4053.

20   Bistoni F, Vecchiarelli A, Cenci E, Puccetti P, Marconi P, Cassone A: Evidence for macrophage-mediated protection against lethal Candida albicans infection. Infect Immun 1986;51:668–674.

21   Cenci E, Romani L, Vecchiarelli A, Puccetti P, Bistoni F: Role of L3T4$^+$ lymphocytes in protective immunity to systemic Candida albicans infection in mice. Infect Immun 1989;57:3581–3587.

22   Cenci E, Romani L, Vecchiarelli A, Puccetti P, Bistoni F: T cell subsets and IFN-γ production in resistance to systemic candidosis in immunized mice. J Immunol 1990;144:4333–4339.

23   Romani L, Mocci S, Cenci E, Rossi R, Puccetti P, Bistoni F: Candida albicans-specific Lyt-2$^+$ lymphocytes with cytolytic activity. Eur J Immunol 1991;21:1567–1570.

24   Cenci E, Romani L, Mencacci A, Spaccapelo R, Schiaffella E, Puccetti P, Bistoni F: Interleukin-4 and interleukin-10 inhibit nitric oxide-dependent macrophage killing of Candida albicans. Eur J Immunol 1993;23:1034–1038.

25   Tonnetti L, Spaccapelo R, Cenci E, Mencacci A, Puccetti P, Coffman RL, Bistoni F, Romani L: Interleukin-4 and -10 exacerbate candidiasis in mice. Eur J Immunol 1995;25:1559–1565.

26   Puccetti P, Romani L, Bistoni F: A T_H1–T_H2-like switch in candidiasis: New perspectives for therapy. Trends Microbiol 1995;3:237–240.

27   Mencacci A, Cenci E, Spaccapelo R, Tonnetti L, Romani L, Puccetti P, Bistoni F: Rationale for cytokine and anti-cytokine therapy of Candida albicans infection. J Mycol Méd 1995;5:25–30.

28   Romani L, Bistoni F, Mencacci A, Cenci E, Spaccapelo R, Puccetti P: IL12 in Candida albicans infections. Res Immunol 1995;146:532–538.

29   Ashman RB, Papadimitriou JM: Production and function of cytokines in natural and acquired immunity to Candida albicans infection. Microbiol Rev 1995;59:646–672.

30   Savolainen J, Koivikko A, Kalimo K, Nieminen E, Viander M: IgE, IgA and IgG antibodies and delayed skin responses towards Candida albicans antigens in atopics with and without saprophytic growth. Clin Exp Allergy 1990;20:549–554.

31   Witkin SS, Jeremias J, Ledger WJ: Vaginal eosinophils and IgE antibodies to Candida albicans in women with recurrent vaginitis. J Med Vet Mycol 1989;27:57–58.

32   Regulez P, Garcia Fernandez JF, Moragues MD, Schneider J, Quindos G, Ponton J: Detection of anti-*Candida albicans* IgE antibodies in vaginal washes from patients with acute vulvovaginal candidiasis. Gynecol Obstet Invest 1994;37:110–114.

33   Savolainen J, Lammintausta K, Kalimo K, Viander M: *Candida albicans* and atopic dermatitis. Clin Exp Allergy 1993;23:332–339.

34   Back O, Scheynius A, Johansson SG: Ketoconazole in atopic dermatitis: Therapeutic response is correlated with decrease in serum IgE. Arch Dermatol Res 1995;287:448–451.

35   Terada N, Konno A, Shirotory K, Fujisawa T, Atsuta J, Ichimi R, Kikuchi Y, Takaki S, Takatsu K, Togawa K: Mechanism of eosinophil infiltration in the patient with subcutaneous angioblastic lymphoid hyperplasia with eosinophilia (Kimura's disease). Mechanism of eosinophil chemotaxis mediated by candida antigen and IL-5. Int Arch Allergy Immunol 1994;104:18–20.

36   Lilic D, Cant AJ, Abinun M, Calvert JE, Spickett GP: Chronic mucocutaneous candidiasis. I. Altered antigen-stimulated IL-2, IL-4, IL-6 and interferon-gamma (IFN-γ) production. Clin Exp Immunol 1996;105:205–212.

37   Lilic D, Calvert JE, Cant AJ, Abinun M, Spickett GP: Chronic mucocutaneous candidiasis. II. Class and subclass of specific antibody responses in vitro and in vivo. Clin Exp Immunol 1996; 105:212–219.

38   Odds FC: *Candida* and Candidosis, ed 2. London, Baillière-Tindall, 1988.

39   Reiner SL, Locksley RM: Lessons from *Leishmania*: A model for investigations of CD4$^+$ subset differentiation. Infect Agents Dis 1992;1:33–42.

40   Sher A, Gazzinelli RT, Oswald IP, Clerici M, Kullberg M, Pearce EJ, Berzofsky JA, Mosmann TR, James SL, Morse HC III: Role of T-cell derived cytokines in the downregulation of immune response in parasitic and retroviral infection. Immunol Rev 1992;127:183–204.

41   Reed SG, Scott P: T-cell and cytokine responses in leishmaniasis. Curr Opin Immunol 1993;5: 524–531.

42   Cutler JE: Putative virulence factors of *Candida albicans*. Annu Rev Microbiol 1991;45:187–218.

43   Hostetter MK: Adherence molecules in pathogenic fungi. Curr Opin Infect Dis 1996;9:141–145.

44   Coleman DC, Bennett DE, Sullivan DJ, Gallagher PJ, Henman MC, Shanley DB, Russell RJ: Oral *Candida* in HIV infection and AIDS: New perspectives/new approaches. Crit Rev Microbiol 1993; 19:61–82.

45   Fidel PL Jr, Sobel JD: The role of cell-mediated immunity in candidiasis. Trends Microbiol 1994; 2:202–206.

46   Francis P, Walsh TJ: Current approaches to the management of fungal infections in cancer patients: Part 1. Oncology 1992;6:81–92.

47   Pfaller MA: Epidemiology of candidiasis. J Hosp Infect 1995;30:329–338.

48   Brummer E, Morrison CJ, Stevens DA: Recombinant and natural gamma-interferon activation of macrophages in vitro: Different dose requirements for induction of killing activity against phagocytizable and nonphagocytizable fungi. Infect Immun 1985;49:724–730.

49   Marodi L, Schreiber S, Anderson DC, MacDermott RP, Korchak HM, Johnston RB Jr: Enhancement of macrophage candidacidal activity by interferon-γ. Increased phagocytosis, killing, and calcium signal mediated by a decreased number of mannose receptors. J Clin Ivest 1993;91:2596–2601.

50   Roilides E, Uhlig K, Venzon D, Pizzo PA, Walsh TJ: Neutrophil oxidative burst in response to blastoconidia and pseudohyphae of *Candida albicans*: Augmentation by granulocyte colony-stimulating factor and interferon-γ. J Infect Dis 1992;166:668–673.

51   Stevenhagen A, Van Furth R: Interferon-γ activates the oxidative killing of *Candida albicans* by human granulocytes. Clin Exp Immunol 1993;91:170–175.

52   Kullberg BJ, Van't Wout JW, Hoogstraten C, Van Furth R: Recombinant interferon-γ enhances resistance to acute disseminated *Candida albicans* infection in mice. J Infect Dis 1993;168:436–443.

53   Ausiello CM, Urbani F, Gessani S, Spagnoli GC, Gomez M, Cassone A: Cytokine gene expression in human peripheral blood mononuclear cells stimulated by mannoprotein constituents from *Candida albicans*. Infect Immun 1993;61:4105–4111.

54   Jones-Carson J, Vazquez-Torres A, van der Heyde HC, Warner T, Wagner RD, Balish E: γ/δ T cell-induced nitric oxide production enhances resistance to mucosal candidiasis. Nat Med 1995;1:552–557.

55   Romagnani S: Regulation of the development of type 2 T-helper cells in allergy. Curr Opin Immunol 1994;6:838–846.

56   Adorini L, Magram J, Trembeau S: The role of endogenous IL12 in the induction of Th1-cell-mediated autoimmune diseases. Res Immunol 1995;146:645–651.

57   Nelson RD, Shibata N, Podzorski RP, Herron MJ: *Candida* mannan: Chemistry, suppression of cell-mediated immunity, and possible mechanisms of action. Clin Microbiol Rev 1991;4:1–19.

58   Li SP, Lee SI, Wang Y, Domer JE: *Candida albicans* mannan-specific, delayed-hypersensitivity CD8+ cells are genetically restricted effectors and their production requires CD4 and I-A expression. Int Arch Allergy Immunol 1996;109:334–343.

59   Sadick MD, Heinzel FP, Holaday BJ, Pu RT, Dawkins RS, Locksley RM: Cure of murine leishmaniasis with anti-interleukin-4 monoclonal antibody: Evidence for a T cell-dependent, interferon gammma-independent mechanism. J Exp Med 1990;171:115–127.

60   Powrie F, Menon S, Coffman RL: Interleukin-4 and interleukin-10 synergize to inhibit cell-mediated immunity in vivo. Eur J Immunol 1993;23:3043–3049.

61   Sher A, Coffman RL: Regulation of immunity to parasites by T cells and T cell-derived cytokines. Annu Rev Immunol 1992;10:385–409.

62   Kaufmann SHE, Reddehase MJ: Infection of phagocytic cells. Curr Opin Immunol 1989;2:43–49.

63   Stein M, Keshav S, Harris N, Gordon S: Interleukin-4 potently enhances murine macrophage mannose receptor activity: A marker of alternative immunologic macrophage activation. J Exp Med 1992;176:287–292.

64   Liew FY, Li Y, Severn A, Millot S, Schmidt J, Salter M, Moncada S: A possible novel pathway of regulation by murine Th2 cells of a Th1 cell activity via the modulation of the induction of nitric oxide synthase on macrophages. Eur J Immunol 1991;21:2489–2494.

65   Fidel PL Jr, Lynch ME, Sobel JD: *Candida*-specific cell-mediated immunity is demonstrable in mice with experimental vaginal candidiasis. Infect Immun 1993;61:1990–1995.

66   Cantorna MT, Balish E: Role of CD4+ lymphocytes in resistance to mucosal candidiasis. Infect Immun 1991;59:2447–2455.

67   Fidel PL Jr, Lynch ME, Sobel JD: *Candida*-specific Th1-type responsiveness in mice with experimental vaginal candidiasis. Infect Immun 1993;61:4202–4207.

68   Fidel PL Jr, Lynch ME, Redondo-Lopez V, Sobel JD, Robinson R: Systemic cell-mediated immune reactivity in women with recurrent vulvovaginal candidiasis. J Infect Dis 1993;168:1458–1465.

69   Romani L, Mencacci A, Tonnetti L, Spaccapelo R, Cenci E, Wolf S, Puccetti P, Bistoni F: Interleukin-12 but not interferon-γ production correlates with induction of T helper type-1 phenotype in murine candidiasis. Eur J Immunol 1994;24:909–915.

70   Romani L, Mencacci A, Tonnetti L, Spaccapelo R, Cenci E, Puccetti P, Wolf SF, Bistoni F: IL-12 is both required and prognostic in vivo for T helper type 1 differentiation in murine candidiasis. J Immunol 1994;152:5167–5175.

71   Romani L, Mencacci A, Cenci E, Spaccapelo R, Toniatti C, Puccetti P, Bistoni F, Poli V: Impaired neutrophil response and CD4+ T helper cell 1 development in interleukin-6-deficient mice infected with *Candida albicans*. J Exp Med 1996;183:1345–1355.

72   Romani L, Mencacci A, Cenci E, Spaccapelo R, Schiaffella E, Tonnetti L, Puccetti P, Bistoni F: Natural killer cells do not play a dominant role in CD4+ subset differentiation in *Candida albicans*-infected mice. Infect Immun 1993:61:3769–3774.

73   Schmitt E, Hoehn P, Huels C, Goedert S, Palm N, Rüde E, Germann T: T helper type 1 development of naive CD4+ T cells requires the coordinate action of interleukin-12 and interferon-γ and is inhibited by transforming growth factor-β. Eur J Immunol 1994;24:793–798.

74   Seder RA, Paul WE: Acquisition of lymphokine-producing phenotype by CD4+ cells. Annu Rev Immunol 1994;12:635–673.

75   Bradley LM, Dalton DK, Croft M: A direct role for IFN-γ in regulation of Th1 cell development. J Immunol 1996;157:1350–1358.

76   Bianchi R, Grohmann U, Belladonna ML, Silla S, Fallarino F, Ayroldi E, Fioretti MC, Puccetti P: IL-12 is both required and sufficient for initiating T cell reactivity to a class I-restricted tumor peptide (P815AB) following transfer of P815AB-pulsed dendritic cells. J Immunol 1996;157:1589–1597.

77   Trinchieri G, Scott P: Interleukin-12: A proinflammatory cytokine with immunoregulatory functions. Res Immunol 1995;146:423–431.

78   Klein RS, Harris CA, Small CB, Moll B, Lesser M, Friedland GH: Oral candidiasis in high-risk patients as the initial manifestation of the acquired immunodeficiency syndrome. N Engl J Med 1984;311:354–358.

79   Imam N, Carpenter CJ, Mayer KH, Fisher A, Stein M, Dauforth SB: Hierarchical pattern of mucosal *Candida* infection in HIV-seropositive women. Am J Med 1990;89:142–146.

80   Smith PD, Eisner MS, Manischewitz JF, Gill VJ, Masur H, Fox CF: Esophageal disease in AIDS is associated with pathologic processes rather than mucosal human immunodeficiency virus type 1. J Infect Dis 1993;167:547–552.

81   Coogan MM, Sweet SP, Challacombe SJ: Immunoglobulin A (IgA), IgA1, and IgA2 antibodies to *Candida albicans* in whole and parotid saliva in immunodeficiency virus infection and AIDS. Infect Immun 1994;62:892–896.

82   Moore RD, Chaisson RE: Natural history of opportunistic disease in an HIV-infected urban clinical cohort. Ann Intern Med 1996;124:633–642.

83   McCarthy GM: Host factors associated with HIV-related oral candidiasis. A review. Oral Surg Oral Med Oral Pathol 1992;73:181–186.

84   Cannon RD, Holmes AR, Mason AB, Monk BC: Oral *Candida*: Clearance, colonization, or candidiasis? J Dent Res 1995;74:1152–1161.

85   Clerici M, Shearer GM: A Th1 to Th2 switch is a critical step in the etiology of HIV infection. Immunol Today 1993;14:107–111.

86   Romagnani S, Maggi E: Th1 versus Th2 responses in AIDS. Curr Opin Immunol 1994;4:616–622.

87   Mosmann T: Cytokine patterns during the progression to AIDS. Science 1994;265:193–194.

88   Graziosi C, Pantaleo G, Gantt KR, Fortin J-P, Demarest JF, Cohen OJ, Sékaly RP, Fauci AS: Lack of evidence for the dichotomy of Th1 and Th2 predominance in HIV-infected individuals. Science 1994;265:248–252.

89   Clerici M, Lucey DR, Berzofsky JA, Pinto LA, Wynn TA, Blatt SP, Dolan MJ, Hendrix CW, Wolf SF, Shearer GM: Restoration of HIV-specific cell-mediated immune responses by interleukin-12 in vitro. Science 1993;262:1721–1724.

90   De Bernardis F, Chiani P, Ciccozzi M, Pellegrini G, Ceddia T, D'Offizzi G, Quinti I, Sullivan PA, Cassone A: Elevated aspartic proteinase secretion and experimental pathogenicity of *Candida albicans* isolates from oral cavities of subjects infected with human immunodeficiency virus. Infect Immun 1996;64:466–471.

91   Cassone A, Palma C, Djeu JY, Aiuti F, Quinti I: Anticandidal activity and interleukin-1β and interleukin-6 production by polymorphonuclear leukocytes are preserved in subjects with AIDS. J Clin Microbiol 1993;31:354–357.

92   Domer JE: Intragastric colonization of infant mice with *Candida albicans* induces systemic immunity demonstrable upon challenge as adults. J Infect Dis 1988;157:950–958.

93   D'Andrea A, Rengaraju M, Valiante NM, Chehimi J, Kubin M, Aste-Amezaga M, Chan SH, Kobayashi M, Young D, Nickbarg E, Chizzonite R, Wolf SF, Trinchieri G: Production of natural killer cell stimulatory factor (NKSF/IL-12) by peripheral blood mononuclear cells. J Exp Med 1992;176:1378–1398.

94   Trinchieri G: Interleukin-12: A cytokine produced by antigen-presenting cells with immunoregulatory functions in the generation of T helper cells type 1 and cytotoxic lymphocytes. Blood 1994; 84:4008–4027.

95   Ma X, D'Andrea A, Kubin M, Aste-Amezaga M, Sartori A, Monteiro J, Showe J, Wysocka M, Trinchieri G: Production of IL-12. Res Immunol 1995;146:432–438.

96   Cassatella MA, Meda L, Gasperini S, D'Andrea A, Ma X, Trinchieri G: Interleukin-12 production by human polymorphonuclear leukocytes. Eur J Immunol 1995;25:1–5.

97   Cassatella MA: The production of cytokines by polymorphonuclear neutrophils. Immunol Today 1995;16:21–26.

98   Bodey GP, Anaissie EJ: Chronic systemic candidiasis. Eur J Clin Microbiol Infect Dis 1989;8:855–857.

99 Romani L, Mencacci A, Cenci E, Del Sero G, Bistoni F, Puccetti P: An immunoregulatory role for neutrophils in CD4$^+$ T helper subset selection in mice with candidiasis. J Immunol 1997;158: 2356–2362.

100 Ramani L, Mencacci A, Cenci E, Spaccapelo R, Del Sero G, Nicoletti I, Trinchieri G, Bistoni F, Puccetti P: Neutrophil production of IL-12 and IL-10 in candidiasis and efficacy of IL-12 therapy in neutropenic mice. J Immunol 1997;158:5349–5356.

101 Heufler C, Koch F, Stanzl U, Topar G, Wysocka M, Trinchieri G, Enk A, Steinman RM, Romani N, Schuler G: Interleukin-12 is produced by dendritic cells and mediates T helper 1 development as well as interferon-γ production by T helper cells. Eur J Immunol 1996;26:659–668.

102 D'Andrea A, Aste-Amezaga M, Valiante NM, Ma X, Kubin M, Trinchieri G: Interleukin-10 (IL-10) inhibits human lymphocyte interferon-γ production by suppressing natural killer cell stimulatory factor/IL-12 synthesis in accessory cells. J Exp Med 1993;178:1041–1048.

103 Heinzel FP, Schoenhaut DS, Rerko RM, Rosser LE, Gately MK: Recombinant interleukin-12 cures mice infected with Leishmania major. J Exp Med 1993;177:1505–1509.

104 Sypek JP, Chung CL, Mayor SE, Subramanyan JM, Goldman SJ, Sieburth DS, Wolf SF, Schaub RG: Resolution of cutaneous leishmaniasis: Interleukin-12 initiates a protective T helper type 1 immune response. J Exp Med 1993;177:1797–1802.

105 Afonso LC, Sharton TM, Vieira LQ, Wysocka M, Trincheiri G, Scott P: The adjuvant effect of interleukin-12 in a vaccine against Leishmania major. Science 1994;263:235–237.

106 Gazzinelli RT, Hieny S, Wynn TA, Wolf S, Sher A, Interleukin-12 is required for the T-lymphocyte-independent induction of interferon-γ by an intracellular parasite and induces resistance in T-cell-deficient hosts. Proc Natl Acad Sci USA 1993;90:6115–6119.

107 Finkelman FD, Madden KB, Cheever AW, Katona IM, Morris SC, Gately MK, Hubbard BR, Gause WC, Urban JF Jr: Effects of interleukin-12 on immune response and host protection in mice infected with intestinal nematode parasites. J Exp Med 1994;179:1563–1572.

108 Wynn TA, Eltoum I, Oswald IP, Cheever AW, Sher A: Endogenous interleukin-12 (IL-12) regulates granuloma formation induced by eggs of Schistosoma mansoni and exogenous IL-12 both inhibits and prophylactically immunizes against egg pathology. J Exp Med 1994;179:1551–1561.

109 Tripp CS, Wolf SF, Unanue ER: Interleukin-12 and tumor necrosis factor α are costimulators of interferon γ production by natural killer cells in severe combined immunodeficiency mice with listeriosis, and interleukin-10 is a physiologic antagonist. Proc Natl Acad Sci USA 1993;90:3725–3729.

110 Sedegah M, Finkelman F, Hoffman SL: Interleukin-12 induction of interferon γ-dependent production against malaria. Proc Natl Acad Sci USA 1994;91:10700–10702.

111 Clemons KV, Brummer E, Stevens DA: Cytokine treatment of central nervous system infection: Efficacy of interleukin-12 alone and synergy with conventional antifungal therapy in experimental cryptococcosis. Antimicrob Agents Chemother 1994;38:460–464.

112 Gazzinelli RT, Giese NA, Morse HC III: In vivo treatment with interleukin-12 protects mice from immune abnormalities observed during murine acquired immunodeficiency syndrome (MAIDS). J Exp Med 1994;180:2199–2208.

113 Manetti R, Parronchi P, Giudizi MG, Piccinni MP, Maggi E, Trinchieri G, Romagnani S: Natural killer cell stimulatory factor (interleukin-12 [IL-12]) induces T helper type 1 (Th1)-specific immune responses and inhibits the development of IL-4 producing Th cells. J Exp Med 1993;177:1199–1204.

114 Morris SC, Madden KB, Adamovicz JJ, Gause WC, Hubbard BR, Gately MK, Findelman FD: Effects of IL-12 on in vivo cytokine expression and Ig isotype selection. J Immunol 1994;152: 1047–1056.

115 Wang ZE, Zheng S, Corry DB, Dalton DK, Seder RA, Reiner SL, Locksley RM: Interferon-γ-independent effects of interleukin-12 administered during acute or established infection due to Leishmania major. Proc Natl Acad Sci USA 1994;91:12932–12936.

116 Finkelman FD, Madden KB, Cheever AW, Katona IM, Morris SC, Gately MK, Hubbard BR, Gause WC, Urban JF Jr: Effects of interleukin-12 on immune response and host protection in mice infected with intestinal nematode parasites. J Exp Med 1994;179:1563–1572.

117 Kawakami K, Tohyama M, Xie Q, Saito A: IL-12 protects mice against pulmonary and disseminated infection caused by Cryptococcus neoformans. Clin Exp Immunol 1996;104:208–214.

118 Khoo SK, Denning DW: Invasive aspergillosis in patients with AIDS. Clin Infect Dis 1994;19(S1): 41–48.

119 Kurup VP, Seymour BWP, Choi H, Coffman RL: Particulate *Aspergillus fumigatus* antigens elicit a Th2 resposne in BALB/c mice. J Allergy Clin Immunol 1994;93:1013–1020.

120 Romani L, Puccetti P, Bistoni F: Interleukin-12 in infectious diseases. Clin Microbiol Rev, in press.

121 Wheat J: Histoplasmosis: Recognition and treatment. Clin Infect Dis 1994;19(S1):19–27.

122 Zhou P, Sieve MC, Bennett J, Kwon-Chung KJ, Tewari RP, Gazzinelli RT, Sher A, Seder RA: IL-12 prevents mortality in mice infected with *Histoplasma capsulatum* through induction of IFN-γ. J Immunol 1995;155:785–795.

123 Magee DM, Cox RA: Roles of interferon gamma and interleukin-4 in genetically determined resistance to *Coccidioides immitis*. Infect Immun 1995;63:3514–3519.

124 Magee DM, Cox RA: Interleukin-12 regulation of host defenses against *Coccidioides immitis*. Infect Immun 1996;64:3609–3613.

125 Hoashi M, Imayama S, Hori Y, Kashiwagi S: An AIDS patient with atopic dermatitis-like eruption responsive to systemic anti-fungal treatment. J Dermatol 1992;19:972–975.

126 Elmets CA: Management of common superficial fungal infections in patients with AIDS. J Am Acad Dermatol 1994;31:S60–S63.

127 Lacour M: Acute infections in atopic dermatitis: A clue for a pathogenic role of a Th1/Th2 imbalance? Dermatology 1994;188:255–257.

128 Walsh TJ, Heimenz J, Pizzo PA: Evolving risk factors for invasive fungal infections: All neutropenic patients are not the same. Clin Infect Dis 1994;18:793–798.

Luigina Romani, MD, PhD, Section of Microbiology,
Department of Experimental Medicine and Biochemical Sciences, University of Perugia,
Via del Giochetto, IH 06122 Perugia (Italy)
Fax (75) 585 3400, E-mail: lromani@unipg.it

Adorini L (ed): IL-12. Chem Immunol. Basel, Karger, 1997, vol 68, pp 136–152

....

Identification and Characterization of Protozoan Products That Trigger the Synthesis of IL-12 by Inflammatory Macrophages

Ricardo T. Gazzinelli[a,b,d], *Maristela M. Camargo*[a,b], *Igor C. Almeida*[f], *Yasu S. Morita*[e], *Mónica Giraldo*[a,b], *Alvaro Acosta-Serrano*[e], *Sara Hieny*[d], *Paul T. Englund*[e], *Michael A.J. Ferguson*[f], *Luiz R. Travassos*[e], *Alan Sher*[d]

[a] Biochemistry and Immunology Department, UFMG, Belo Horizonte and
[b] Laboratory of Chagas' Disease, CPqRR, FIOCRUZ, Belo Horizonte,
[c] Discipline of Cellular Biology, UNIFESP, São Paulo, Brazil;
[d] Laboratory of Parasitic Diseases, National Institute of Allergy and Infectious Diseases, NIH, Bethesda, Md.,
[e] Department of Biological Chemistry, Johns Hopkins University, Baltimore, Md., USA, and
[f] Department of Biochemistry, University of Dundee, UK

Importance of IL-12 in Resistance to Intracellular Protozoa

Cell-mediated immunity (CMI) provides a major host defense against microbial infection. However, excessive CMI elicited by microorganisms can cause severe host-tissue damage and death. The elucidation of pathways involved in the activation of this cellular component of the immune system is therefore of crucial importance in designing new strategies for prophylaxis and immunotherapy of infectious diseases. A variety of microbial pathogens, including the intracellular protozoa *Toxoplasma gondii* and *Trypanosoma cruzi*, are good stimuli of CMI and have served as important models for defining specific molecules and lymphocyte subpopulations engaged in its induction and regulation. Recent studies indicate that IL-12 is a key cytokine for initiation of CMI as well as an important mediator in regulating disease outcome [1, 2]. Our laboratories [3–6] and others [7–10] have demonstrated that both *T. gondii* and *T. cruzi* induce IL-12 synthesis by macrophages in vivo and in vitro. Upon stimulation with IL-12 and other costimulatory monokines (e.g. TNF-α, IL-1β and IL-15) [3, 11, 12], NK cells produce high levels of IFN-γ, which further enhances IL-12 synthesis by macrophages previously stimulated by interaction with these protozoa. In addition, IFN-γ stimulates macrophage effector function forming an important barrier against microbial infection prior to the establishment of the adoptive T-cell response [13, 14]. It is of interest that both *T. gondii* and *T. cruzi* elicit a nonspecific immunity [3, 15–17] that limits coinfection and growth of nonrelated pathogens [18–21] as well as the development of certain tumors [22].

In addition to mediating innate resistance against intracellular pathogens before the induction of T-cell-mediated immunity, the early stimulation of macrophages and NK cells appear to have an important role in directing the development of CMI [14, 23]. Thus, upon exposure to either *T. gondii* or *T. cruzi* (or parasite products), IL-12 and IFN-γ, produced by macrophages and NK cells respectively, will favor the differentiation of T-helper (Th) precursor cells into Th1 lymphocytes [24, 25], which mediate CMI. Once differentiated, Th1 cells no longer require IL-12 to maintain their pattern of cytokine secretion and host resistance [4, 26].

In most instances, the nonspecific resistance induced by these protozoa appears to be dependent on activated macrophages. These cells bear several different receptors that recognize microbial components and induce phagocytosis as well as the release of cytokines [23]. This review summarizes our attempts to identify, isolate and characterize putative molecules from *T. gondii* tachyzoites or *T. cruzi* trypomastigotes that trigger the synthesis of IL-12 by macrophages. Defining the chemical nature and structure of such protozoan products may allow us to design artificial compounds that could be used as selective adjuvants for inducing CMI.

The Ability to Trigger IL-12 Synthesis by Inflammatory Macrophages Is Parasite- as well as Parasite-Stage-Specific

A large variety of microorganisms have been shown to signal macrophages to initiate the synthesis of proinflammatory cytokines [13, 14, 23]. Initially, in our studies we decided to perform a comparative study among different species of intracellular protozoan parasites to assess their ability to elicit IL-12 synthesis by inflammatory macrophages. We used *T. gondii* and *T. cruzi* as parasites that induce a strong IL-12 response in vivo resulting in development of CMI independent of the host genetic background. A second group of protozoa tested were different species of *Leishmania*, parasites that appear to evade early induction of IL-12 synthesis both in vivo and in vitro [27, 28]. During infection with *Leishmania* sp. the ability to induce CMI appears to be mainly dependent on the host genetic background or other immunoregulatory influences, such as pregnancy [29] or concomitant infections [30].

To study the ability of different parasite protozoa to trigger monokine synthesis, we have been using murine peritoneal macrophages obtained 4–5 days post-intraperitoneal injection with thioglycollate. In order to prevent contamination with other cell types, we let the macrophages adhere for 2–4 h, and then remove nonadherent cells [4, 31, 32]. The adherent macrophage-enriched cell populations are primed with IFN-γ and exposed to different microbial stimuli. Most in vitro studies indicate that IFN-γ is required for optimal IL-12 synthesis by macrophages [3, 4, 32, 33]. However, from our in vivo experiments using IFN-γ knockout mice it is clear that high levels of IL-12 synthesis can be induced by *T. gondii* infection in the absence of IFN-γ [34]. A possible explanation for this discrepancy is that the major initial source of IL-12 in vivo is not macrophages but dendritic cells or neutrophils. We are currently investigating this hypothesis in our laboratories.

As shown in figure 1, exposure to *T. gondii* tachyzoites or *T. cruzi* trypomastigotes induces the expression of IL-12(p40) mRNA by macrophages. In contrast, when the same macrophage populations are exposed to *Leishmania* sp., no IL-12(p40) response is observed. In fact, recent studies have demonstrated that the in vitro infection of macrophages with *Leishmania* promastigotes results in a selective inhibition of IL-12 synthesis [28]. Because priming with IFN-γ appears to be required for maximal expression of the IL-12(p40) gene in macrophages [33], we repeated the previous experiment with macrophages pretreated with IFN-γ. While the presence of exogenous IFN-γ amplified the transcription of IL-12(p40) by macrophages exposed to tachyzoites or trypomastigotes, it failed to alter the expression of the same gene when exposed to promastigotes of *Leishmania major*. Consistent with this finding are studies demonstrating that treatment or vaccination of susceptible mice with exogenous recombinant IL-12 redirects the differentiation of lymphocytes from a Th2 to a Th1 phenotype, resulting in healing of *L. major* infection [35–37]. In conclusion, the data summarized above clearly indicate that the ability to trigger IL-12 synthesis by macrophages is parasite-specific.

Because of the ease in obtaining different stages of *T. cruzi* we also analyzed the ability of different developmental forms of *T. cruzi* to trigger the synthesis of proinflammatory cytokines by the same macrophages. Interestingly, we found that parasite stages associated with the invertebrate host, i.e. epimastigotes and metacyclic trypomastigotes, were unable to initiate the synthesis of IL-12 and other monokines by the inflammatory macrophages [32]. In contrast, intracellular amastigotes obtained from disrupted tissue culture fibroblasts and trypomastigotes derived from either tissue culture or

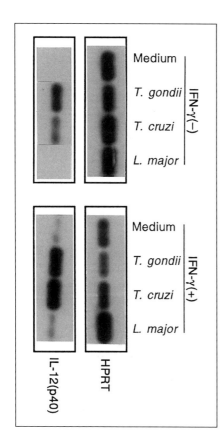

Medium

T. gondii | IFN-γ(–)

T. cruzi

L. major

Medium

T. gondii | IFN-γ(+)

T. cruzi

L. major

IL-12(p40)   HPRT

Fig. 1. Induction of IL-12(p40) mRNA expression by inflammatory macrophages exposed to live forms of *T. gondii, T. cruzi* or *L. major*. Thioglycollate-elicited macrophages were incubated in the presence or absence of IFN-γ and infected with either tachyzoites, trypomastigotes or promastigotes from *T. gondii, T. cruzi* or *L. major*, respectively. After 6 h of incubation, total RNA was extracted from macrophage cultures and expression of the housekeeping gene hypoxanthine phosphoribosyl transferase (HPRT) and the p40 gene from IL-12 heterodimer measured by reverse transcriptase polymerase chain reaction.

infected mouse blood were potent inducers of monokine synthesis by inflammatory macrophages. In addition to triggering the synthesis of IL-12, the exposure of macrophages to amastigotes or trypomastigotes also stimulated the expression of other monokines such as TNF-α, IL-1β, IL-6 and IL-10 [6, 32, 38, 39].

In addition to enhancing the synthesis of IL-12(p40)/IL-12(p70) by macrophages triggered with microbial products, IFN-γ appears to strongly influence both quantitatively and qualitatively the pattern of cytokines expressed by macrophages stimulated by protozoan pathogens. Thus, as noted above, macrophage priming with IFN-γ dramatically enhances IL-12(p40) gene expression as well as IL-12 (p40 and p70) protein secretion by macrophages. A less pronounced effect of IFN-γ is observed on TNF-α production. In contrast, IL-1β and IL-10 expression in macrophages appear to be inhibited by IFN-γ

[13, 28]. In agreement, our recent data obtained with *T. cruzi* parasites clearly show that during macrophage stimulation with live amastigotes or trypomastigotes, but not with invertebrate host-derived parasite forms (i.e. epimastigotes or metacyclic trypomastigotes), costimulation with IFN-γ potentiates the synthesis of IL-12(p40) [32]. A less dramatic effect of IFN-γ priming was observed in terms of TNF-α synthesis by macrophages exposed to live amastigotes or trypomastigotes.

The observations that only parasite stages derived from the vertebrate host are able to initiate the synthesis of IL-12 led us to postulate that trypomastigote and amastigote forms of *T. cruzi* or *T. gondii* tachyzoites may have evolved the capacity to initiate the synthesis of cytokine synthesis by macrophages as a mechanism for establishing CMI and maintaining a mutually beneficial balance between vertebrate host defense mechanisms and parasite growth. Thus, induction of the immune response would protect the host against parasite overgrowth, pathology, as well as mortality. Consistent with this hypothesis, neutralization of endogenous IL-12 during experimental infection with either *T. cruzi* or *T. gondii* results in a dramatic increase of susceptibility and vertebrate host death due to parasitic infection [4, 6, 7, 9, 10]. It is noteworthy that *T. cruzi* and *T. gondii* are facultative macrophage residents, and can live in many types of nonphagocytic nucleated cells. Thereby, macrophage activation by IFN-γ does not lead, necessarily, to parasite elimination. In contrast, in the case of *Leishmania* sp. which reside primarily inside macrophages, the suppression of macrophage activation and IL-12 induction appears to be a crucial strategy for establishing infection although at late stages IL-12 induction appears to be required for parasite control.

Characterization of Parasite Molecules Responsible for Initiating Monokine Synthesis by Inflammatory Macrophages

Our next goal was to isolate the parasite molecules responsible for inducing IL-12 synthesis by inflammatory macrophages. We began by preparing *T. gondii* tachyzoite or *T. cruzi* trypomastigote extracts and submitting these preparations to centrifugation at 20,000 *g* for 30 min. In the case of tachyzoites the activity was detected in both the pellet and supernatant fractions [3, 31, 40]. In contrast, for the trypomastigote stage of *T. cruzi* the activity was retained mainly in the pellet, suggesting that components of parasite membranes were primarily responsible for induction of IL-12 synthesis by inflammatory macrophages (fig. 2) [32]. Therefore, for our work on the latter parasite we decided to use a protocol developed by McConville and Blackwell [41] and modified by Almeida et al. [42] that allows the fractionation of membrane components

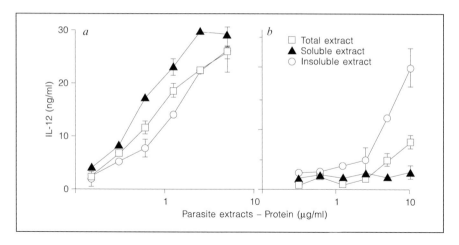

Fig. 2. Induction of IL-12(p40) protein synthesis by inflammatory macrophages exposed to total parasite extracts, soluble fraction and insoluble fraction obtained from *Toxoplasma* tachyzoites (*a*) or *T. cruzi* trypomastigotes (*b*). Thioglycollate-elicited macrophages primed with IFN-γ were incubated with different concentrations of parasite preparations and tissue culture supernatants harvested after 48 h and the levels of IL-12 p40 measured by sandwich ELISA.

based on their degree of hydrophobicity. Each fraction was tested individually in the macrophage stimulation assay. Importantly, the ability of *T. cruzi* trypomastigote molecules (or extracts) to induce IL-12 synthesis in the absence of IFN-γ is minimal. Therefore, we utilized macrophages primed with IFN-γ in all assays for IL-12 induction.

Figure 3 shows a scheme of the methodology [adapted from 42] employed to isolate glycosylphosphatidylinositol (GPI)-anchored glycoproteins from *T. cruzi.* A pellet of $10^{10}-10^{11}$ parasites is prepared and submitted to organic extraction with chloroform, methanol and water. The resulting organic phase obtained from the above extraction is dried under a nitrogen stream and submitted to a partition with butan-1-ol and water. The fractions recovered in the organic and aqueous phases are termed F1 and F2, respectively. The F1 fraction contains highly hydrophobic molecules from parasite membranes such as phospholipids, phosphatidylinositols (PIs) and glycosylinositolphospholipids (GIPLs), whereas the F2 fraction contains other less hydrophobic molecules which are linked to the parasite membranes. The pellet obtained from initial extraction with chloroform, methanol and water is then submitted to 9% butan-1-ol extraction. The soluble material is termed F3 and the pellet F4. While fraction F3 consists mainly of parasite surface glycoproteins, the F4 besides cell debris contains proteins and other molecules not solubilized

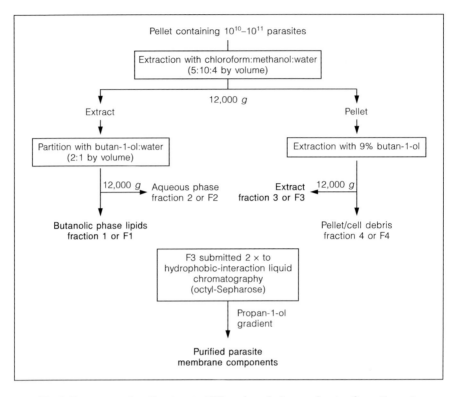

Fig. 3. Strategy used to fractionate GPI-anchored glycoconjugates from *T. cruzi* membranes.

by the sequential organic extractions. The cytokine stimulatory activity was enriched in fractions F3 and F1 when compared with total parasite extracts or insoluble pellets (F4) from trypomastigotes extracts. The aqueous fraction (F2) obtained after butanol/H₂O partition of the organic extract had low activity (not shown).

The strong cytokine stimulatory activity present in fraction F1 suggests the involvement of highly hydrophobic molecules such as phospholipids and/or GIPLs. In contrast, fraction F3 contains hydrophilic glycosylated molecules that are associated with the parasite membranes. Most protozoan parasite surface glycoproteins are thought to be anchored to the parasite membrane through a GPI structure. Therefore, we employed hydrophobic-interaction chromatography on octyl-Sepharose column (Pharmacia Biotech, Sweden) as the next purification step. The F3 fraction was lyophilized, resuspended in 100 mM ammonium acetate, 5% propan-1-ol, and applied to the octyl-Se-

Table 1. Protease treatment is required for extraction by organic solvents of parasite glycolipids which induce TNF-α and IL-12 synthesis by inflammatory macrophages

	Proteinase K treatment	Aqueous phase	Organic phase
Octyl-Sepharose purified			
T. gondii fraction	No	+ + + +	–
T. cruzi GPI-mucins	No	+ + + +	–
Octyl-Sepharose purified			
T. gondii fraction	Yes	+	+ + +
T. cruzi GPI-mucins	Yes	+	+ + +

+ + + + = High activity; + = low activity and – = no activity in inducing cytokine synthesis by inflammatory macrophages primed with IFN-γ.

pharose column, which was further eluted with a propan-1-ol gradient (5–60%). The fractions containing the trypomastigote GPI-anchored glycoproteins were identified with anti-Gal antibodies, pooled and submitted to butan-1-ol:water partition to remove any remaining phospholipids. The aqueous phase was, then, dried and re-submitted to the octyl-Sepharose chromatography and eluted using a shallow propan-1-ol gradient (20–45%). The material eluted from the second run in the octyl-Sepharose column, which has previously been shown to be highly enriched in GPI-anchored glycoconjugates, was highly active in inducing IL-12 synthesis by inflammatory macrophages primed with IFN-γ. The maximal activity was reached at concentrations of approximately 50–100 ng/ml.

Using a similar procedure with soluble tachyzoite antigens or membranes treated with protease, extracted with butanol and separated on octyl-Sepharose, we have been able to partially purify a glycolipid-containing fraction from *T. gondii* tachyzoites which stimulates the synthesis of high levels of IL-12 by inflammatory macrophages primed with IFN-γ.

The data summarized schematically in table 1 strongly suggest that in the case of both trypomastigote glycoconjugates or the tachyzoite-soluble components eluted from octyl-Sepharose, GPI anchors or related protein-linked glycoproteins are largely responsible for the induction of proinflammatory cytokines by macrophages. Thus, after butanol:water partition and before digestion of the material with Proteinase K, all the activity is recovered in the aqueous phase. In contrast, most of the activity is recovered in the butanol phase after digestion with Proteinase K. As discussed below, further analysis of the glycoconjugates to characterize the structural requirements for macrophage activation, suggested that unsaturated acyl fatty acid chains and periodate-sensitive units from GPI anchors are crucial elements for the infective trypomastigote form to initiate IL-12 synthesis by macrophages [31, 32].

Surface GPI-Anchored Mucin-Like Glycoproteins Isolated from *T. cruzi* Trypomastigotes Are Potent Inducers of Monokine Synthesis by Inflammatory Macrophage

Although we are currently in the process of purifying the bioactive tachyzoite components eluted from the octyl-Sepharose column, the monokine-inducing substances isolated from trypomastigotes have recently been characterized as GPI-anchored mucin-like glycoproteins (GPI-mucins) [42]. These molecules are the major surface antigens in this developmental stage of *T. cruzi* and are composed of carbohydrate chains *O*-linked to serine or threonine residues on a polypeptide backbone which is anchored to the trypomastigote membrane via a GPI structure [42]. Further characterization of the GPI anchors from these glycoproteins reveals that the lipid tail is composed of a glycerol containing one alkyl and one acyl chain. The most striking feature of the PI moieties of trypomastigote GPI-mucins is the presence of two unsaturated acyl chains (oleic/C18:1 and linoleic/C18:2) that together account for 75% of the PI structure and so far have not been detected in GPI anchors from other *T. cruzi* developmental stages [32]. Interestingly, the F1 fraction that displays the cytokine stimulatory activity is also rich in PIs containing linoleic (C18:2) fatty acid chains [unpubl. data].

Although our experiments suggest that the GPI anchor is the active moiety of GPI-mucins, we cannot discard a role for the polypeptide backbone with the carbohydrate branch as a potentiating factor for GPI-mucin activity. Nevertheless, our results suggest that mucin-like glycoproteins from *T. cruzi* do not by themselves contain the activity when separated from GPI anchors. Thus, protein digestion or treatment with specific exo-glycosidases fails to eliminate the cytokine stimulatory activity from GPI-mucins. In contrast, periodate oxidation completely abolishes the biological activity of these molecules. It is noteworthy that periodate treatment also eliminates the activity present on GPI anchors purified from GPI-mucins (as well as the monokine-inducing activities expressed by *T. gondii* tachyzoites [31]). Thus, it is likely that the targets of periodate treatment are the carbohydrate and/or inositol structures in the GPI anchors themselves. Finally, our results show that the acyl chain from GPI-mucins appears to be important in triggering IL-12 synthesis by macrophages, since alkaline hydrolysis which eliminates the ester-linked fatty

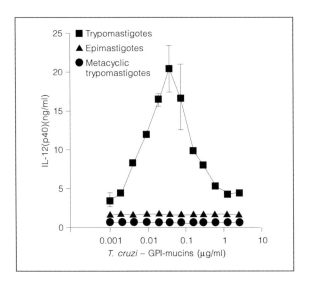

Fig. 4. Induction of IL-12(p40) protein synthesis by inflammatory macrophages exposed to GPI-mucins extracted from different developmental stages of *T. cruzi*. Thioglycollate-elicited macrophages primed with IFN-γ were incubated with different concentrations of parasite GPI-mucins and tissue culture supernatants harvested after 48 h and the levels of IL-12 p40 measured by sandwich ELISA.

acid from the GPI anchors also destroys most of the activity of these molecules on macrophages.

All of the different developmental stages of *T. cruzi* are covered by mucin-like glycoproteins which are distinct not only in their carbohydrate composition but also at the level of the lipid tail from their GPI anchors [32, 43, 44]. Consistent with the experiments performed with live parasites, only the GPI-mucins from trypomastigotes (fig. 4) or amastigotes (not shown) activate monokine synthesis by IFN-γ-primed macrophages. In contrast, mucin-like molecules from epimastigotes or metacyclic trypomastigotes (fig. 4) are unable to induce this response [32].

Different Protozoa Share GPI-Anchored Surface Molecules Capable of Inducing Monokine Synthesis by Inflammatory Macrophages

The findings summarized in table 2 compare the ability of GPI-anchored surface molecules obtained from different parasitic protozoa to induce mono-kine (TNF-α and/or IL-12) synthesis by inflammatory macrophages. Con-

Table 2. Protozoan parasite products which induce the synthesis of IL-12 and other proinflammatory cytokines by murine inflammatory macrophages

	Live parasite	Parasite extracts	Parasite molecules
Trypanosoma cruzi			
Epimastigotes	−	−	− (GPI-mucins)
Metacyclic trypomastigotes	−	−	− (GPI-mucins, GIPLs)
Amastigotes	+	+	+ (GPI-mucins)
Trypomastigotes	+	+	+ (GPI-mucins)
Toxoplasma gondii			
Tachyzoites	+	+	+ (protein-associated glycolipids)
Leishmania donovani			
Promastigotes	−	−	− (LPG and GIPLs)
Leishmania major			
Promastigotes	−	−	− (LPG)
Leishmania mexicana			
Promastigotes	−	−	− (LPG)
Plasmodium falciparum			
Merozoites	?	+	+ (MSP-1, MSP-2 and PIs)
Trypanosoma brucei			
Trypomastigotes	?	+	+ (membrane form of VSG)

Results summarized from 27, 28, 31, 32, 44, 54–58.

sistent with their capacity of *Leishmania* species to evade the induction of CMI glycolipids (e.g. LPG and GIPLs) obtained from membranes of these parasites are poor inducers of cytokine synthesis. The latter observations are supported by studies demonstrating that macrophage infection with different species of *Leishmania* results in inhibition of several functions displayed by activated macrophages, such as microbicidal activity, cytokine secretion and apoptosis [45–51]. At least in some systems these inhibitory effects of *Leishmania* infection can be mimicked by LPG [46, 48] or GIPLs [51] isolated from parasite membranes. In fact, LPGs isolated from *Leishmania* have a unique GPI anchor containing a monoalkylglycerol with a long (24:0 or 26:0) saturated fatty acid chain [52, 53] which may, at least in part, be responsible for their inhibitory activity on macrophage functions [46, 48], through the suppression of protein kinase C (PKC) activity. It is noteworthy that potent inhibitory effects of monoalkylglycerol on PKC activity have been demonstrated in other systems [54].

The results summarized in table 2 also show that in contrast to the molecules obtained from *Leishmania* sp., GPI anchors and/or PIs isolated from *Plasmodium falciparum* [55–57] and from *Trypanosoma brucei* [58] possess an activity that is similar to those described above for GPI-anchored molecules from *T. cruzi* trypomastigotes (or amastigotes), and to the uncharacterized glycolipid fraction from *T. gondii* tachyzoites, in potently inducing proinflammatory cytokine synthesis by macrophages. Interestingly, acute infection with *Plasmodium* sp. is characterized by a systemic increase in monokine (e.g. TNF-α, IL-6 and IL-1) synthesis which resembles septic shock. Studies performed by two different groups suggest that lipid-containing components from *P. falciparum* membranes are important activators of monokine synthesis by macrophages. In one approach, Schofield and co-workers [55–57] have demonstrated a role for GPI anchors isolated from the major merozoite surface molecules (MSP-1 and MSP-2) in triggering the cytokine secretion by macrophages. In a different set of experiments, Bate and Kwiatkowski [59] described a similar activity expressed by PI-containing molecules isolated from the same developmental forms of *P. falciparum*. The active moiety is currently being purified and appears to be distinct from the GPI anchors characterized by the first group of investigators [D. Kwiatkowski, pers. commun.]. In contrast to *Leishmania* LPGs, the merozoite surface proteins (MSP-1 and MSP-2) from *P. falciparum* appear to be strong activators of protein kinases, and some of their activities are apparently blocked by treatment of macrophages with specific inhibitors of protein phosphorylation such as Genistein and Tyrphostin [55–57]. The same group demonstrated that GPI anchors isolated from the Variant Surface Glycoprotein (VSG) of *T. Brucei* bloodstream trypomastigotes have potent TNF-α-inducing activity on mouse macrophages [58]. In the case of *T. brucei* VSG and *P. falciparum* MSP-1 and MSP-2, GPI anchors possess a diacyl-glycerol containing C14:0 or C16:0 fatty acid chains which appears to be important for the cytokine-inducing activity of these glycolipids [55–62].

While there is growing evidence implicating protozoan GPI structures as important mediators of monokine induction, major questions remain unanswered. In particular, it will be important to determine whether triggering by these molecules involves specific receptors and to identify the signalling pathways involved. A further question relates to the structural requirements that make some, but not all, GPI anchors able to trigger monokine synthesis in macrophages. The studies discussed above suggest the involvement of both the glycan core and fatty acid chains. A comparative study involving GPI anchors from different protozoan parasites would be very informative in correlating similarities in structure with biological activity in inducing cytokine synthesis by macrophages. A second strategy would be to compare the activity of the entire GPI anchor with different fragments (e.g. glycan core, PI or lipid tails) from the same GPI anchor in terms of their ability to trigger monokine production.

Other Microbial Products with IL-12-Inducing Activity

In addition to the eukaryotic glycolipids discussed above, IL-12-inducing components have been identified in a number of bacterial pathogens. While LPS is clearly a dominant IL-12 inducer in gram-negative bacteria, lipoteichoic acid (LTA) has recently been identified as a potent stimulator of the cytokine in gram-positive species [63]. Interestingly, the induction of IL-12 by LTA can be blocked with anti-CD14 antibodies suggesting that LTA and LPS activate IL-12 expression by a common pathway. Although protozoan glycolipid anchors, LPS and LTA have common structural features, an entirely unrelated class of IL-12 inducers are the unmethylated CpG dinucleotides. These motifs which are abundant in bacterial DNA but suppressed in most eukaryotes stimulate high levels of IL-12 and IL-6 production as well as IFN-γ synthesis by NK cells [64, 65]. Since B cells are a major target for this form of stimulation [65], an entirely different cellular pathway for IL-12 triggering may be involved than that utilized in the macrophage/monocyte-based responses discussed above. The in vivo importance of DNA-induced IL-12 production in innate defense against bacterial infection has not been formally evaluated although exogenously administered CpG dinucleotides have been shown to protect mice against *Listeria* infection in vivo [64].

In addition to glycolipids and nucleotides, peptide structures may also serve as IL-12 inducers. At present the major example is a 45-kD recombinant antigen obtained from a *Leishmania brasiliensis* library that stimulates IL-12 as well as Th1 lymphokine synthesis by peripheral blood mononuclear cells from parasite-infected as well as healthy human subjects [66].

Conclusions

The studies summarized in this review indicate that protein-associated glycolipids derived from intracellular protozoa may be of crucial importance in determining the induction of IL-12 and other proinflammatory cytokines by macrophages. Because IL-12 has been shown to be a key cytokine in potentiating natural immunity as well as determining the nature of the adaptive immune response, it is likely that the interaction of these molecules with macrophages plays a major role in determining the parasite:host equilibrium and disease outcome during protozoan infections. Thus, membrane-associated glycolipids obtained from different species of *Leishmania* are unable to trigger or inhibit the synthesis of IL-12 by macrophages, a finding consistent with the need for this parasite to evade CMI early in infection. In contrast, as documented here, *T. gondii* tachyzoites or *T. cruzi* trypomastigotes produce related glycolipids which are potent inducers of IL-12 synthesis by inflammatory macrophages. We propose that the latter two parasites that can invade many types of nucleated vertebrate host cells, and therefore are potentially highly virulent, induce IL-12 synthesis by macrophages in order to regulate their own numbers thereby ensuring both host and parasite survival. The newly developed techniques for disrupting genes in protozoa [67] may provide a powerful approach for testing this hypothesis.

Acknowledgements

R.T.G. is recipient of Biotechnology Career Fellowship from the Rockfeller Foundation and a Research Fellowship from CNPq and is funded by grants from PADCT/CNPq (62.0106/95-6-SBIO) and CNPq (522.056/95-4). M.M.C. and L.T.R. were supported by fellowships from CNPq, I.C.A. by a fellowship from FAPESP, Brazil, and A.A.S. by CONICIT, Venezuela. Y.S.M. and P.T.E. were funded by an NIH grant (AI27608).

References

1   Trinchieri G: Interleukin-12: A pro-inflammatory cytokine with immuno-regulatory functions that bridge innate resistance and antigen-specific adaptative immunity. Annu Rev Immunol 1995;13:252–276.
2   Biron CA, Gazzinelli RT: IL-12 effects on immune responses to microbial infections: A key mediator in regulating disease outcome. Curr Opin Immunol 1995;7:485–496.
3   Gazzinelli RT, Hieny S, Wynn T, Wolf S, Sher A: IL-12 is required for the T-cell independent induction of IFN-γ by an intracellular parasite and induces resistance in T-deficient hosts. Proc Natl Acad Sci USA 1993;90:6115–6119.
4   Gazzinelli RT, Wysocka M, Hayashi S, Denkers EY, Hieny S, Caspar P, Trinchieri G, Sher A: Parasite-induced IL-12 stimulates early IFN-γ synthesis and resistance during acute infection with *Toxoplasma gondii*. J Immunol 1994;153:2533–2543.
5   Gazzinelli RT, Wysocka M, Hieny S, Scharton-Kersten T, Cheever A, Kühn R, Müller W, Trinchieri G, Sher A: In absence of endogenous IL-10 mice acutely infected with *Toxoplasmic gondii* succumb to a lethal immune response dependent on CD4+ T cells and accompanied by overproduction of IL-12, IFN-γ, TNF-α. J Immunol 1996;157:798–805.
6   Aliberti JCS, Cardoso MAG, Martins GA, Gazzinelli RT, Vieira LQ, Silva JS: IL-12 mediates resistance to *Trypanosoma cruzi* in mice and is produced by murine macrophages in response to live trypomastigotes. Infect Immun 1996;64:1961–1967.
7   Khan IA, Matsuura T, Kasper LH: Interleukin-12 enhances murine survival against acute toxoplasmosis. Infect Immun 1994;62:1639–1642.
8   Hunter CA, Subauste CS, van Cleave VH, Remington J: Production of gamma interferon by natural killer cells from *Toxoplasma gondii*-infected SCID:mice regulation by interleukin-10, interleukin-12 and tumor necrosis factor-alpha. Infect Immun 1994;62:2818–2824.

9   Hunter CA, Candolfi CA, Subauste C, van Cleave VH, Remington J: Studies on the role of IL-12 in murine toxoplasmosis. Immunology 1995;84:16–20.

10 Hunter CA, Slifer T, Araujo F: Interleukin-12-mediated resistance to *Trypanosoma cruzi* is dependent on tumor necrosis factor-alpha and gamma interferon. Infect Immun 1996;64:2381–2386.

11 Hunter CA, Chizzonite R, Remington J: IL-1β is required for IL-12 to induce production of IFN-γ by NK cells. J Immunol 1995;155:4347–4354.

12 Carson WE, Ross ME, Baiocchi RA, Marien MJ, Boiani N, Grabstein K, Caligiuri M: Endogenous production of interleukin 15 by activated human monocytes is critical for optimal production of interferon-γ by natural killer cells in vitro. J Clin Invest 1995;96:2578–2582.

13 Gazzinelli RT, Amichay D, Scharton-Kersten T, Grunvald E, Farber JM, Sher A: Role of macrophage-derived cytokines in the induction and regulation of cell-mediated immunity to *Toxoplasma gondii*. Curr Top Microb Immunol 1996;219:127–140.

14 Gazzinelli RT: Molecular and cellular basis of interleukin-12 activity in prophylaxis and therapy against infectious diseases. Mol Med Today 1996;2:258–267.

15 Hauser WE Jr, Sharma SD, Remington J: Augmentation of NK cell activity by soluble and particulate fractions of *Toxoplasma gondii*. J Immunol 1983;131:458–463.

16 Hatcher FM, Kuhn RE: Spontaneous lytic activity against allogeneic tumor cells and depression of specific cytotoxic responses in mice infected with *Trypanosoma cruzi*. J Immunol 1981;126: 2436–2442.

17 Hatcher FM, Kuhn RE, Cerrone MC, Burton RC: Increased natural killer cell activity in experimental American trypanosomiasis. J Immunol 1981;1127:1126–1130.

18 Ruskins J, Remington J: Immunity and intracellular infection: Resistance to bacteria in mice infected with a protozoan. Science 1968;160:72–74.

19 Mahmoud AAF, Warren KS, Strickland GT: Acquired resistance to infection with *Schistosoma mansoni* induced by *Toxoplasma gondii*. Nature 1976;263:56–57.

20 Ortiz-Ortiz L, Ortega T, Capin R, Martinez T: Enhanced mononuclear phagocytic activity during *Trypanosoma cruzi* infection in mice. Int Arch Allergy Appl Immunol 1976;50:232–242.

21 Kierszenbaum F, Sonnenfeld G: Characterization of the antiviral activity produced during *Trypanosoma cruzi* infection and protective effects of exogenous interferon against experimental Chagas' disease. J Parasitol 1982;68:194–198.

22 Hibbs JB, Lambert LH, Remington J: Resistance to murine tumours conferred by chronic infection with intracellular protozoa, *Toxoplasma gondii* and *Besnoitia jellisoni*. J Infect Dis 1971;124:587–592.

23 Fearon DT, Locksley RM: The instructive role of innate immunity in the acquired immune response. Science 1996;272:50–54.

24 Hsieh CS, Macatonia SE, Tripp CS, Wolf S, O'Garra A, Murphy KM: Development of Th1 CD4 + T cells through IL-12 produced by *Listeria*-induced macrophages. Science 1993;260:547–549.

25 Seder RA, Gazzinelli RT, Sher A, Paul WE: IL-12 acts directly on CD4 + T cells to enhance priming for IFN-γ production and diminishes IL-4 inhibition of such priming. Proc Natl Acad Sci USA 1993;90:10188–10192.

26 Tripp CS, Kanagawa O, Unanue E: Secondary response to *Listeria* infection requires IFN-γ but is partially independent of IL-12. J Immunol 1995;155:3427–3432.

27 Reiner SL, Zheng SC, Wang ZE, Stowring L, Locksley RM: *Leishmania* promastigotes evade interleukin-12 induction by macrophages and stimulate a broad range of cytokines from CD4(+) T cells during initiation of infection. J Exp Med 1994;179:447–456.

28 Carrera L, Gazzinelli RT, Badolato R, Hieny S, Muller W, Kuhn R, Sacks DL: *Leishmania* promastigotes selectively inhibit interleukin-12 induction in bone marrow-derived macrophages from susceptible and resistant mice. J Exp Med 1996;183:515–526.

29 Krishnan L, Guilbert LJ, Russell AS, Wegmann TG, Mosmman T, Belosevic M: Pregnancy impairs resistance of C57BL/6 mice to *Leishmania major* infection and causes decreased antigen-specific IFN-γ responses and increased production of helper 2 cytokines. J Immunol 1996;156:644–652.

30 Oliveira MAP, Santiago HC, Lisboa CR, Ceravolo IP, Gazzinelli RT, Vieira LQ: Different species of *Leishmania* induce IL-12 and IFN-γ production by murine cells distinctively from *Trypanosoma cruzi* and *Toxoplasma gondii*. Mem Inst Oswaldo Cruz 1996;91(suppl):168.

31 Grunvald E, Chiaramonte M, Hieny S, Wysocka M, Trinchieri G, Vogel SN, Gazzinelli RT, Sher A: Biochemical characterization and protein kinase C dependency of monokine inducing activities in *Toxoplasma gondii*. Infect Immun 1996;64:2010–2018.

32 Camargo MM, Almeida IC, Pereira MES, Ferguson MAJ, Travassos LR, Gazzinelli RT: GPI-anchored mucin-like glycoproteins isolated from *Trypanosoma cruzi* trypomastigotes initiate the synthesis of pro-inflammatory cytokines by macrophages. J Immunol 1997;158:5890–5901.

33 Ma X, Chow JM, Gri G, Carra G, Gerosa F, Wolf SF, Dzialo R, Trinchieri G: The interleukin-12 p40 promoter is primed by interferon-γ in monocytic cells. J Exp Med 1996;183:147–157.

34 Scharton-Kersten TM, Wynn TA, Denkers EY, Bala S, Grunvald E, Hieny S, Gazzinelli RT, Sher A: In the absence of endogenous IFN-γ, mice develop unimpaired IL-12 responses to *Toxoplasma gondii* while failing to control acute infection. J Immunol 1996;157:4045–4054.

35 Heinzel FP, Schoenhaut DS, Rerko RM, Rosser LE, Gately MK: Recombinant interleukin-12 cures mice infected with *Leishmania major*. J Exp Med 1993;177:1505–1509.

36 Sypek JP, Chung CL, Mayor SEH, Subramanyam JM, Goldman SJ, Sieburth DS, Wolf SF, Schaub RG: Resolution of cutaneous leishmaniasis: Interleukin-12 initiates a protective T helper type 1 immune response. J Exp Med 1993;177:1797–1802.

37 Afonso LCC, Scharton TM, Vieira LQ, Wysocka M, Trinchieri G, Scott P: The adjuvant effect of interleukin-12 in a vaccine against *Leishmania major*. Science 1994;263:235–237.

38 Silva JS, Vespa GNR, Cardoso MAG, Aliberti JCS, Cunha FQ: Tumor necrosis factor alpha mediates resistance to *Trypanosoma cruzi* infection in mice by inducing nitric oxide production in infected gamma interferon-activated macrophages. Infect Immun 1995;63:4862–4867.

39 Van Voorhis WC: Coculture of human peripheral blood mononuclear cells with *Trypanosoma cruzi* leads to proliferation of lymphocytes and cytokine production. J Immunol 1992;148:239–248.

40 Sher A, Oswald IP, Hieny S, Gazzinelli RT: *Toxoplasma gondii* induces a T-independent IFN-γ response in natural killer cells that requires both adherent accessory cells and tumor necrosis factor-α. J Immunol 1993;150:3982–3989.

41 McConville MJ, Blackwell JM: Developmental changes in the glycosylated phosphatidylinositols of *Leishmania donovani*. J Biol Chem 1991;266:15170–15179.

42 Almeida IC, Ferguson MAJ, Schenkman S, Travassos LR: Lytic anti-α-galactosyl antibodies from patients with chronic Chagas' disease recognize novel O-linked oligosaccharides on mucin-like glycosyl-phosphatidylinositol-anchored glycoproteins of *Trypanosoma cruzi*. Biochem J 1994;304: 793–802.

43 Serrano AA, Schenkman S, Yoshida N, Mehlert A, Richardson JM, Ferguson MAJ: The lipid structure of the glycosylphosphatidylinositol-anchored mucin-like sialic acid acceptors of *Trypanosoma cruzi* changes during parasite differentiation from epimastigotes to infective metacyclic trypomastigote forms. J Biol Chem 1995;270:27244–27253.

44 Schenkman S, Ferguson MAJ, Heise N, Almeida MLC, Mortara R, Yoshida N: Mucin-like glycoproteins linked to the membrane by GPI anchor are the major acceptor of sialic acid in a reaction catalyzed by trans-sialidase in metacyclic forms of *Trypanosoma cruzi*. Mol Biochem Parasitol 1993; 59:293–303.

45 Reiner NE, Ng W, Wilson CB, McMaster WR, Burchett S: Modulation of in vitro monocyte responses to *Leishmania donovani*. J Clin Invest 1990;85:1914–1924.

46 Descoteaux A, Matlashewski G, Turco SJ: Inhibition of macrophage protein kinase C-mediated protein phosphorylation by *Leishmania donovani* lipophosphoglycan. J Immunol 1992;149:3008–3015.

47 Descoteaux A, Turco SJ, Sacks DL, Matlashewski G: *Leishmania donovani* lipophosphoglycan selectively inhibits signal transduction in macrophages. J Immunol 1991;146:2747–2753.

48 Frankenburg S, Leibovici V, Mansbach N, Turco SJ, Rosen G: Effects of glycolipids of *Leishmania* parasites on human monocyte activity. Inhibition by lipophosphoglycan. J Immunol 1990;145: 4284–4289.

49 Moore KJ, Labrecque S, Matlashewski G: Alteration of *Leishmania donovani* infection levels by selective impairment of macrophage signal transduction. J Immunol 1993;150:4457–4465.

50 Moore KJ, Matlashewski G: Intracellular infection by *Leishmania donovani* inhibits macrophage apoptosis. J Immunol 1994;152:2930–2937.

51   Proudfoot L, O'Donnell CA, Liew FY: Glycoinositolphospholipids of *Leishmania major* inhibit nitric oxide synthesis and reduce leishmanicidal activity in murine macrophages. Eur J Immunol 1995;25:745–750.

52   McConville MJ, Turco SJ, Ferguson MAJ, Sacks DL: Developmental modification of lipophosphoglycan during the differentiation of *Leishmania major* promastigotes to an infectious stage. EMBO J 1992;11:3593–3600.

53   Orlandi PA, Turco SJ: Structure of the lipid moiety of the *Leishmania donovani* lipophosphoglycan. J Biol Chem 1987;262:10384–10391.

54   Kramer IM, van der Bend RL, Tool AT, van Blitterswijk WJ, Roos D, Verhoeven AJ: 1-O-hexadecyl-2-Q-methylglycerol, a novel inhibitor of protein kinase C, inhibits respiratory burst in human neutrophils. J Biol Chem 1989;264:5876–5884.

55   Schofield L, Hackett F: Signal transduction in host cells by a glycosylphosphatidylinositol toxin of malaria parasites. J Exp Med 1993;177:145–153.

56   Schofield L, Novakovic P, Gerold P, Schwarz RT, McConville MJ, Tachado SD: Glycosylphosphatidylinositol toxin of *Plasmodium* up-regulates intercellular adhesion molecule-1, vascular cell adhesion molecule-1 and E-selectin expression in vascular endothelium cells and increases leukocyte and parasite cytoadherence via tyrosine kinase-dependent signal transduction. J Immunol 1996; 156:1886–1896.

57   Tachado SD, Gerold P, McConville MJ, Baldwin T, Quilici B, Schwarz RT, Schofield L: Glycosylphosphatidylinositol toxin of *Plasmodium* induces nitric oxide synthase expression in macrophages and vascular endothelium cells by a protein tyrosine kinase-dependent and protein kinase C-dependent signaling pathway. J Immunol 1996;156:1897–1907.

58   Tachado SD, Schofield L: Glycosylphosphatidylinositol toxin of *Trypanosoma brucei* regulates IL-1α and TNF-α expression in macrophages by protein tyrosine kinase mediated signal transduction. Biochem Biophys Res Commun 1995;205:984–991.

59   Bate CAW, Kwiatkowski D: A monoclonal antibody that recognizes phosphatidylinositol inhibits induction of tumor necrosis factor alpha by different strains of *Plasmodium falciparum*. Infect Immun 1994;62:5261–5266.

60   Gerold P, Dieckmann-Schuppert A, Schwarz RT: Glycosylphosphatidylinositol synthesized by asexual erythrocytic stages of the malarial parasite, *Plasmodium falciparum*. Candidates for plasmodial glycosylphosphatidylinositol membrane anchor precursors and pathogenic factors. J Biol Chem 1994;269:2597–2606.

61   Gerold P, Schofield L, Blackman MJ, Holder AA, Schwarz RT: Structural analysis of the glycosylphosphatidylinositol membrane anchor of the merozoite surface proteins-1 and -2 of *Plasmodium falciparum*. Mol Biochem Parasitol 1996;75:131–143.

62   Ferguson MAJ, Howans SW, Dwek RA, Rademacher TW: Glycosyl-phosphatidylinositol moiety that anchors *Trypanosoma brucei* variant surface glycoprotein to the membrane. Science 1988;239:753–759.

63   Cleveland MG, Gorham JD, Murphy TL, Tuomanen E, Murphy KM: Lipoteichoic acid preparations of gram-positive bacteria induce interleukin-12 through a CD-14-dependent pathway. Infect Immun 1996;64:1906–1912.

64   Krieg AM: An innate immune defense mechanism based on the recognition of CpG motifs in microbial DNA. J Lab Clin Med 1996;128:128–133.

65   Klinman DM, Yi AK, Beaucage SL, Conover J, Krieg AM: CpG motifs in bacteria DNA rapidly induce lymphocytes to secrete interleukin-6, interleukin-12 and interferon-gamma. Proc Natl Acad Sci USA 1996;93:2879–2883.

66   Skeiky YAW, Guderian JA, Benson DR, Bacelar O, Carvalho E, Kubin M, Badaro R, Trinchieri G, Reed SG: A recombinant *Leishmania* antigen that stimulates human peripheral blood mononuclear cells to express a Th1-type cytokine profile and to produce IL-12. J Exp Med 1995;181: 1527–1537.

67   Beverley SM: Hijacking the cell: Parasites in the driver's seat. Cell 1996;87:787–789.

Dr. R.T. Gazzinelli, Laboratory of Chagas' Disease – CPqRR, Fundação Oswaldo Cruz, Av. Augusto de Lima 1715, 30190-002 Belo Horizonte, MG (Brazil)

Adorini L (ed): IL-12. Chem Immunol. Basel, Karger, 1997, vol 68, pp 153–174

....

Antitumor Activities of IL-12 and Mechanisms of Action

Michael R. Shurin, Clemens Esche, Jean-Marie Péron, Michael T. Lotze

Biologic Therapeutics Program, University of Pittsburgh Cancer Institute, Pittsburgh, Pa., USA

Introduction

Interleukin-12 (IL-12) serves as a bridge between the adoptive and the innate immune response. It facilitates a number of immune mechanisms including activation and generation of CTL, stimulation of NK activity, increase in macrophage function and promotion of Th1 cell generation [1–3]. It suggests that IL-12 is one of the key cytokines involved in the development of antitumor immunity and makes it attractive as an anticancer agent.

As can be seen in figure 1, the number of articles devoted to the antitumor activity of IL-12 remarkably increases every year. Such growing interest of tumor biologists and immunologists in this cytokine results from studies with experimental tumors which have shown that IL-12 is one of the most powerful antitumor cytokines identified to date. Stimulated by these intriguing results in multiple animal models, several clinical trials have been initiated to evaluate the antitumor effect of systemic and local delivery of IL-12 in cancer patients. However, at present, it is too early to make conclusions whether IL-12 has a significant antitumor role in any of these trials. Additionally, data regarding the role of exogenous and endogenous IL-2 in cellular and intracellular mechanisms of tumor immunity, clearly suggests that recombinant IL-12 protein provides a new tool to explore the key regulatory role of the immune system in tumor development, growth and regression.

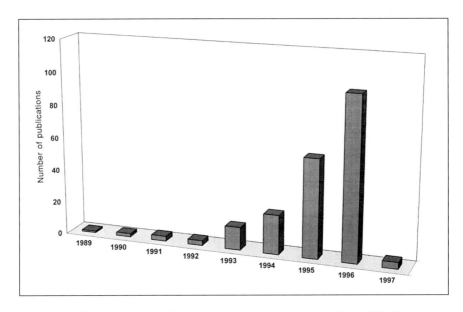

Fig. 1. The number of publications related to the antitumor activity of IL-12 in animal models and human clinical trials.

In vitro Studies

After isolation and purification of a novel cytokine termed natural killer cell stimulatory factor (NKSF, or IL-12), Kobayashi et al. [4] observed that NKSF could enhance NK cell lysis of lymphoma cell line targets. Later, Lieberman et al. [5] demonstrated that IL-12 increased the cytotoxic activity of NK cells obtained from healthy donors against colon carcinoma cell lines. Chehimi et al. [6] confirmed this observation and concluded that IL-12 could modulate the cytotoxic capability of both NK and T cells. Similar results have also been reported using human neuroblastoma cell lines, which are usually NK-resistant, but the addition of IL-12 activates NK cells and increases target cell lysis [7]. Mariani et al. [8] studied whether IL-12 and/or IL-2 stimulate NK cells to increase their lytic efficiency against HOS osteosarcoma cell line and concluded that IL-12 was more efficient than IL-2 in augmenting NK cytotoxicity. IL-12 delivery in vitro corrected the apparent defect of PBMC from cancer patients to lyse the NK-sensitive K562 target and enhanced the cytotoxicity against both NK-sensitive and NK-resistant tumor targets in resting PBMC from a patient who had recently undergone allogeneic bone marrow transplantation for hematologic malignancy [9].

Furthermore, IL-12 stimulated specific antiautologous tumor cytotoxic activity and proliferative capacity of TIL in several types of cancer [10, 11], as well as IFN-γ production by T-cells obtained from tumor-bearers [12]. For instance, tumor-infiltrating CD8+ T lymphocytes obtained from breast cancer, renal cancer or neuroblastoma patients and activated with IL-2 and IL-12, revealed greatly augmented cytotoxicity against autologous tumor cells compared with that induced by IL-2 alone [13]. Similar data was reported for ovarian cancer: Lymphocytes obtained from peripheral blood or ascites of ovarian cancer patients and activated by IL-12 were able to lyse autologous tumor cells and the SKOV3 ovarian cancer cell line [14].

Evaluation of NK number and activity in cervical cancer patients revealed that NK cells from poorly responding chemotherapy patients expressed less lytic activity per NK cell and were insensitive to IL-12 stimulation when compared with patients with a better clinical response [15]. This most likely occurred due to reduced expression of IL-12 receptor or altered intracellular signal transduction pathways. IL-12 has also been demonstrated to increase the activity of NK cells, obtained from most hairy cell leukemia patients [16].

Hanagiri et al. [17] carried out a functional evaluation of regional lymph node lymphocytes from patients with lung cancer after in vitro activation with IL-12 and IL-2. They found that IL-12 in culture with low doses of IL-2 (5–10 IU/ml) enhanced proliferation, tumor cytotoxic activity of cells, and production of cytokines, such as IFN-γ, TNF-α and TNF-β. Interestingly, using mixed lymphocyte tumor culture with mastocytoma P815 cells, Gajewski et al. [18] reported that although IL-12 had little effect on the net proliferation of developing effector cells, it increased specific lytic activity 10-fold, acted synergistically with B7-1 in induction of IFN-γ production during primary stimulation, and resulted in a shift toward a Th1 cytokine profile following secondary stimulation.

To summarize the in vitro evaluation of tumoricidal activities of IL-12, we would like to note that it is likely that IL-12 has no direct effect on most tumor cell line growth in cultures [19–21] consistent with the absence of IL-12 receptors on a variety of tumor cell lines [22]. However, it has been recently demonstrated that IL-12 is able to induce apoptosis in myeloid leukemia cells in vitro [23] and modulates adherent properties of human colon cancer cells [24], suggesting that the presence of IL-12 receptors on some tumor cells cannot be ruled out.

Animal Models

IL-12 has been shown to be highly effective in inhibition of tumor growth or complete tumor rejection in a variety of animal tumor models. For instance,

IL-12 significantly suppressed the growth of subcutaneous B16F10 melanoma when treatment was initiated 2 weeks after injection of tumor cells in mice [20]. Likewise, administration of IL-12 resulted in a significant elongation of animal survival in murine Renca renal cell adenocarcinoma and M5076 reticulum cell sarcoma models [20]. Treatment with IL-12 has been shown to inhibit growth of tumor nodules in mice bearing the lethal X5563 B-cell lymphomas [19] and Meth-A sarcoma [25]. In addition, it was shown that both systemic and peritumoral administration of IL-12 prolonged survival, reduced pulmonary metastasis and, in most cases, caused complete tumor regression in murine adenocarcinoma, and several sarcoma models [20, 26–28].

Using aggressive micrometastasizing ovarian carcinoma models, Mu et al. [29] demonstrated that starting 12 days after subcutaneous implantation of tumor cells, several injections of IL-12 at 2- to 3-day intervals caused regression of growing tumors. The strong antitumor effect of IL-12 against liver metastases growth was also demonstrated using another highly metastatic RAW117-H10 lymphoma in mice [30]. Furthermore, IL-12 treatment was also effective for the treatment of established experimental pulmonary and hepatic metastases [20] and inhibited the development of metastases in both lung and lymph nodes, whereas IL-2 did not [29]. Intraperitoneal administration of IL-12 has also demonstrated a high efficacy on the hepatic metastases in a rat model [31]. Hashimoto et al. [32] showed that systemic administration of IL-12 into mice activates NK1$^+$ $\alpha\beta$ T cells with intermediate TCR in the liver and inhibits hepatic metastases of EL-4 lymphoma cells in C57BL/6 and nu/nu mice. The same group later showed that LPS administration into mice induces IL-12 production from Kupffer cells and subsequent production of IFN-γ induces cytotoxic NK1.1$^+$ $\alpha\beta$ T cells in the liver, suggesting a mechanism of antitumor activity in the liver [33]. In fact, it was shown that IL-12-stimulated hepatic mononuclear cells were transferred into tumor-bearing mice, both EL-4 lymphoma metastases in the liver and 3LL lung carcinoma metastases in the lung were inhibited [34].

A strong antitumor effect of IL-12 was also detected in murine fibrosarcoma models [12]. Five injections of IL-12 into tumor-bearing mice induced complete tumor regression when treatment was initiated at early (1–2 weeks), intermediate (4–5 weeks), or even late (7 weeks) stages of tumor growth. Mice which rejected the primary tumor, exhibited complete resistance to a rechallenge with the same tumor. Three or five injections of IL-12 into mice bearing CSA1M fibrosarcoma or OV-HM ovarian carcinoma induced complete tumor regression [35].

In addition to the remarkable antitumor activity of IL-12 in transplantable tumor systems in mice, recent studies detected that immunotherapy with IL-12 dose-dependently delayed appearance and reduced incidence of tumors induced by carcinogenic hydrocarbon 3-methylcholanthrene [36] or methyl-nitrosourea [37].

In spite of the fact that a number of murine tumors are susceptible to IL-12-based immunotherapy at doses of 0.01–1 µg/day, others may appear to be resistant. Martinotti et al. [38] have shown that systemic IL-12 administration had a negligible effect on C26 colon carcinoma growth, whereas the same treatment reduced the size of B16 melanomas in mice.

Although IL-12 given alone to mice bearing 3-day established CT26 adenocarcinoma transduced with a model antigen did not have consistent antitumor activity, a profound therapeutic effect was observed when IL-12 administration was combined with a recombinant vaccinia virus encoding tumor antigen and/or B7-1 [39]. Similarly, a combination of relatively ineffective, when used alone, B7-1 transfection or systemic IL-12 treatment in poorly immunogenic murine SCK mammary carcinoma models, resulted in a significant increase of tumor rejection and dramatically delayed tumor development [40]. Nishimura et al. [41] reported that although B16-BL-6 melanoma cells, which are a highly metastatic subclone of B16 cells, showed resistance to IL-12 gene therapy, combination therapy with the B7-1 gene and systemic IL-2 administration, almost completely inhibited tumor metastases. Additional experiments showed that the synergistic effect of B7-1 and IL-12 was mediated by a rapidly developing systemic response that was dependent on both $CD8^+$ and $CD4^+$ T lymphocytes, as well as IFN-γ production [40]. The efficacy of combined B7-1 and IL-12 therapy in stimulating specific antitumor immune response against a poorly immunogenic, aggressive tumor indicates the importance of further evaluation of different combinations of immunotherapies to increase the usefulness of immunotherapeutic approaches.

In addition, efficacy of IL-12 administration in tumor-bearing animals seems to depend on the day of treatment initiation. Surprisingly, in the TS/A adenocarcinoma model, IL-12 therapy cured more mice when initiated on day 7 rather than on day 1 [42]. Similar data has been reported by Noguchi et al. [25] when they observed that the effect of IL-12 was more pronounced against established than incipient tumors in the Meth-A sarcoma murine model. One interpretation of these findings is that the efficacy of IL-12 as an antitumor cytokine depends on the number of tumor infiltrating NK and T cells. In fact, this notion was recently supported by Colombo et al. [43] who showed that effectivity of IL-12-based treatment in the C26 carcinoma model depends on the presence of NK and $CD8^+$ cells at the site of the tumor.

It is important to mention that IL-12 is able to synergistically increase the antitumor efficacy of a number of vaccines when added as a component of the treatment. Vagliani et al. [42] reported that IL-12 increases the therapeutic activity of an IL-2-transfected tumor cell vaccine. Indeed, coadministration of IL-12 enhanced efficacy of vaccination with mutated p53 peptides [25] and improved the antimetastatic effect of DNA immunization [44]. Furthermore, IL-12 also synergizes with systemic IL-2 in antitumoral activity in a number of murine tumor models, including pulmonary metastases of a colon carcinoma [45]. In addition, the combined vitamin-D_3/IL-12 treatment of Lewis lung carcinoma-bearing mice, which includes the synergistic augmentation of autologous tumor-specific cytolytic activity within the regional lymph nodes, has recently been described [46]. In the Lewis lung carcinoma model, combinations of IL-12 and M-CSF, along with fractionated radiation therapy, resulted in a synergistic antitumor response [47]. Brunda et al. [22] also investigated the activity of IL-12 combined with chemotherapeutic drugs and reported that in the B16F10 melanoma and M5076 reticulum cell sarcoma models, combination of IL-12 with Adriamycin but not Taxol or 5-fluorouracil, caused an improved antitumor efficacy.

Finally, to fill in the picture of IL-12 activity in animals, it is necessary to note several side effects observed after systemic administration of this cytokine. IL-12 has been shown to induce hematologic toxicities, hepatotoxicity and skeletal muscle degeneration in mice [48, 49]. Daily administration of high dose of IL-12 (1 µg) led to anemia, lymphopenia, neutropenia and mild uncomplicated thrombocytopenia. Splenomegaly was caused by extensive extramedullary hematopoiesis involving all three lineages of cells. Histologic examination of the liver showed Kupffer cell hyperplasia and mononuclear cell infiltration in the hepatic parenchyma. Continual administration of high doses of IL-12 induced coagulative necrosis in surrounding tissues with marked elevation in serum transaminases. Muscle toxicity of unknown mechanism characterized by muscle necrosis, calcification and elevation of serum muscle enzymes was also observed in mice receiving high doses of IL-12 (1–10 µg/day). In primates (*Saimiri sciureus*) 2 out of 6 animals which received high doses of IL-12 (50 µg/kg/day for 14 days) developed a vascular leak syndrome associated with pulmonary edema and ascites but no hepatotoxicity or muscle degeneration was observed [48, 49].

Clinical Investigations

The encouraging results in animal models have prompted the evaluation of IL-12 in cancer patients. The first clinical trial of IL-12 protein was started in spring 1994 by the Genetic Institute in association with the Tufts New England Medical Center, the Dana Farber Cancer Institute, the Indiana University School of Medicine and the University of Pittsburgh Cancer Institute as a Phase I dose escalation study. Few side effects observed in this study included mild and reversible hematologic disorders, mild fever well controlled by acetaminophen, asthenia, oral stomatitis limiting therapy at the higher doses and an elevation of the transaminases at the 1,000 ng/kg dose in 3 out of 4 patients [50].

A Phase II trial was therefore started at the dose of 500 ng/kg. It was stopped after almost all patients experienced serious adverse effects, such as gastrointestinal tract bleeding, asthenia, hepatotoxicity [51]. This latter trial omitted the initial dose of IL-12 suggesting that IL-12 'protected' against subsequent IL-12 toxicity. So far, data from Roche Phase I clinical trial demonstrated that after alteration of route and scheme of IL-12 administration, the cytokine has been well tolerated, with no serious adverse events occurring [51]. Furthermore, the clinical trials of systemic administration of rhIL-12 demonstrated a strong effect on leukocyte distribution and cytokine levels. Del Vecchio et al. [52] described an objective response at soft tissue levels (cutaneous/subcutaneous tissue) in 3 out of 10 patients with metastatic melanoma, although side effects (fever, chills, headache, osteoarthromyalgias) have also been observed. Dose-dependent toxicity of systemic IL-12 in human trials was also noted by others [53, 97]. Observed side effects of systemic administration of IL-12 forced clinicians and investigators to evaluate other approaches of IL-12 delivery. Gene therapy is one strategy which can significantly decrease the toxicity associated with systemic administration of IL-12 and which most closely mimics the natural immune response [54].

Gene Therapy: Murine Models and Clinical Trials

Availability of cytokines in the tumor can increase the efficacy and reduce toxicity of immunotherapy. Genetic engineering of cells, including tumor cells, to produce certain cytokines is an effective method to increase local concentration of cytokines at the tumor site. Local secretion and systemic injection of IL-12 may generate the same effect on tumor establishment and growth if the comparable amount of cytokine is available at the tumor site and bloodstream to activate enough T lymphocytes and NK cells and overcome tumor-induced immunosuppression [38, 43]. Genetic modification of either tumor cells or fibroblasts with IL-12 gene to increase the local concentration of IL-12 has been tested both in preclinical and clinical settings.

Using a retroviral vector it has been shown that IL-12-transfected NIH3T3 fibroblasts reduce tumor growth if admixed with poorly immunogenic BL-6 melanoma cells and administered in mice [55]. This treatment induced immunity to subsequent tumor inoculation. Local production of IL-12 by genetically modified fibroblasts was accomplished by histological patterns of tumor necrosis, macrophage infiltration, and encapsulation by fibroblasts, and the delay of tumor appearance was proportional to the amount of secreted cytokine. Similar data have been obtained using the MCA-105 murine sarcoma [56]. Furthermore, it was also shown that injection of IL-12-transduced fibroblasts in mice can effectively eliminate or inhibit growth of established MCA-207 sarcoma in a dose-dependent manner, requiring delivery of >150 ng/kg/dose of IL-12 [57]. The same results were obtained in additional experiments using the poorly immunogenic MCA-102 murine sarcoma cell line [58].

Martinotti et al. [38] demonstrated the transduction of C26 murine colon carcinoma cells with a polycistronic vector encoding p40 and p35 IL-12 subunits and producing 30–80 pg/ml/10^6 cells/72 h IL-12 accompanied with delayed tumor formation evaluated as subcutaneous tumor growth or lung and liver metastases. Interestingly, the depletion of CD4$^+$ cells before inoculation of IL-12-transfected tumor cells resulted in further delay of tumor appearance and allowed tumor regression in 40% of the mice, suggesting that CD4$^+$ T cells may inhibit CD8-mediated immune response against C26 tumor cells [38]. Furthermore, it was shown that in CD4-depleted mice, 1 µg rhIL-12 given systemically over a period of 10 days gave the same antitumor results as 30–80 pg/ml secretion of IL-12 at the tumor site [43]. Improved transfection of the same C26 tumor cells to secrete about 5,000 pg/ml/10^6/48 h IL-12 resulted in a stronger antitumor response. In mice given injection of 5×10^5 cells, an initial tumor take of 100% followed by a complete tumor rejection [43]. Mice that rejected tumors developed specific memory so that a subsequent challenge with C26 cells was rejected. These results suggested that the amount of IL-12 made available locally in the tumor may determine the tumor progression or regression. The same conclusion was made by Obana et al. [59] who demonstrated that the relatively higher IL-12 producer tumor cell line induced immunologic memory in the rejected mice, but the lower producer did not.

Rodolfo et al. [60] evaluated the therapeutic efficacy of IL-12-transfected C26 colon carcinoma cells given subcutaneously in mice bearing lung metastases of syngeneic, histologically related, and antigenically cross-reacting C51 carcinoma. They found that vaccination with IL-12-transfected tumor cells cured 40% of mice and demonstrated a better antimetastatic therapeutic effect as compared with non-transfected or IL-2-transfected counterparts. This effect of IL-12 was related not only to the induction of systemic tumor-specific CTL response, but also to the production of antitumor antibodies, as well as to a faster infiltration of the metastatic lungs by activated T cells and to either high Th1 or low Th2 systemic activation [60].

Meko et al. [61] reported significantly delayed tumor emergence and decreased tumor size in mice that received subcutaneous injection of MCA-101 fibrosarcoma and PAN-02 pancreatic tumor cells infected with nonreplicating, noncytopathic vaccinia virus expressing IL-12. Taking into consideration the documented synergistic effect of IL-12 with B7-1 (see above), Chen et al. [62a] analyzed in vivo the growth rate of P815 mastocytoma cells after their transfection with B7-1, IL-12, or both together. They concluded that B7-1 alone was sufficient for inducing an immune response that can eliminate primary tumor in mice, but both IL-12 and B7-1 were required for rejection of secondary tumors. Similar data was recently reported by Nishimura et al. [37] who showed that cotransfection of B7-1 gene and IL-12 gene into B16-BL6 melanoma cells was the most effective at inhibiting tumor metastases when compared with single transfections of both genes.

The alternative approach to the genetic engineering of tumor cells to produce IL-12, is to deliver the IL-12 gene in vivo. A simple strategy is the transfer of IL-12 cDNA into epidermal cells overlaying intradermal tumor using particle-mediated (gene gun) delivery. Using this approach, Rakhmile-vich et al. [62b] reported a complete rejection of established tumors in mice bearing Meth-A sarcoma, SA-1 sarcoma, Renca carcinoma, or L5178Y lymphoma. This strong antitumor effect, achieved by 1–4 treatments with IL-12 cDNA-coated particles, was CD8-dependent and led to the generation of immunologic memory.

A lot of attention has also been focused in recent years on other methods of direct in vivo cytokine gene delivery, namely using viral vectors such as adenovirus, adeno-associated virus, and poxvirus. These viruses can infect both replicating and nonreplicating cells and allow transient expression of high level of cytokine gene. According to Bramson et al. [63], intratumoral injection of adenovirus carrying IL-12 gene was effective in more than 75% of treated murine tumors. Caruso et al. [64] reported similar results: intratumoral administration of a recombinant adenovirus expressing the mIL-12 gene alone yielded substantial or complete hepatic tumor regression of the poorly immunogenic MCA-26 colon carcinoma in mice. This treatment resulted in significant increase in the animal survival, with 25% of the treated mice still living after 70 days [64].

A high efficacy of IL-12 gene therapy in a number of animal tumor models led us to investigate local delivery of IL-12 in clinic. A Phase I clinical trial of IL-12 gene therapy was initiated in summer 1995 at the University of Pittsburgh Cancer Institute [50]. In this protocol, autologous fibroblasts, genetically engineered with retroviral vector carrying human IL-12 genes p35 and p40, were directly injected in the peritumoral areas of patients with advanced malignancies of various histological types. No untoward effects have been observed in any of the patients enrolled in this protocol. Significant reduction in tumor sizes were observed at the injection site or at the noninjected sites in 3 patients with melanoma and 1 with head and neck cancer [50, 65]. Further evaluation of the clinical effectivity of IL-12 gene therapy in cancer patients is in progress.

Mechanisms of Antitumor Activity of IL-12

A number of biological activities of IL-12 can mediate or contribute to the potent antitumor effect of this cytokine, including stimulation of NK function and IFN-γ synthesis, activation of Th1 response, increase in macrophage function, enhancement of CTL killing, inhibition of angiogenesis, and, probably, modulation of dendritic cell activity (tables 1, 2).

The high efficacy of IL-12-based immunotherapies in a variety of tumor models allowed us to hypothesize that the levels of circulating or local IL-12 in tumor-bearers might not be adequate to retain satisfactory immunological activity. Impaired production of IFN-γ, shown for several tumor models [66, 67], indirectly supports this notion. Recently, it was clearly demonstrated that the production of IL-12 by macrophages from D1-DMBA-3 mammary tumor-bearing mice was down-regulated with progressive tumor growth [21]. Furthermore, incubation of macrophages with tumor-derived factors resulted in significant decrease in p40 chain expression. Thus, these results indicate that the *down-regulation of IL-12 production* in tumor-bearers leads to impaired stimulation of T lymphocyte to generate high levels of IFN-γ, which, in turn, results in an increase in effector function [21]. Indeed, it was shown that PBMC from patients with cutaneous T-cell lymphoma had a defect in IL-12 production and released significantly less IFN-γ in response to PHA stimulation [68]. Intriguingly, IL-12 appears to have the capacity to correct the deficiency in IFN-γ production by PBMC from patients and markedly enhances cell-mediated cytotoxicity [68].

On the other hand, Hegde et al. [69] observed that the subcutaneous transplantation of AK-5, a rat histiocytic tumor, induced the expression of IL-12 message (p35 and p40) by days 6–8 in splenocytes. Similarly, analysis of serum samples from tumor-bearing rats demonstrated the presence of circulating IL-12 around the same time. These results suggest that the ability of the AK-5 tumor to induce the endogenous production of IL-12 may be responsible for keeping the NK cells constantly in an activated state and resultant spontaneous regression of this tumor.

It should be emphasized that the general belief is that a key role in the antitumor mechanism is attributed to *T lymphocytes* and IFN-γ, which is produced by both NK and T cells [12, 70]. In some models, CD4$^+$ T lymphocytes were important for the IL-12 effect on tumors, possibly by activating CTL and NK responses [55, 71]. For example, complete regression of murine

Table 1. Antitumor activity of systemically administered IL-12 in murine tumor models.

Model	Reference (first author)	Note
B16F10 melanoma	Brunda, 1993 [70]	lung metastasis subcutaneous growth
	Brunda, 1996 [49]	Synergy with Adriamycin
Renca renal cell adenocarcinoma	Brunda, 1993 [70]	
	Brunda, 1995 [72]	
	Tannenbaum, 1996 [27]	Combination with IL-2
	Wigginton, 1996 [102]	
MC-38 colon adenocarcinoma	Nastala, 1994 [26, 71]	Lung metastases
	Stern, 1994 [101]	subcutaneous growth
MCA-105 and MCA-207 sarcoma	Nastala, 1994 [26, 71]	
MCA-207	Zitvogel, 1996 [57]	Synergy with dendritic cells
M5076 reticulum cell sarcoma	Brunda, 1993 [70]	
	Brunda, 1996 [49]	Synergy with Adriamycin
X5563 B-cell lymphoma	O'Tolle, 1993 [19]	
Meth-A sarcoma	Noguchi, 1995 [36]	
RC-2 renal cell carcinoma	Onishi, 1996 [28]	
RAW117-H10 lymphoma	Verbik, 1996 [30]	Liver metastases
EL-4 lymphoma	Hashimoto, 1995 [32]	
	Takeda, 1996 [34]	Liver metastasis
Lewis lung carcinoma	Stern, 1994 [101]	Lung metastasis
	Voest, 1995 [85]	
	Takeda , 1996 [34]	
	Teicher, 1996 [47]	
AK-5 histiocytoma	Hegde, 1995 [69]	Rat, role of endogenous IL-12
CSA1M fibrosarcoma	Zou, 1995 [12]	
	Yu , 1996 [35]	
OV-HM ovarian carcinoma	Mu, 1995 [29]	
	Yu, 1996 [35]	Lung and lymph node metastases
	Fujiwara , 1996 [74]	
B16 melanoma	Martinotti, 1995 [38]	
	Teicher, 1996 [47]	Lung metastases
CT26 adenocarcinoma	Rao, 1996 [39]	Synergy with B7-1
	Tannenbaum, 1996 [27]	
SCK mammary carcinoma	Coughlin, 1995 [40]	Synergy with B7-1
	Wysocka, 1996 [49]	
B16-BL-6 melanoma	Nishimura, 1996 [37]	Synergy with B7-1
TS/A adenocarcinoma	Vagliani, 1996 [42]	
C3 sarcoma	Shurin, unpubl. data	
C26 carcinoma	Colombo, 1996 [43]	
3-Methylcholanthrene-induced tumor	Noguchi, 1996 [25]	
Methylnitrosourea-induced tumor	Nishimura, 1996 [37]	
P815 mastocytoma	Fallarino, 1996 [43]	Role of endogenous IL-12
	Bianchi, 1996 [93]	

Table 2. Antitumor activity of paracrine and autocrine delivered IL-12 in murine tumor models.

Model	Reference (first author)	Note
B16-BL6 melanoma	Tahara, 1994 [58], 1996 [55]	IL-12-transfected fibroblasts
	Nishimura, 1996 [41]	Lung metastases; combination with B7-1
MCA-102 sarcoma	Tahara, 1995 [65]	
	Zitvogel, 1995 [91]	IL-12-transfected fibroblasts
MC-38 colon carcinoma	Zitvogel, 1995 [91]	IL-12-transfected fibroblasts
MCA-105 sarcoma	Pappo, 1995 [56]	IL-12-transfected fibroblasts
MCA-207 fibrosarcoma	Tahara, 1995 [65]	
	Zitvogel, 1995 [91]	IL-12-transfected fibroblasts
	Zitvogel, 1996 [100]	Synergy with B7-1
C26 colon carcinoma	Martinotti, 1995 [38]	
	Colombo, 1996 [43]	
P815 mastocytoma	Chen, 1996 [62]	Synergy with B7-1
A20 B lymphoma	Nishimura, 1996 [41]	
C-51 colon carcinoma	Rodolfo, 1996 [60]	Vaccination with syngenic C26 tumor cells transfected with IL-12
TS/A mammary adeno-carcinoma	Zitvogel, 1996 [100]	Synergy with B7-1
MCA-26 colon carcinoma	Caruso, 1996 [64]	Intratumoral administration of a recombinant adenovirus expressing IL-12
MCA-101 fibrosarcoma	Meko, 1996 [61]	Infection of tumor cells with vaccinia virus
PAN-02 pancreatic tumor		expressing IL-12
MCA-205 fibrosarcoma	Zitvogel, 1996 [92]	IL-12-engineered dendritic cells
Renca adenocarcinoma	Rakmilevich, 1996 [62]	Gene gun-induced IL-12 transfection of
Meth-A sarcoma		epidermal cells overlying intradermal
SA-1 sarcoma		tumors
L5178Y lymphoma		
B16 melanoma		
P815 mastocytoma		

tumors after IL-12 administration was shown to be associated with massive infiltration of T cells and Mac-1$^+$ cells [35]. Furthermore, Mac-1$^+$ and CD8$^+$ cells have been shown to infiltrate murine Renca carcinoma and CT26 colon adenocarcinoma tumors from animals undergoing IL-12 treatment within 24 h of initiation of therapy [27]. The fast accumulation of these cells at the tumor site may be related to the appearance of the *chemokine IP-10*, whose mRNA was detected in the tumor coincidently with the IFN-γ production, since it has been reported to be chemotactic for monocytes and activated T lymphocytes [27]. Another important finding of the same authors is the detection of mRNA encoding cytolytic T-cell effector molecules *perforin* and *granzyme B* in the tumor tissue from IL-12-treated animals within 6 days. However, T lymphocytes do not always support the antitumor action of IL-12, as we have already mentioned, but can actually inhibit IL-12 efficacy in several tumor models [38].

Several authors reported that neutralizing anti-IFN-γ antibodies can abolish the antitumor effect of IL-12 in a variety of animal tumor models [12, 35, 71, 72], suggesting that *IFN-γ* is required for the optimal antitumor efficacy of IL-12. There is a notion that progressive tumor growth is accompanied by the decreased lymphokine-producing capacity of cells [12, 73]. Addition of IL-12 to spleen cell cultures generated from 4- to 10-week-old tumor-bearing mice caused a striking enhancement in the production of IFN-γ compared with cultures of these cells in the absence of IL-12 or normal spleen cells in the presence of IL-12. More importantly, IFN-γ mRNA expression was observed in fresh tumor masses from tumor-bearing mice receiving IL-12 treatment [12].

Thus, it is likely that the antitumoral activity of IL-12 is mediated through the release of IFN-γ at the site of the tumor [74]. IFN-γ can stimulate macrophages to produce and release TNF-α and activate iNOS expression to synthesize *NO*. In fact, increase in serum IFN-γ and nitrogen oxides, exceeding those observed with IL-2 treatment, has been demonstrated in mice treated with recombinant IL-12 [71]. Similarly, it has been recently noted that IL-12 administration to either control or tumor-bearing mice induced progressive increase in serum NO levels [75]. Furthermore, IL-12 therapy resulted in overcoming the suppressed NO synthesis by the tumor-bearer's macrophages and delayed tumor growth. Therefore, it is conceivable that NO plays a significant role in the antitumor activity of IL-12. In fact, Sotomayor et al. [66] demonstrated that macrophages obtained from D1-DMBA-3 tumor-bearing mice have a suppressed ability to produce NO, which may be related to the low levels of IFN-γ in these animals. But on other hand, there is data demonstrating that IFN-γ is capable of stimulating the expression of iNOS mRNA in some tumor cell lines, for instance, the murine CSA1M fibrosarcoma [35]. Interestingly, IFN-γ stimulated CSA1M cells to produce large amounts of NO which functioned to inhibit their own growth in vitro. The role of NO and other macrophage-derived factors, as well as biology and functional characteristics of tumor-infiltrating macrophages, are discussed in other recent reviews [76–78].

In addition to these mechanisms of IFN-γ action on the immunity, there is data highlighting the important role of a direct effect of IFN-γ on tumor cells [79]. It was shown that in vitro exposure of several types of tumor cell lines to IFN-γ resulted in moderate to potent inhibition of tumor cell growth [35]. IFN-γ is known to stimulate the up-regulation of *MHC molecules on tumor cells* and to increase tumor immunogenicity. For instance, both murine and human tumor cell lines transfected with IFN-γ gene exhibited increased surface expression of HLA class I molecules when tested by FACS and Western blot [80]. Similarly, IFN-γ induces expression of HLA class II on tumor cell lines [81]. Evaluation of 52 ex vivo tumor samples containing ovarian, lung, breast, and colon carcinomas, has demonstrated that in vitro exposure to IFN-γ and TNF-α elevated the level of MHC class I expression in 24 of 52 tumors [82]. Recently, it was shown that IFN-γ can stimulate surface expression of both HLA class I and II in several neuroblastoma cell lines [Dr. Galina V. Shurin, pers. commun.].

Apart from this, an additional mechanism of antitumor activity of IFN-γ has been proposed [83, 84, 98]. According to this, growth inhibition of tumor cells is mediated by the activation of *indoleamine 2,3-dioxygenase* enzyme which catalyzes the oxygenative decyclization of *L*-tryptophan and results in depletion of this essential amino acid in culture or microenvironment. In reference to Yu et al. [35], indoleamine 2,3-dioxygenase mRNA and IFN-γ mRNA were detected in murine OV-HM ovarian carcinoma during administration of IL-12, which actually accompanied complete tumor regression. Additionally, it has been recently reported that treatment of B16F10 melanoma tumor cells in vitro with IFN-γ increases Adriamycin (chemotherapeutics)-induced *apoptosis*, consistently with improved antitumor effect of combined IL-12 and Adriamycin in murine models [22]. Taken together, these reports suggest an additional mechanism of direct action of IFN-γ on tumor cells and regulation of their proliferation.

Repeated observation of antitumor activity of IL-12 in T-cell-deficient mice and an absence of a direct effect on tumor cells suggest that IL-12 may possess *anti-angiogenetic properties* that account for the antitumor effect in vivo. In fact, Voest et al. (85) demonstrated that five injections of 1 µg/day IL-12 almost completely inhibited neovascularization in C57BL/6, SCID, and NK-deficient beige mice in a model of basic fibroblast growth factor-induced corneal neovascularization. This potent suppression of angiogenesis was prevented by administration of IFN-γ-neutralizing antibodies. This fact together with the observation that injection of IFN-γ reproduced the antiangiogenic effect of IL-12 suggests that suppression of neovascularization was mediated through IFN-γ. It has been also shown that IFN-γ is able to inhibit the angiogenesis at the tumor site through induction of IFN-γ-inducible protein 10 (IP-10) [27, 85]. Using intradermal inoculation of human tumor cell lines in x-ray immunosuppressed mice, Majewski et al. [86] found that systemic treatment with mIL-12 significantly decreased tumor-induced angiogenesis in a time- and dose-dependent manner. This effect of IL-12 was also mediated through the induction of IFN-γ synthesis [86].

Using a murine colon 26 carcinoma model, Mori et al. [87] found that IL-12 inhibited tumor growth and also suppressed the induction of cancer cachexia. The anticachectic activity, determined as an alleviation of body weight and adipose tissue and reduction of hypoglycemia and serum IL-6 levels, was observed even at low doses of IL-12, insufficient to inhibit tumor growth. In athymic mice bearing the same tumor, IL-12 was no longer anti-cachectic and did not induce IFN-γ. This data suggested that the anticachectic activity of IL-12 is T-cell dependent and results from at least two mechanisms, the down-regulation of *IL-6 levels* and stimulation of IFN-γ release [87].

Interestingly, exogenous systemic administration of IFN-γ cannot replace IL-12 in complete elucidation of the antitumor effect of this cytokine [20, 70]. In addition, the antitumor effect of IL-12 in the Renca tumor model was reduced in nude mice compared with euthymic mice, but an approximately 10-fold higher level of serum IFN-γ was induced in nude than in euthymic animals [70]. These studies demonstrated that induction of high serum levels of IFN-γ is not solely sufficient to mediate an antitumor effect of IL-12. One explanation is that the IFN-γ receptor is ubiquitariously expressed whereas the expression of IL-12 receptor is restricted to T cells and NK cells [88], which are present at the tumor site. For instance, it has been demonstrated that neither IL-12 alone nor IL-2 transfection alone inhibits the growth of C26 murine colon adenocarcinoma. Only the combination of IL-2 gene trans-fection, which increases the number and activity of tumor-infiltrating leuko-cytes, with IL-12 administration resulted in significant antitumor immunity [42]. The reverse combination is also effective since it has been shown that the administration of systemic or local IL-2 significantly increases antitumor efficacy of IL-12 gene therapy [56]. On other side, it has been reported that IL-12 is effective in NK-deficient mice bearing B16F10 melanoma [20] and NK-depleted mice with MCA-207 or Renca tumors, suggesting that NK cells are not essential for the antitumor activity of IL-12. It is important to mention that in one study, however, the IL-12-based therapy revealed a strong antitumor effect in T- and B-cell-deficient SCID mice injected with a X5563 B-cell lymphoma [19].

The Role of Dendritic Cells

It is important to mention that the relationship between *dendritic cells* (DC), known to be key cells in induction of antitumor immunity [89], and IL-12 also plays a significant role in the mechanisms of antitumor activity of DC. It has been documented that the neutralization of IL-12 in vivo in mice immunized with tumor peptide-pulsed DC, blocks the induction of specific

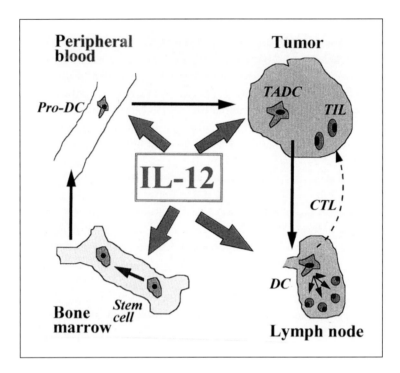

Fig. 2. Relationship between DC and IL-12 in the antitumor activities. IL-12 synergizes with a number of growth factors to stimulate proliferation and differentiation of hematopoietic progenitor and stem cells and increases generation of DC as well. IL-12 likely increases survival of DC and their ability to stimulate proliferation of T lymphocytes. In addition, IL-12 produced by DC at the tumor site may protect TIL and DC from tumor-induced inhibition and apoptosis.

immune response to tumor peptide [90–92]. Additionally, evaluating the immune responses in mice immunized with P815 mastocytoma-specific peptide, the same authors concluded that the exogenous IL-12 required both CD4[+] and CD8[+] cells and the immune response initiated by IL-12 relied on later production of IL-12 by the host [90]. Similarly, Fallarino et al. [93] using IL-12 neutralization in vivo concluded that *endogenous IL-12* is vital for the rejection of murine tumors, supporting a role for endogenous administration of this cytokine to favor a Th1-like phenotype in the immunotherapy of cancer. IL-12 is produced by monocytes, macrophages, keratinocytes, peripheral blood neutrophils and EBV-transfected B cells. Recently, it was documented that DC are another important source of IL-12. Scheicher et al. [94] demonstrated that phagocytosis of antigens by progenitor DC results in de novo synthesis of both IL-12 chains. Macatonia et al. [95] confirmed IL-12 production by DC by positive immunofluorescence staining with Abs specific for the inducible p40 subunit. In this way, DC can drive Th1 development in the absence of IL-4. Heufler et al. [96] demonstrated that murine as well as human DC can produce IL-12 mRNA and protein in response to conventional stimuli. In addition, DC can express IL-12 in response to antigen-specific interaction with T cells. This fact has not been described for other antigen presenting cells so far and raises the question whether DC can promote Th1 development without exogenous stimuli in vivo, too (fig. 2).

Recently, the ability of IL-12 to enhance efficacy of tumor peptide therapy has been shown using a mouse model [92]. IL-12 was engineered into DC using retroviral-mediated or plasmid-based transfection methods resulting in up to 25 ng rhIL-12/10^6 cells/48 h. These engineered cells are capable of promoting enhanced antitumor, antigen-specific CTL responses compared to non-transduced DC. Together, these observations indicate that IL-12 treatment stimulates IFN-γ production, which, in turn, induces expression of various genes directly in tumor cells or in tumor-infiltrating immune cells. Thus, the effectiveness of IL-12 therapy in humans or in animal models directly depends on our ability to further define and understand these mechanisms.

Conclusion

In summary, IL-12 is a cytokine with profound antitumor activity. However, it is clear that different schedules and modalities of immunotherapy, as well as local and systemic levels of available IL-12, determine the strength of the subsequent antitumor immune response and overall tumor rejection or progressive growth. Thus, further evaluation of the experimental and clinical usage of IL-12, as well as mechanisms of its action on the cells of the immune system and tumor cells, is of great interest and obvious importance.

References

1   Trinchieri G: Interleukin-12: A proinflammatory cytokine with immunoregulatory functions that bridge innate resistance and antigen-specific adaptive immunity. Annu Rev Immunol 1995;13:251–276.
2   Germann T, Rüde E: Interleukin-12. Int Arch Allergy Immunol 1995;108:103–112.
3   Stern AS, Magram J, Presky DH: Interleukin-12, an integral cytokine in the immune response. Life Sci 1996;58:639–654.
4   Kobayashi M, Fitz L, Ryan M, Hewick RM, Clark SC, Chan S, Loudon R, Sherman F, Perussia B, Trinchieri G: Identification and purification of natural killer cell stimulatory factor, a cytokine with multiple biologic effects on human lymphocytes. J Exp Med 1989;170:827–845.

5   Lieberman MD, Sigal RK, Williams NN, Daly JM: Natural killer cell stimulatory factor augments natural killer cell and antibody-dependent tumoricidal response against colon carcinoma cell lines. J Surg Res 1991;50:410–415.

6   Chehimi J, Valiante NM, D'Andrea A, Rengaraju M, Rosado Z, Kobayashi M, Perussia B, Wolf SF, Starr SE, Trinchieri G: Enhancing effect of natural killer cell stimulatory factor (NKSF/interleukin-12) on cell-mediated cytotoxicity against tumor-derived and virus-infected cells. Eur J Immunol 1993;23:1826–1830.

7   Rossi AR, Pericle F, Rasleigh S, Janiec J, Djeu JY: Lysis of neuroblastoma cell lines by human natural killer cells activated by interleukin-2 and interleukin-12. Blood 1994;83:1323–1328.

8   Mariani E, Tarozzi A, Meneghetti A, Tadolini M, Facchini A: Lytic activity of IL-2 and IL-12-stimulated NK cells against HOS osteosarcoma cell line. Boll Soc Ital Biol Sper 1996;72:21–27.

9   Soiffer RJ, Robertson MJ, Murray C, Cochran K, Ritz J: Interleukin-12 augments cytolytic activity of peripheral blood lymphocytes from patients with hematologic and solid malignancies. Blood 1993;82:2790–2796.

10 Andrews JV, Schoof DD, Bartagnolli MM, Peoples GE, Goedegebuure PS, Eberlein TJ: Immunomodulatory effects of interleukin-12 on human tumor-infiltrating lymphocytes. J Immunother 1993; 14:1–10.

11 Zeh HJ, Hurd S, Storkus WJ, Lotze MT: Interleukin-12 promotes the proliferation and cytolytic maturation of immune effectors: Implications for the immunotherapy of cancer. J Immunother 1993;14:155–161.

12 Zou JP, Yamamoto N, Fujii T, Takenaka H, Kobayashi M, Herrmann SH, Wolf SF, Fujiwara H, Hamaoka T: Systemic administration of rIL-2 induces complete tumor regression and protective immunity: Response is correlated with a striking reversal of suppressed IFN-gamma production by antitumor T cells. Int Immunol 1995;7:1135–1145.

13 Kuge S, Watanabe K, Malino K, Tokuda Y, Mitomi T, Kawamura N, Habu S, Nishimura T: Interleukin-12 augments the generation of autologous tumor-reactive CD8$^+$ cytotoxic T lymphocytes from tumor-infiltrating lymphocytes. Jpn J Cancer Res 1995;86:135–139.

14 DeCesare SL, Michelini-Norris B, Blanchard DK, Barton DP, Cavanagh D, Roberts WS, Fiorica JV, Hoffmann MS, Djeu JY: Interleukin-12-mediated tumoricidal activity of patient lymphocytes in an autologous in vitro ovarian cancer assay system. Gynecol Oncol 1995;57:86–95.

15 Marana HR, Andrade JM, Silva JS: Natural killer cells and interleukin-12 in patients with advanced cervical cancer under neoadjuvant chemotherapy. Braz J Med Biol Res 1996;29:473–477.

16 Bigda J, Mysliwska J, Dziadziuszko R, Bigda J, Mysliwski A, Hellmann A: Interleukin-12 augments natural killer-cell mediated cytotoxicity in hairy cell leukemia. Leuk Lymphoma 1993; 10:121–125.

17 Hanagiri T, Takenoyama M, Yshimatsu T, Hirashima C, Yoshino I, Nakanishi K, Nagashima A, Nomoto K, Yasumoto K: Effects of interleukin-12 on in vitro culture with interleukin-2 of regional lymph node lymphocytes from lung cancer patients. Cancer Immunol Immunother 1996;43:87–93.

18 Gajewski TF, Renauld JC, Van Pel A, Boon T: Costimulation with B7-1, IL-6 and IL-12 is sufficient for primary generation of murine antitumor cytolytic T lymphocytes in vitro. J Immunol 1995;154: 5637–5648.

19 O'Toole M, Wolf S, O'Brien C, Hubbard B, Hermann S: Effect of in vivo IL-12 administration on murine tumour cell growth. J Immunol 1993;150:294A.

20 Brunda MJ, Luistro L, Hendrzak JA, Fountoulakis M, Garotta G, Gately MK: Role of interferon-γ in mediating the antitumor efficacy of interleukin-12. J Immunother 1995;17:71–77.

21 Handel-Fernandez ME, Gheng X, Herbert LM, Lopez DM: Down-regulation of IL-12, not a shift from a T helper–1 to a T helper-2 phenotype, is responsible for impaired IFN-gamma production in mammary tumor-bearing mice. J Immunol 1997;158:280–286.

22 Brunda MJ, Luistro L, Rumennik L, Wright RB, Wigginton JM, Wiltrout RH, Hendrzak JA, Palleroni AV: Interleukin-12: Murine models of a potent antitumor agent. Ann NY Acad Sci 1996; 795:266–276.

23 Stine KC, Warren BA, Becton DL: Apoptosis induced by interleukin-12 measured by DNA electrophoresis and in situ end labeling in leukemia. Ann NY Acad Sci 1996;795:420–421.

24 Hiscox S, Hallett MB, Puntis MCA, Jiang WG: Inhibition of cancer cell motility and invasion by interleukin-12. Clin Exp Metastasis 1995;13:877–889.

25 Noguchi Y, Jungbluth A, Richards EC, Old L: Effect of interleukin 12 on tumor induction by 3-methylcholanthrene. Proc Natl Acad Sci USA 1996;93:11798–11801.
26 Nastala CL, Edington HD, McKinney TG, Tahara H, Nalesnik MA, Brunda MJ, Gately MK, Wolf SF, Schreiber RD, Storkus WJ, Lotze MT: Recombinant IL-12 administration induces tumor regression in association with IFN-gamma production. J Immunol 1994;153:1697–1706.
27 Tannenbaum CS, Wicker N, Armstrong D, Tubbs R, Finke J, Bukowski RM, Hamilton TA: Cytokine and chemokine expression in tumors of mice receiving systemic therapy with IL-12. J Immunol 1996;156:693–699.
28 Onishi T, Ohishi Y, Iuzuka N, Suzuki Y, Hosobe T, Nakajo H, Makino H, Saotome H: Study on anti-tumor effects of interleukin-12 for spontaneously arose murine renal cell carcinoma. Jpn J Urol 1996;87:1175–1182.
29 Mu J, Zou JP, Yamamoto N, Tsutsui T, Tai XG, Kobayashi M, Herrmann S, Fujiwara H, Hamaoka T: Administration of recombinant interleukin-12 prevents outgrowth of tumor cells metastasizing spontaneously to lung and lymph nodes. Cancer Res 1995;55:4404–4408.
30 Verbik DJ, Stinson WW, Brunda MJ, Kessinger A, Joshi SS: In vivo therapeutic effects of interleukin-12 against highly metastatic residual lymphoma. Clin Exp Metastasis 1996;14:219–229.
31 Okuno K, Jinnai H, Lee YS, Kaneda K, Yasutomi M: Interleukin-12 augments the liver-associated immunity and reduces liver metastases. Hepatogastroenterology 1996;43:1196–1202.
32 Hashimoto W, Takeda K, Anzai R, Ogasawara K, Sakihara H, Sugiura K, Seki SS, Kumagai K: Cytotoxic NK1.1 Ag$^+$ $\alpha\beta$ T cells with intermediate TCR induced in the liver of mice by IL-12. J Immunol 1995;154:4333–4340.
33 Takahashi M, Ogasawara K, Takeda K, Hashimoto W, Sakihara H, Kumagai K, Anzai R, Satoh M, Seki S: LPS induces NK1.1$^+$ $\alpha\beta$ T cells with potent cytotoxicity in the liver of mice via production of IL-12 from Kupffer cells. J Immunol 1996;156:2436–2442.
34 Takeda K, Seki S, Ogasawara K, Anzai R, Hashimoto W, Sugiura K, Takahashi M, Satoh M, Kumagai K: Liver NK1.1$^+$ CD4$^+$ $\alpha\beta$ T cells activated by IL-12 as a major effector in inhibition of experimental tumor metastasis. J Immunol 1996;156:3366–3373.
35 Yu W, Yamamoto N, Takenaka H, Mu J, Tai XG, Zou JP, Ogawa M, Tsutsui T, Wijesuriya R, Yoshida R, Herrmann S, Fujiwara T: Molecular mechanisms underlying IFN-γ-mediated tumor growth inhibition induced during tumor immunotherapy with rIL-12. Int Immunol 1996;8:855–865.
36 Noguchi Y, Richards EC, Chen Y, Old LJ: Influence of IL-12 on p53 peptide vaccination against established Meth-A sarcoma. Proc Natl Acad Sci USA 1995;92:2219–2223.
37 Nishimura T, Watanabe K, Yahata T, Uede T, Saiki I, Herrmann SH, Kobayashi M, Habu S: The application of IL-12 to cytokine therapy for tumors. Ann NY Acad Sci 1996;795:375–378.
38 Martinotti A, Stoppacciaro A, Vagliani M, Melani C, Spreafico F, Wysocka M, Parmiani G, Trinchieri G, Colombo MP: CD4 T cells inhibit in vivo the CD8-mediated immune response against murine colon carcinoma cells transduced with interleukin-12 genes. Eur J Immunol 1995;25:137–146.
39 Rao JB, Chamberlain RS, Bronte V, Carroll MW, Irvine KR, Moss B, Rosenberg SA, Restifo NP: IL-12 is an effective adjuvant to recombinant vaccinia virus-based tumor vaccines: Enhancement by simultaneous B7-1 expression. J Immunol 1996;156:3357–3365.
40 Coughlin CM, Wysocka M, Kurzawa HL, Lee WM, Trinchieri G, Eck SL: B7-1 and interleukin-12 synergistically induce effective antitumor immunity. Cancer Res 1995;55:4980–4987.
41 Nishimura T, Watanabe K, Yahata T, Ushaku L, Ando K, Kimura M, Saiki I, Uede T, Habu S: Application of interleukin-12 to antitumor cytokine and gene therapy. Cancer Chemother Pharmacol 1996;38(suppl):27–34.
42 Vagliani M, Rodolfo M, Cavallo F, Parenza M, Melani C, Parmiani G, Forni G, Colombo MP: Interleukin-12 potentiates the curative effect of a vaccine based on interleukin-2 transduced tumor cells. Cancer Res 1996;56:467–470.
43 Colombo MP, Vagliani M, Spreafico F, Parenza M, Chiodoni C, Melani C, Stoppacciaro A: Amount of interleukin-12 available at the tumor site is critical for tumor regression. Cancer Res 1996;56:2531–2534.
44 Irvine KR, Rao JB, Rosenberg SA, Restifo NP: Cytokine enhancement of DNA immunization leads to effective treatment of established pulmonary metastases. J Immunol 1996;156:238–245.

45 Leder GH, Oppenheim M, Rosenstein M, Lotze MT, Beger HG: Addition of interleukin-12 to low dose interleukin-2 treatment improves antitumor efficacy in vivo. Z Gastroenterol 1995;33:499–505.

46 Prechel MM, Lozano Y, Wright MA, Ihm J, Young MRI: Immune modulation by interleukin-12 in tumor-bearing mice receiving vitamin D_3 treatments to block induction of immunosuppressive granulocyte/macrophage progenitor cells. Cancer Immunol Immunother 1996;42:213–220.

47 Teicher BA, Ara G, Menon K, Schaub RG: In vivo studies with interleukin-12 alone and in combination with monocyte colony-stimulating factor and/or fractionated radiation treatment. Int J Cancer 1996;65:80–84.

48 Gately MK, Gubler U, Brunda MJ, Nadeau RR, Andersson TD, Lipman JM, Sarmiento U: Interleukin-12: A cytokine with therapeutic potential in oncology and infectious diseases. Ther Immunol 1994;1:187–196.

49 Brunda MJ, Luistro L, Rumennik L, Wright RB, Dvorozniak M, Aglione A, Wigginton JM, Wiltrout RH, Hendrzak JA, Palleroni AV: Antitumor activity of interleukin-12 in preclinical models. Cancer Chemother Pharmacol 1996;38(suppl):16–21.

50 Lotze MT, Zitvogel L, Campbell R, Robbins PD, Elder E, Haluszczak C, Martin D, Whiteside TL, Storkus WJ, Tahara H: Cytokine gene therapy of cancer using interleukin-12: Murine and clinical trials. Ann NY Acad Sci 1996;795:440–454.

51 Lamont AG, Adorini L: IL-12: A key cytokine in immune regulation. Immunol Today 1996;17: 214–217.

52 Del Vecchio M, Mortarini R, Rimassa L, Fowst C, Anichini A, Parmiani G, Cascinelli N, Bajetta E: Preliminary experience with rHu IL-12 in the treatment of metastatic melanoma. J Clin Oncol 1996;14:1748–1752.

53 Marshall E: Cancer trial of interleukin-12 halted. Science 1995;268:1555.

54 Tahara H, Zitvogel L, Storkus WJ, Elder EM, Kinzler D, Whiteside TL, Robbins PD, Lotze MT: Antitumor effects in patients with melanoma, head and neck carcinoma and breast cancer in Phase I/II clinical trials of interleukin-12 gene therapy using direct injection of tumors with genetically engineered autologous fibroblasts. Proc ASCO 1997, in press.

55 Tahara H, Zitvogel L, Storkus WJ, Robbins PD, Lotze MT: Murine models of cancer cytokine gene therapy using interleukin-12. Ann NY Acad Sci 1996;795:275–283.

56 Pappo I, Tahara H, Robbins PD, Gately MK, Wolf SF, Barnea A, Lotze MT: Administration of systemic or local interleukin-2 enhances the anti-tumor effects of interleukin-12 gene therapy. J Surg Res 1995;58:218–226.

57 Zitvogel L, Mayordomo JI, Tjandrawan T, DeLeo AB, Clarke MR, Lotze MT: Therapy of murine tumors with tumor peptide-pulsed dendritic cells: Dependence on T cells, B7 costimulation and T helper cell 1-associated cytokines. J Exp Med 1996;183:87–97.

58 Tahara H, Zeh H Jr, Storkus WJ, Pappo J, Watkins SC, Gubler U, Wolf SF, Robbins PD, Lotze MT: Fibroblasts genetically engineered to secrete interleukin-12 can suppress tumor growth and induce antitumor immunity to a murine melanoma in vivo. Cancer Res 1994;54:182–189.

59 Obana S, Miyazawa H, Hara E, Tamura T, Nariuchi M, Fujimoto S, Yamamoto H: Induction of anti-tumor immunity by mouse tumor cells transfected with mouse interleukin-12 gene. Jpn J Med Sci Biol 1995;48:221–236.

60 Rodolfo M, Zilocchi C, Melani C, Cappetti B, Arioli I, Parmiani G, Colombo MP: Immunotherapy of experimental metastases by vaccination with interleukin gene-transduced tumor cell vaccines. J Immunol 1996;157:5536–5542.

61 Meko JB, Tsung K, Norton JA: Cytokine production and anti-tumor effect of a nonreplicating, noncytopathic recombinant vaccinia virus expressing interleukin-12. Surgery 1996;120:274–282.

62a Chen PW, Geer DC, Podack ER, Ksander BR: Tumor cells transfected with B7-1 and interleukin-12 cDNA induce protective immunity. Ann NY Acad Sci 1996;795:325–327.

62b Rakhmilevich AL, Turner J, Ford MJ, McCabe D, Sun WH, Sondel PM, Grota K, Yang NS: Gene gun-mediated skin transfection with interleukin-12 gene results in regression of established primary and metastatic murine tumors. Proc Natl Acad Sci USA 1996;93:6291–6296.

63 Bramson J, Hitt M, Gallichan WS, Rosenthal KL, Gauldie J, Graham FL: Construction of a double recombinant adenovirus vector expressing a heterodimeric cytokine: In vitro and in vivo production of biologically active interleukin-12. Hum Gene Ther 1996;7:333–342.

64   Caruso M, Nguyen KP, Kwong YL, Bisong X, Kosai KI, Finegold M, Woo S, Chen SH: Adenovirus-mediated interleukin-12 gene therapy for metastatic colon carcinoma. Proc Natl Acad Sci USA 1996;93:11302–11306.

65   Tahara H, Zitvogel L, Storkus WJ, Zeh H, McKinney HG, Schreiber TG, Gubler U, Robbins PD, Lotze MT: Effective eradication of established murine tumors with IL-12 gene therapy using a polycistronic retroviral vector. J Immunol 1995;154:6466–6474.

66   Sotomayor EM, Cheng XF, Fu YX, Hawkins A, Calderon-Higginson C, Lopez DM: Impaired activation of tumoricidal function in macrophages from mammary tumor bearers: The role of IFN-γ. Int J Oncol 1993;3:719–722.

67   Ghosh P, Komschlies KL, Cippitelli M, Longo DL, Subleski J, Ye J, Sica A, Young H, Wiltrout RH, Ochoa AC: Gradual loss of T-helper 1 populations in spleen of mice during progressive tumor growth. J Natl Cancer Inst 1995;87:1478–1483.

68   Rook AH, Kubin M, Fox FE, Niu Z, Cassin M, Vowels BR, Gottlieb SL, Vonderhuid EC, Lessin SR, Trinchieri G: The potential therapeutic role of interleukin-12 in cutaneous T-cell lymphoma. Ann NY Acad Sci 1996;795:310–318.

69   Hegde SP, Bright JJ, Kausalya S, Khar A: AK-5 tumor-induced expression of interleukin-12: Role of IL-12 in NK-mediated AK-5 regression. Cell Immunol 1995;162:241–247.

70   Brunda MJ, Luistro L, Warrier RR, Wright RB, Hubbard BR, Murphy M, Wolf SF, Gately MK: Antitumor effect and antimetastatic activity of interleukin-12 against murine tumors. J Exp Med 1993;178:1223–1230.

71   Nastala CL, McKinney TJ, Edington HD, Tahara H, Storkus WJ, Lotze MT: Interleukin-12 induces specific antitumor immunity in animals bearing established subcutaneous murine sarcoma. Surg Forum 1994;45:492–494.

72   Brunda MJ, Gately MK: Interleukin-12: Potential role in cancer therapy; in DeVita VT, Hellman S, Rosenberg SA (eds): Important Adv Oncol 1995. Philadelphia, Lippincott, 1995, pp 3–18.

73   Ghosh P, Sica A, Young HA, Ye J, Franco JL, Wiltrout RH, Longo DL, Rice NR, Komschlies KL: Alterations in NFκB/Rel family proteins in splenic T-cells from tumor-bearing mice and reversal following therapy. Cancer Res 1994;54:2969–2972.

74   Fujiwara H, Hamaoka T: Antitumor and antimetastatic effects of interleukin-12. Cancer Chemother Pharmacol 1996;38(suppl):22–26

75   Wigginton JM, Kuhns DB, Back TC, Brunda MJ, Wiltrout RH, Cox GW: Interleukin-12 primes macrophages for nitric oxide production in vivo and restores depressed nitric oxide production by macrophages from tumor-bearing mice: Implications for the antitumor activity of interleukin-12 and/or interleukin-2. Cancer Res 1996;56:1131–1136.

76   Mantovani A: Tumor-associated macrophages in neoplastic progression: A paradigm for the in vivo function of chemokines. Lab Invest 1994;71:5–16.

77   Cui S, Reichner JS, Mateo RB, Albina JE: Activated murine macrophages induce apoptosis in tumor cells through nitric oxide-dependent or -independent mechanisms. Cancer Res 1994;54: 2462–2467.

78   Sagar SM, Singh G, Hodson DI, Whitton AC: Nitric oxide and anti-cancer therapy. Cancer Treat Rev 1995;21:159–181.

79   Dighe AS, Richards E, Old LS, Schreiber RD: Enhanced in vivo growth and resistance to rejection of tumor cells expressing dominant negative IFN-gamma receptors. Immunity 1994;1:447–456.

80   Howard B, Burrascano M, McCallister T, Chong K, Gangavalli R, Severinsson L, Jolly DJ, Darrow T, Vervaert C, Abdel-Wahab Z: Retrovirus-mediated gene transfer of the human gamma-IFN gene: A therapy for cancer. Ann NY Acad Sci 1994;716:167–187.

81   Lu Y, Boss JM, Hu SX, Xu HJ, Blanck G: Apoptosis-independent retinoblastoma protein rescue of HLA class II messenger RNA IFN-gamma inducibility in non-small cell lung carcinoma cells. Lack of surface class II expression associated with a specific defect in HLA-DRA induction. J Immunol 1996;156:2495–2502.

82   Vegh Z, Wang P, Vanky F, Klein E: Selectively down-regulated expression of major histocompatibility complex class I alleles in human solid tumors. Cancer Res 1993;53(suppl):2416–2420.

83   Ozaki Y, Edelstein MP, Duch DS: Induction of indoleamine 2,3-dioxygenase: A mechanism of the antitumor activity of interferon-γ. Proc Natl Acad Sci USA 1988;85:1242.

84   Burke F, Balkwill FR: Cytokines in animal models of cancer. Biotherapy 1996;8:229–241.
85   Voest EE, Kenyon BM, O'Reilly MS, Truitt G, D'Amato RJ, Folkmann J: Inhibition of angiogenesis in vivo by interleukin-12. J Natl Cancer Inst 1995;87:581–586.
86   Majewski S, Marczak M, Szmurlo A, Jablonska S, Bollag W: Interleukin-12 inhibits angiogenesis induced by human tumor cell lines in vivo. J Invest Dermatol 1996;106:1114–1118.
87   Mori K, Fujimot-Ouchi K, Ishikawa T, Sekiguchi F, Ishitsuka H, Tanaka Y: Murine interleukin-12 prevents the development of cancer cachexia in a murine model. Int J Cancer 1996;67:849–855.
88   Trinchieri G: Interleukin-12: A cytokine produced by antigen-presenting cells with immunoregulatory functions in the generation of T-helper cells type 1 and cytotoxic lymphocytes. Blood 1994; 84:4008–4027.
89   Shurin MR: Dendritic cells presenting tumor antigen. Cancer Immunol Immunother 1996;43: 158–164.
90   Bianchi R, Grohmann U, Belladonna ML, Silla S, Fallarino F, Ayroldi E, Fioretti MC, Puccetti P: IL-12 is both required and sufficient for initiating T cell reactivity to a class I-restricted tumor peptide (P815AB) following transfer of P815AB-pulsed dendritic cells. J Immunol 1996;157:1589–1597.
91   Zitvogel L, Tahara H, Robbins PD, Storkus WJ, Clarke MR, Nalesnik MA, Lotze MT: Cancer immunotherapy of established tumors with IL-12. Effective delivery by genetically engineered fibroblasts. J Immunol 1995;155:1393–1403.
92   Zitvogel L, Couderc B, Mayordomo JL, Robbins P, Lotze MT, Storkus WJ: IL-12-engineered dendritic cells serve as effective tumor vaccine adjuvants in vivo. Ann NY Acad Sci 1996;795: 284–293.
93   Fallarino F, Uyttenhove C, Boon T, Gajewski T: Endogenous IL-12 is necessary for rejection of P815 tumor variants in vivo. J Immunol 1996;156:1095–1100.
94   Scheicher C, Mehlig M, Dienes HP, Reske K: Uptake of microparticle-absorbed protein antigen by bone-marrow derived dendritic cells results in up-regulation of interleukin-1α and interleukin-12 p40/p35 and triggers prolonged, efficient antigen presentation. Eur J Immunol 1995;25:1566–1572.
95   Macatonia SE, Hosken NA, Litton M, Vieira P, Hsieh C, Culpepper JA, Wysocka M, Trinchieri G, Murphy KM, O'Garra A: Dendritic cells produce IL-12 and direct the development of Th1 cells from naive CD4$^+$ T cells. J Immunol 1995;154:5071–5079.
96   Heufler C, Koch F, Stanzl U, Topar G, Wysocka M, Trinchieri G, Enk A, Steinmann RM, Romani N, Schuler G: Interleukin-12 is produced by dendritic cells and mediates T helper 1 development as well as interferon-γ production by T helper 1 cells. Eur J Immunol 1996;26:659–668.
97   Cohen J: IL-12 deaths: Explanation and a puzzle. Science 1995;270:908.
98   Fujiwara H, Clark SC, Hamaoka T: Cellular and molecular mechanisms underlying IL-12-induced tumor regression. Ann NY Acad Sci 1996;795:294–309.
99   Wysocka M, Coughlin CM, Kurzawa HL, Trinchieri G, Eck SL, Lee WMF: Mechanism of the induction of anti-tumor immunity by B7.1 and interleukin-12. Ann NY Acad Sci 1996;795:429–433.
100 Zitvogel L, Robbins PD, Storkus WJ, Clarke MR, Maeurer MJ, Campbell RL, Davis CG, Tahara H, Schreiber RD, Lotze MT: Interleukin-12 and B7.1 co-stimulation cooperate in the induction of effective antitumor immunity and therapy of established tumors. Eur J Immunol 1996;26:1335–1341.
101 Stern LL, Tarby CM, Tamborini B, Truitt GA: Preclinical development of IL-12 as an anticancer drug: Comparison to IL-12. Proc Am Assoc Cancer Res 1994;35:520A.
102 Wigginton JM, Komschlies KL, Back TC, Franco JL, Brunda MJ, Wiltrout RH: Administration of interleukin-12 pulse interleukin-2 and the rapid and complete eradication of murine renal carcinoma. J Natl Cancer Inst 1996;88:38–43.

Michael R. Shurin, MD, PhD, University of Pittsburgh Cancer Institute, Division of Surgical Oncology, 300 Kaufmann Bldg, 3471 Fifth Ave, Pittsburgh, PA 15213 (USA)
Tel. (412) 692-4995, Fax (412) 692-2520, E-mail: mshu@med.pitt.edu

Adorini L (ed): IL-12. Chem Immunol. Basel, Karger, 1997, vol 68, pp 175–197

....

Targeting IL-12, the Key Cytokine Driving Th1-Mediated Autoimmune Diseases

Luciano Adorini[a], *Francesca Aloisi*[b], *Francesca Galbiati*[a],
Maurice K. Gately[c], *Silvia Gregori*[a], *Giuseppe Penna*[a],
Francesco Ria[d], *Simona Smiroldo*[a], *Sylvie Trembleau*[a]

[a] Roche Milano Ricerche, Milano, Italia;
[b] Istituto Superiore di Sanità, Roma, Italia;
[c] Hoffmann-La Roche, Inc., Nutley, N.J., USA;
[d] Università Cattolica del Sacro Cuore, Roma, Italia

The Th1/Th2 Dichotomy

CD4[+] [1, 2] as well as CD8[+] [3] T cells can be distinguished, based on their pattern of cytokine production, into three major types: Th1, Th2, and Th0. The distinction between type 1 and type 2 has actually been proposed to represent a fundamental dichotomy for all T-cell subsets [4]. Th1 cells are characterized by secretion of interferon-γ (IFN-γ), IL-2, and TNF-β, and they promote cell-mediated immunity able to eliminate intracellular pathogens. Conversely, Th2 cells selectively produce IL-4 and IL-5, and are involved in the development of humoral immunity protecting against extracellular pathogens. Th0 cells, which could either represent precursors of Th1/Th2 cells or a terminally differentiated subset, are not restricted in their lymphokine production. The development of Th1 and Th2 cells is influenced by several factors, but two are most important: cytokines and ligand-TCR interaction. Decisive roles in the polarization of T cells are played by IL-12 and IL-4, guiding T-cell responses towards the Th1 or Th2 phenotype, respectively [5, 6]. The avidity of interaction between peptide-class II ligands and TCR also controls the cytokine secretion profile. As demonstrated by using different antigen doses in vitro [7, 8] and in vivo [9, 10] and by altered peptide ligands [11], lower avidity interactions appear to favor Th2 cell development.

Polarized Th1 and Th2 subsets can be generated from CD4$^+$ populations in vitro [12], can be recovered from primed animals [13] and are found in patients suffering from autoimmune or allergic diseases [4]. However, polarized Th1 and Th2 cells represent extremes in a spectrum. Detection of intracytoplasmic cytokine production by polarized Th1 and Th2 cell populations analyzed at the single-cell level has confirmed the existence of defined Th1 and Th2 cells, selectively producing IFN-γ or IL-4, respectively, but has also revealed intermediate patterns [14]. Within this spectrum, discrete subsets of differentiated T cells secreting a mixture of Th1 and Th2 cytokines, for example IFN-γ and IL-10, have been identified [15]. Molecular mechanisms to explain the polarization of Th1 and Th2 subsets, based on the differential expression of the receptors for IFN-γ and IL-12, do exist. The ability of IFN-γ to inhibit the proliferation of Th2 but not of Th1 cells may be related to lack of IFN-γR β chain expression in Th1 cells [16]. However, IFN-γR β chain loss also occurs in IFN-γ-treated Th2 cells, and therefore does not appear to represent a Th1 cell-specific differentiation event [17]. Conversely, developmental commitment to the Th2 lineage results from rapid loss of IL-12 signaling in Th2 cells [18]. The inability of Th2 cells to respond to IL-12 appears to be due to selective down-regulation of IL-12R β2 subunit [19, 20]. These findings are therefore consistent with a general model in which selective modulation of IL-12 signaling plays an important role in the acquisition of distinct Th cell phenotypes.

The reciprocal regulation between Th cell subsets is another driving force polarizing CD4$^+$ T cells into differentiated Th1 or Th2 cells. IL-12 promotes the development of Th1 cells [12, 21, 22] and inhibits IL-4-induced IgE synthesis [23]. IFN-γ amplifies the IL-12-dependent development of Th1 cells [24] and inhibits Th2 cell proliferation [25]. Conversely, IL-4 and IL-10 inhibit lymphokine production by Th1 clones [26]. In addition, IL-10 [27], IL-4 and IL-13 [28] suppress the development of Th1 cells through down-regulation of IL-12 production by monocytes. However, the reciprocal regulation of IL-12 and IL-4 is not only negative. For example, IL-12 administered to mice after the establishment of a *Leishmania major*-specific Th2 response actually enhances rather than suppresses IL-4 production [29].

IL-12 Production by Antigen-Presenting Cells

IL-12 is a key cytokine in immunoregulation [30]. The powerful activity of IL-12 requires a tight control, which is exerted at different levels. The primary control is exerted on IL-12 production by antigen-presenting cells (APC), a major factor driving the response towards the Th1 or Th2 phenotype.

Normal Mature B Cells Present Antigen to CD4$^+$ T Cells but Fail to Produce IL-12: Selective APC for Th2 Cell Development?

Among the different APC populations capable of presenting peptide-class II MHC complexes, dendritic cells (DC) and B cells have been studied extensively, but their relative role in the presentation of protein antigen and CD4$^+$ T-cell priming in vivo is still controversial. Using mice lacking B cells, presentation to CD4$^+$ T cells of antigenic complexes derived from processing of protein antigen administered in adjuvant was found in some studies to require B cells [31], whereas in others B cells were found not critical [32]. Similarly, administration of soluble protein to normal mice was found to lead to selective expression of antigenic complexes either by antigen-specific B cells [33] or by DC [34].

To address this point, we have compared the relative capacity of DC and B cells, recruited in lymph nodes during the inflammatory response induced by adjuvant administration, to present protein antigen administered in different forms. Immune lymph node cells (LNC) from mice immunized with hen egg-white lysozyme (HEL) in adjuvant display HEL peptide-MHC class II complexes able to stimulate, in the absence of any further antigen addition, specific T-hybridoma cells [35, 36]. Using this read-out system, we have compared expression by DC and B cells of antigenic complexes derived from processing of native HEL, either given subcutaneously in adjuvant or in soluble form intravenously. Following subcutaneous administration of HEL in adjuvant, DC are the only APC expressing detectable HEL peptide-class II complexes [37]. Conversely, when HEL is administered in soluble form intravenously to mice previously injected with adjuvant only, lymph node B cells are much more efficient than DC in the presentation of HEL peptides [38]. These results demonstrate that protein antigen injected in soluble form is presented best by B cells, whereas the same protein is presented only by lymph node DC when administered in adjuvant. Therefore, different protocols of protein antigen administration lead to expression of peptide-class II complexes by different APC.

Although IL-12 was discovered as a product of EBV-transformed B cells [39, 40], secretion of IL-12 by normal B cells is still unclear. B cells, even when activated to induce similar levels of T-cell proliferation as DC, still drive a Th0-type response, with relatively low levels of IFN-γ being produced even upon neutralization of IL-4 [8]. The low level of IFN-γ produced by Th cells does not appear to be IL-12-dependent, suggesting that normal B cells do not produce this cytokine [41]. Actually, B cells have been shown to inhibit IL-

12 production [42]. Conversely, other MHC class II$^+$ APC have been shown to be major producers of IL-12. Among them macrophages secrete high levels of p75 when stimulated by bacteria as *Staphylococcus aureus* or by bacterial products such as lipopolysaccharide plus IFN-γ [43]. In addition, macrophages have been shown to direct, via secretion of IL-12, the development of antigen-specific T cells towards the Th1 phenotype [12]. Macatonia et al. [44] have shown IL-12 production by DC, and IL-12 p75 has been found to be secreted by DC upon contact with T cells [45–47].

We have studied antigen presentation and IL-12 production ex vivo by APC obtained from an inflammatory site, since IL-12 is likely to be produced in higher amounts at the site of inflammation by professional APC. DC were found to be unique among APC in the capacity to present efficiently peptide-class II complexes formed in vivo and to simultaneously secrete substantial amounts of IL-12 p75. IL-12 secretion by DC is strongly up-regulated by ligand-TCR and CD40-CD40L interactions with CD4$^+$ T cells, which are established through cognate interaction during antigen presentation. The feedback from antigen-specific T cells leading to increased IL-12 secretion is much more efficient in DC than in Mϕ, in contrast to bacterial stimuli which induce similar levels of IL-12 secretion in both cell types. The efficient presentation of antigenic complexes derived from proteins present in inflammatory sites and the production of IL-12 may account for the capacity of DC recruited in immune lymph nodes to prime naive CD4$^+$ T cells in vivo. We have recently shown that IL-12 administration to nonobese diabetic (NOD) mice results in acceleration of autoimmune diabetes, associated with massive infiltration of lymphoid cells, including N418$^+$ cells, into the pancreas [48]. Considering the efficiency of DC in antigen presentation and their capacity to produce IL-12, it is likely that pancreatic DC play a role in the induction of diabetogenic Th1 cells [49] and therefore may represent an interesting target to treat organ-specific autoimmune diseases.

Conversely, B cells fail to secrete IL-12 following either antigen-specific interaction with T cells or nonspecific stimulation (fig. 1). The capacity of B cells to present antigen in vivo, at least under some conditions [38, 50], but not to secrete IL-12, may play a role in selectively priming Th2 cells. Several lines of evidence suggest that antigen presentation by B cells may skew the development of CD4$^+$ cells towards the Th2 pathway [51–53]. Induction of experimental allergic encephalomyelitis (EAE), a Th1-mediated autoimmune disease, has been prevented by targeting the autoantigen to B cells [54], and this prevention has been found to be associated with the priming of antigen-specific Th2 cells [55]. IgD targeting on the B-cell surface by bivalent antibody fragments results in B-cell activation [56], which might be a prerequisite for priming of Th2 cells [55]. In addition, lack of spontaneous recovery from EAE

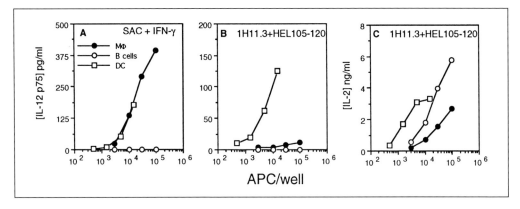

Fig. 1. B cells fail to secrete IL-12 in vitro. Mφ (90% Mac-1[+]) were obtained by peritoneal cavity lavage of thioglycollate-injected BALB/c mice. Another group of BALB/c mice was immunized with CFA into the hind footpads. Six days later popliteal lymph nodes were collected and APC populations separated. Large B cells (>95% B220[+]) were obtained from immune LNC by a combination of Percoll centrifugation and magnetic cell sorting. The DC-enriched population obtained from low buoyant density cells was further depleted of T and B cells using appropriate magnetic beads. The indicated numbers of Mφ, B cells and DC-enriched N418[+] APC were cultured in the presence of SAC (1:5,000) and IFN-γ (50 U/ml) in complete medium (*A*). In *B* and *C*, the indicated numbers of APC were cultured with the I-E[d]-restricted HEL108-116-specific T-cell hybridoma 1H11.3 in the presence of 0.3 μM HEL peptide 105-120. The concentrations of IL-12 p75 (*A, B*) and IL-2 (*C*) in 24-hour culture supernatants were determined by two-sites sandwich ELISA.

in B-cell-deficient mice has been attributed to the absence of B cells capable of driving Th2 responses [57]. Therefore, antigen presentation by APC lacking the capacity to secrete IL-12, such as B cells, could favor Th2 development. Since B cells, in vivo, can present more effectively protein rather than peptide antigen to CD4[+] T cells [33], this may also explain why soluble protein but not peptide administration diverts the immune response of TCR transgenic CD4[+] cells to the Th2 pathway [58].

Selective induction of Th2 cell responses by APC unable to secrete IL-12 is not restricted to B cells. Keratinocytes, the most abundant cell type in the skin, when activated express class II molecules and can function as APC. Activated T cells stimulated by keratinocytes, in contrast to professional APC, produce almost exclusively Th2-type cytokines and very little IFN-γ. This immune deviation appears to result from the inability of keratinocytes to secrete IL-12, because IFN-γ production is restored by exogenous IL-12 [59].

Thus, autoantigen presentation by IL-12-deficient APC could effectively induce immune deviation to the Th2 phenotype. It would be interesting to

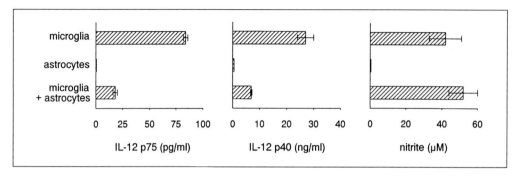

Fig. 2. Inhibitory effect of astrocytes on IL-12 production by activated microglia. Microglia, astrocyte and astrocyte/microglia cultures were established from neonatal mouse forebrains. Cell cultures were stimulated for 24 h with LPS and IFN-γ, levels of IL-12 p40 and p75 in culture supernatants were quantified by specific ELISA. Coculture of astrocytes with microglia (1:1) inhibits IL-12 p40 and p75 secretion by microglia. Conversely, microglial secretion of nitrite, a stable metabolite of nitric oxide, is not affected, indicating that microglial secretory activities are not aspecifically suppressed by astrocytes.

evaluate antigen targeting to non-IL-12-producing APC in the treatment of established Th1-mediated autoimmune diseases.

Astrocytes Inhibit IL-12 Secretion by Central Nervous System (CNS) Microglia: Regulation of IL-12 Secretion by APC-APC Interaction

To elucidate mechanisms regulating IL-12 production in an immune privileged site such as the CNS, recent studies have investigated IL-12 production by two CNS glial cell populations, microglia and astrocytes. Microglia, a CNS APC morphologically and functionally related to the monocyte/macrophage lineage, synthesize and secrete heterodimeric IL-12 [60, 61]. Conversely, astrocytes, a CNS APC of neuroectodermal origin, fail to produce IL-12 p75 and secrete only minimal amounts of p40 molecules. Interestingly, astrocytes actively suppress IL-12 secretion by microglia (fig. 2) [61]. These findings demonstrate a novel mode of IL-12 regulation at the APC level in the absence of T cells.

Since IL-12 promotes IFN-γ secretion by T cells [62] and IFN-γ in turn stimulates antigen presentation by microglia [63], it is likely that this cytokine network provides a positive feedback loop for induction of Th1 responses and microglia activation during infection or inflammation. The primary reason for heterodimeric IL-12 secretion by microglia is probably to promote immune responses against neurotropic infectious agents. IL-12 can exert its protective activity by stimulating NK and T cells, and inducing IFN-γ secretion by these cell types [5]. As a consequence of intercerebral IL-12 production, an immunostimulatory loop that perpetuates chronic inflammation within the brain can be established via induction of Th1 cells.

Conversely, the anti-inflammatory cytokine IL-10 is a powerful inhibitor of IL-12 microglial production, both at the mRNA and protein level [61]. This parallels the capacity of IL-10 to inhibit IL-12 production as well as other costimulatory surface molecules (e.g. CD80/CD86) or soluble cytokines (e.g. TNF-α, IL-1β) by professional APC such as macrophages and DC [27, 64, 65]. As microglia is the major intracerebral source of IL-10, this could represent an autocrine negative feedback mechanism able to interrupt an immunostimulatory circuit. Prevention of EAE by IL-10 administration [66] and increase of IL-10 mRNA and IL-10 expressing cells in the brain during the recovery phase of active EAE [67] are consistent with a role of IL-10 in down-regulating CNS inflammation.

Astrocytes and microglia differ markedly in their ability to provide co-stimulatory signals for T-cell activation [68]. In addition, unlike microglia, astrocytes fail to secrete IL-12 [61]. In this respect, astrocytes are similar to nonprofessional APC such as keratinocytes, which fail to secrete IL-12 and promote Th2 rather than Th1 responses [59]. IFN-γ-activated mouse astrocytes can present antigen and, quite interestingly, are very efficient in stimulating Th2-type cytokine secretion [F. Aloisi et al., manuscript in preparation]. The finding that astrocytes inhibit IL-12 p75 secretion by IFN-γ/LPS-stimulated microglia suggests a possible mechanism for inhibition of Th1 responses by astrocytes [61]. Astrocytes also down-regulate secretion of TNF-α by LPS-stimulated microglia, but do not reduce or even increase IL-10 secretion by microglia [F. Aloisi, unpubl. data]. These data raise the possibility that astrocytes inhibit synthesis of proinflammatory cytokines while enhancing deactivating mechanisms in microglia. This, in conjunction with inhibition of IL-12 secretion, may limit spreading of inflammation in the brain parenchyma.

Th1 and Th2 Cells in Autoimmune Diseases

The relative role of Th1 and Th2 cells in autoimmune diseases is currently very actively explored. At present, the results indicate a critical role of Th1 cells in the pathogenesis of many organ-specific autoimmune diseases. Conversely, the role of Th2 cells is still unclear, although indirect evidence for their protective capacity has been provided.

Experimental Models

Th1 cells are considered to be involved in the induction of several experimental autoimmune diseases [49, 69–71]. Evidence for this is based on adoptive transfer experiments demonstrating that CD4$^+$ cells producing Th1-type lymphokines can transfer disease, both in EAE [72] and in insulin-dependent diabetes mellitus (IDDM) [73–75] models. However, cytokine regulation is complex, for example TNF-α and IL-10 have opposite effects on IDDM depending on the developmental stage of the immune system [76, 77]. This could also explain why, in some cases, β-cell destruction in IDDM has been associated with Th2 rather than Th1 cells [78, 79].

The reciprocal regulation between T-cell subsets predicts a role for Th2 cells in inhibition of autoimmune diseases. Regulatory T cells that suppress the development of EAE produce Th2-type cytokines [80] and recovery from EAE is associated with increased Th2 cytokines in the CNS [81]. In addition, administration of IL-4 to mice with EAE ameliorates the disease [51]. These results clearly suggest that activation of Th2 cells may prevent EAE. A role for Th2 cells has also been proposed for inhibition of IDDM development. Evidence for a protective role of Th2 cells is provided by the reduced IDDM incidence following IL-4 [82] or IL-10 [83] administration to NOD mice. A role for Th2 cells regulating the onset of IDDM is also suggested by their capacity to inhibit the spontaneous onset of diabetes in rats [84] and by the correlation between protection from IDDM and IL-4 production in double-transgenic mice on BALB/c background [85]. Transgenic NOD mice that express IL-4 in their pancreatic β cells are protected from insulitis and IDDM, a direct indication that Th2 cytokines can prevent destructive autoimmunity [86].

However, Th2 cells transgenic for a TCR derived from a clone able to transfer IDDM, when injected into neonatal NOD mice, invaded the islets but neither provoked disease nor did they provide substantial protection [75]. Similar results were also obtained by adoptive transfer of nontransgenic Th1 and Th2 cell lines into neonatal mice [87]. Therefore, these data do not support the concept that Th2 cells afford protection from IDDM, at least in the effector phase of the disease. Rather, they are in accord with the observation that transgenic expression by islet cells of IL-10 [77, 88], an inhibitory lymphokine of Th1 cells, actually promotes insulitis and IDDM.

Collectively, these results point to a critical role of Th1 cells in the induction of autoimmune diseases, whereas the influence of Th2 cells is still controversial. In any case, whether or not Th2 cells exert a direct protective role, diversion away from proinflammatory Th1 cells should be effective in reducing the chronic inflammatory response which is typical of organ-specific autoimmune diseases.

Human Diseases

Th1 cells appear to be involved also in human organ-specific autoimmune diseases. CD4$^+$ T-cell clones isolated from lymphocytic infiltrates of Hashimoto's thyroiditis or Graves' disease exhibit a clear-cut type 1 phenotype [89]. In addition, most T-cell clones derived from peripheral blood or cerebrospinal fluid of multiple sclerosis (MS) patients show a Th1 lymphokine profile [90]. Expression of IL-12 p40 mRNA has been detected in acute MS lesions, particularly from early disease cases [91], suggesting that IL-12 up-regulation may be an important event in disease initiation. T cells from MS patients induce CD40L-dependent IL-12 secretion in the progressive but not in the relapsing-remitting form of the disease, suggesting a link to disease pathogenesis [92].

Involvement of Th1 cells has also been suggested in other human autoimmune diseases. Insulitis in IDDM patients has been shown to comprise a large number of IFN-γ-producing lymphocytes [93]. T-cell clones derived from the synovial membrane of rheumatoid arthritis (RA) patients also display a Th1 phenotype as they produce, upon activation, large amounts of IFN-γ and no or very little IL-4 [94]. Another study has shown that most CD4$^+$ and CD8$^+$ clones recovered from synovial fluid of RA patients display a Th1 phenotype [95]. Interestingly, in situ hybridization for T-cell cytokine expression demonstrates a Th1-like pattern in most synovial samples from RA patients, whereas samples from patients with reactive arthritis, a disorder with similar synovial pathology but driven by persisting exogenous antigen, express a Th0 phenotype [96].

The situation is less clear in most systemic autoimmune disorders. In general, heterogeneous cytokine profiles are found in the serum or target organs of patients with systemic autoimmunity, such as systemic lupus, Sjögren's syndrome, and primary vasculitis [4].

The Role of IL-12 in Th1-Mediated Autoimmune Diseases

IL-12 is a heterodimer composed of two covalently linked glycosylated chains, p35 and p40, encoded by distinct genes [97, 98]. This cytokine, produced predominantly by activated monocytes and dendritic cells but also by other cell types such as neutrophiles [99], enhances proliferation and cytolytic activity of NK and T cells, and stimulates their IFN-γ production [100]. Most importantly, IL-12 induces the development of Th1 cells in vitro [12, 21] and in vivo [22]. In addition, IL-12 is a potent cofactor stimulating growth, IFN-γ synthesis, and cell adhesion of already differentiated Th1 cells [101]. The key role of IL-12 in the induction of Th1 cell-mediated autoimmune diseases is clearly documented in several experimental models.

Insulin-Dependent Diabetes Mellitus

Administration of IL-12 induces rapid onset of IDDM in 100% of NOD female mice, whereas only about 60–70% of control littermates eventually develop IDDM [48]. This effect is not due to toxicity of IL-12 for pancreatic β cell, as shown by the normal appearance of islet cells and by the absence of IDDM in BALB/c mice treated with IL-12. Acceleration of IDDM in genetically susceptible NOD mice is accompanied by increased Th1 cytokine production by islet-infiltrating $CD4^+$ and $CD8^+$ T cells, and by selective destruction of islet β cells, suggesting a causal link between IL-12, Th1 cell induction, and development of IDDM.

Conversely, following a protocol developed by O'Hara and Henderson [102], we could confirm that intermittent administration of IL-12 (once weekly for 12 weeks) to NOD mice delays and reduces IDDM development [S. Trembleau et al., unpubl. data]. Data explaining these opposite effects of IL-12 are not yet available. However, it is conceivable that intermittent administration of IL-12, while still favoring Th1 induction, may be unable to sustain Th1 cell development. Thus, the aborted induction of a Th1 response, possibly coupled to the emergence of regulatory Th2 cells, may result in delay of Th1-mediated disease progression. This result should not be considered a surprising paradox, but rather an expected property of Th1/Th2 cell regulation.

To determine the role of endogenous IL-12 in IDDM development, mice deficient in IL-12 were generated by targeted disruption of the gene encoding the p40 subunit [103] and backcrossed to the NOD background. Spleen cells from IL-12$^{-/-}$ NOD mice produce neither IL-12 p40 nor IL-12 p75 when stimulated with lipopolysaccharide (LPS) or SAC plus IFN-γ, and fail to produce IFN-γ after stimulation with SAC or LPS. Conversely, spleen cells from IL-12$^{-/-}$ NOD mice secrete IFN-γ when stimulated with plate-bound anti-TCR mAb, indicating their capacity to produce IFN-γ. In agreement with the results obtained in vitro, IL-12$^{-/-}$ NOD mice, after LPS administration, do not produce detectable IL-12 p40 or IL-12 p75, and show a 95% reduction of serum IFN-γ levels. Antigen priming in IL-12$^{-/-}$ NOD mice gives rise to antigen-specific T cells that are able to secrete IL-2, IL-4, IL-5 and IL-10 in amounts comparable to littermate controls, but are defective in IFN-γ secretion. Preliminary results show a reduced incidence of IDDM in IL-12$^{-/-}$ NOD mice as compared to controls, indicating that endogenous IL-12 is required for IDDM development [S. Trembleau et al., manuscript in preparation].

Experimental Allergic Encephalomyelitis

IL-12 administration significantly increases the severity of EAE [104]. Similarly, mice treated with IL-12 in vivo following the transfer of proteolipid protein (PLP)-stimulated LNC develop a more severe and prolonged form of EAE, as compared to vehicle-treated controls. Most importantly, administration of anti-IL-12 antibodies substantially reduces the incidence and severity of adoptively transferred EAE, suggesting that endogenous IL-12 plays a key role in its pathogenesis [105]. Consistent with its role in promoting the activation and differentiation of pathogenic Th1 cells, IL-12 was detected in the brain of rats with EAE just before the development of clinical signs [67].

Collagen-Induced Arthritis

Treatment of DBA/1 mice with IL-12 enhances the autoimmune response to type II collagen resulting in severe, destructive arthritis. IFN-γ production by collagen-specific CD4$^+$ T cells as well as synthesis of complement-fixing antibodies of IgG2a and IgG2b isotypes is strongly up-regulated, suggesting that IL-12-induced Th1 cells may have a crucial role in the pathogenesis of this form of arthritis [106]. This is confirmed by the reduced incidence and severity of collagen-induced arthritis in IL-12-deficient mice, although in a few mice severe disease developed in spite of a highly reduced Th1 response [107]. Surprisingly, injection of high doses of IL-12 in DBA/1 mice immunized with collagen and mycobacteria ameliorates disease, suggesting that some initial events in the induction of collagen-induced arthritis can be suppressed by high doses of IL-12 [108].

Experimental Colitis

A Th1-mediated experimental colitis can be induced by rectal administration of the haptenizing reagent 2,4,6-trinitrobenzene sulfonic acid (TNBS) [109]. This disease can be treated by administration of anti-IL-12 antibodies even late after onset, suggesting that endogenous IL-12 may be required not only for induction but also for progression of experimental colitis [109]. Administration of anti-CD40L antibodies during the induction phase of the Th1 response prevents IFN-γ production by lamina propria CD4$^+$ T cells, and also clinical and histological evidence of disease. Disease prevention is caused by inhibition of IL-12 secretion, as demonstrated by immunohistochemistry [110]. Experimental colitis can also be inhibited by oral administration of haptenized colonic proteins (HCP) before rectal administration of TNBS. This form of oral tolerance appears to be due to the generation of mucosal T cells producing TGF-β and Th2-type cytokines. The suppressive effect of orally administered HCP is abrogated by the concomitant administration of anti-TGF-β or IL-12, suggesting a reciprocal relationship between IL-12 and TGF-β on tolerance induction in TNBS-induced colitis [111].

Favoring the Development of Th2 Cells by IL-12 Antagonist Administration Inhibits IDDM Development

IL-12 may thus have a primary role in the induction of several organ-specific autoimmune diseases [49], rendering IL-12 antagonists attractive candidates for immunointervention. IL-12 is not only a differentiation factor essential for the development of Th1 cells, but also a costimulus for activation of effector Th1 cells [64, 101], suggesting that administration of IL-12 antagonists may represent a strategy not only to prevent but possibly also to treat Th1-mediated autoimmune diseases.

A natural antagonist of IL-12 is the IL-12 p40 molecule itself. The mouse p40 chain specifically antagonizes mouse IL-12 p75 [112], and the primary inhibitory species is a disulfide-linked homodimeric form of IL-12 p40, termed $(p40)_2$ [113]. Based on competitive binding assays performed under high affinity binding conditions, mouse $(p40)_2$ appears to bind to the mouse IL-12R with an affinity similar to that of IL-12, but it does not trigger biologic activity and specifically inhibits IL-12-mediated responses. The p40 homodimer is 25- to 50-fold more potent than the p40 monomer as an IL-12R antagonist. This is parallelled by a similar capacity to inhibit IL-12-dependent activities, such as induction of IFN-γ synthesis by spleen cells. Human p40 also exists in dimeric and monomeric form [114], and human $(p40)_2$ binds to a human T-cell line expressing high affinity IL-12R at least 20-fold better than the monomer. However, unlike mouse $(p40)_2$ which binds to the mouse IL-12R with an affinity comparable to IL-12 itself, human $(p40)_2$ binds to the human IL-12R with an affinity 5- to 10-fold lower than human IL-12, and human $(p40)_2$ is correspondingly less potent than mouse $(p40)_2$ in inhibiting IL-12 bioactivity. Collectively, the available data demonstrate that both mouse and human $(p40)_2$ bind to the IL-12R and act as competitive antagonists of IL-12.

Evidence for p40 molecules as natural antagonists of IL-12 is suggested by the observation that p40 is produced in large excess over IL-12 both in vitro [43, 115] and in vivo [116, 117], and that p40 levels remain high for a long time after stimulation, whereas IL-12 production rapidly decreases [116, 117]. After LPS stimulation in vitro mouse peritoneal exudate cells produce IL-12, p40 and $(p40)_2$ molecules [M. Gately, unpubl. data]. The naturally occurring $(p40)_2$ can be visualized by Western blot analysis, purified and shown to inhibit IL-12-induced T-cell proliferation. Therefore, it is conceivable that $(p40)_2$ acts as an endogenous regulator of IL-12 activity. In addition to its ability to act as a competitive antagonist of IL-12 in vitro, mouse $(p40)_2$ can also inhibit IL-12 functions in vivo, as demonstrated by dose-dependent inhibition of endotoxin-induced IFN-γ production and of Th1 development in response to antigen priming [118a].

The IL-12 antagonist (p40)$_2$ can inhibit endogenous IL-12 activity and deviate the default Th1 development of naive TCR transgenic CD4$^+$ cells to the Th2 pathway [118b]. The same in vitro treatment does not modify the cytokine profile of polarized Th1 cells, but prevents further recruitment of CD4$^+$ cells into the Th1 subset. To assess the effect of (p40)$_2$ on Th1- and Th2-mediated responses in vivo, serum immunoglobulin isotypes were determined after (p40)$_2$ administration. Three-week-old NOD mice were injected daily with vehicle or 3 mg/kg (p40)$_2$. After 62 days of continuous treatment, mice were bled and the concentration of total serum antibodies of IgM, IgG2a, IgG1 and IgE isotypes was measured by ELISA. The amount of IgM remained unchanged between the two groups, whereas IgG1 and IgE were highly increased, and IgG2a decreased in mice treated with (p40)$_2$ as compared to vehicle. The isotype profile in (p40)$_2$-treated mice clearly indicates an increase in Th2 and a decrease in Th1 *helper* activity.

Administration of (p40)$_2$ to 3-week-old NOD mice results in a deviation of pancreas-infiltrating CD4$^+$ cells to Th2/Th0 phenotype (fig. 3). To evaluate a possible relationship between this immune deviation and IDDM development, NOD female mice were injected daily with (p40)$_2$ or vehicle from 3 to 12 weeks of age and glycemia levels were monitored afterwards. By 44 weeks of age, spontaneous IDDM developed in 100% of control mice but its incidence was significantly reduced and delayed in mice treated with (p40)$_2$ (fig. 3). Mice treated with (p40)$_2$ or vehicle from 3 to 12 weeks of age were also injected with cyclophosphamide at week 8 and 10. The (p40)$_2$ treatment nearly abrogated the development of cyclophosphamide-accelerated IDDM: only 1 out of 10 mice developed IDDM during the follow-up period whereas out of 10 vehicle-treated mice, 9 became diabetic. In the spontaneous IDDM model, the intracytoplasmic cytokine profile of pancreas-infiltrating cells from diabetic normoglycemic NOD mice has been compared. No major differences were observed between diabetic and normoglycemic mice in control groups: CD4$^+$ cells produced only IFN-γ and their percentage was slightly higher in diabetic mice. Conversely, among (p40)$_2$-injected mice, normoglycemic, as compared to diabetic mice, displayed a reduced number of Th1 cells. Moreover, pancreas-infiltrating cells from normoglycemic mice contained 21% of Th2 cells producing IL-4 only, and 5% of Th0 cells producing both IL-4 and IFN-γ, whereas diabetic mice had only 4 and 2%, respectively (fig. 3). Thus, protection from IDDM is associated with a deviation to the Th2 phenotype.

The effect of (p40)$_2$ administration was also studied in adult NOD mice, which display florid insulitis characterized by a high percentage of IFN-γ- and no IL-4-producing cells. NOD mice were treated continuously with (p40)$_2$ from 9 weeks of age onwards, using two protocols of administration, 3 mg/kg daily or twice weekly. In both cases administration of (p40)$_2$ delayed and

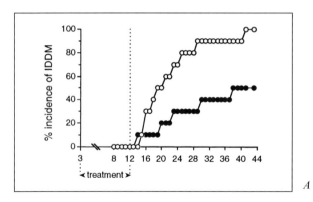

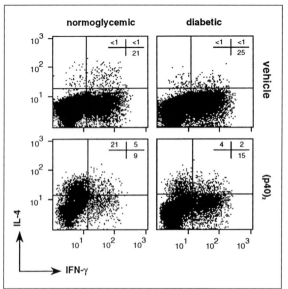

Fig. 3. (p40)$_2$ administration to 3-week-old NOD mice reveals a correlation between immune deviation to Th2 and protection from IDDM. NOD mice (10/group) were injected daily with vehicle alone (○) or containing 3 mg/kg (p40)$_2$ (●) from 3 to 12 weeks of age. *A* Spontaneous IDDM development was monitored by weekly measurement of blood glucose levels. *B* Purified pancreas-infiltrating cells were obtained from individual mice at the age of 14 weeks from the experiment described in *A*. All cells were restimulated for 4 h with PMA and ionomycin and analyzed by flow cytometry for IFN-γ (abscissa) and IL-4 (ordinate) production. Acquisition was performed on CD4$^+$ cells. Percentages of positive cells, set according to the isotype controls (not shown), are shown in the top right-end corner of each quadrant.

reduced the incidence of spontaneous IDDM but did not affect cyclophosphamide-accelerated IDDM. Intracytoplasmic staining of pancreas-infiltrating CD4$^+$ cells from (p40)$_2$-treated mice never showed more than 4% of IL-4-producing cells. This would suggest that partial protection from IDDM is associated with partial deviation to the Th2 phenotype. Collectively, the results show that deviation to Th2 of pancreas-infiltrating cells in NOD mice is more efficient when treatment is started at 3 weeks of age as compared to adult mice, and that progression to overt disease is more effectively controlled when treatment is initiated before the onset of insulitis.

In conclusion, (p40)$_2$ administration favors Th2 development, which is associated with protection from disease. Administration of the IL-12 antagonist before the onset of insulitis nearly abrogates IDDM. However, treatment initiated after the onset of insulitis, when Th1 cells already infiltrate the pancreatic islets, is less effective. This is consistent with the observation that polarized TCR transgenic Th1 cells do not reverse their phenotype when restimulated by antigen in the presence of (p40)$_2$, but their further recruitment is prevented. We are currently trying to analyze whether Th2 cells are directly responsible for protection from IDDM or whether the immune deviation away from Th1 cells actually accounts for the decreased IDDM incidence.

Prospects

The results reviewed highlight the critical role of Th1 cells in autoimmune diseases and suggest targeting IL-12 to control disease induction and progression. The IL-12 p40 and p35 promoters have been cloned and their detailed analysis is well under way [see Ma et al., this volume]. Regulation of IL-12R expression also contributes mechanisms and targets for effective control of IL-12 activities [19, 20].

Regulation of the Th1/Th2 balance can be effectively induced not only by IL-12 targeting, but also by antigen administration. The emerging picture of different Th subset development following different modes or doses of antigen administration allows the integration of the Th1/Th2 paradigm into the concept of immune deviation [49, 71, 119]. Immune deviation can be exemplified by autoantigen-specific therapy of IDDM in NOD mice. Autoantigens in IDDM are fairly well known [120] and the definition of a peptide-binding motif for I-A^{g7}, the class II MHC molecule of NOD mice, should facilitate identification of autoantigenic epitopes relevant to the pathogenesis and immunotherapy of this disease [121]. Among autoantigens in IDDM, glutamic acid decarboxylase (GAD) appears to be most important, because responses to GAD are detected before responses to other autoantigens, including insulin, heat-shock protein, peripherin and carboxypeptidase H [122, 123]. Intravenous or intrathymic administration of GAD to 3-week-old NOD mice, which do not yet display insulitis, prevents T-cell proliferation to GAD, as well as the development of intra-islet infiltration and IDDM in mice when adult. The reduction in the number of IFN-γ-secreting GAD-specific T cells [122] associated to the persistent production of autoantibodies to GAD [123] suggests that parenteral GAD administration can indeed induce a biased shift towards a Th2 response. Evidence for induction of a protective Th2 response has recently been obtained by nasal administration of GAD peptides to NOD mice [124]. These data indicate that nasal administration of GAD65 peptides induces a Th2 cell response that inhibits the spontaneous development of autoreactive Th1 responses and the progression of β-cell autoimmunity in NOD mice.

Additional approaches to immune deviation are also emerging, such as DNA vaccination. The TCR variable chain Vβ8.2 is expressed on pathogenic T cells that induce EAE in H-2^u mice immunized with myelin basic protein (MBP) [125]. Vaccination of these mice with naked DNA encoding Vβ8.2 protects them from EAE, and protection has been found associated to a shift from a Th1 to a Th2 response [126].

Collectively, these results suggest that immune deviation towards the Th2 phenotype may be effective in treating Th1-mediated autoimmune diseases, but the most effective manipulation of Th1 and Th2 cells in autoimmunity may eventually rely on a combination of antigen- and cytokine-based approaches. Ideally, they could be used to target specifically autoreactive T cells, diverting them from autoaggression by changing their lymphokine production profile. This strategy, which has been successfully applied to immunotherapy of parasitic diseases [22, 127], may complement attempts at treating human autoimmune diseases based on self antigen administration. A critical point for the clinical applicability of these approaches is the possibility to modify the Th1/Th2 balance in ongoing autoimmune diseases. This appears to be the case, at least in part, as demonstrated by administration of the IL-12 antagonist (p40)$_2$ to adult NOD mice. It may thus be possible to develop immune deviation protocols for the treatment of established autoimmune diseases.

References

1   Mosmann TR, Cherwinski H, Bond MW, Giedlin MA, Coffmann RL: Two types of murine helper T cell clone. I. Definition according to profile of lymphokine activities and secreted proteins. J Immunol 1986;136:2348–2357.
2   Del Prete G, De Carli M, Mastromauro C, Biagiotti R, Macchia D, Falagiani P, Ricci M, Romagnani S: Purified protein derivative of *Mycobacterium tuberculosis* and excretory-secretory antigen(s) of *Toxocara canis* expand in vitro human T cells with stable and opposite (type 1 T helper or type 2 T helper) profile of cytokine production. J Clin Invest 1991;88:346–350.

3   Erard F, Wild M-T, Garcia-Sanz JA, Le Gros G: Switch of CD8 T cells to noncytolytic CD8⁻CD4⁻ cells that make T$_H$2 cytokines and help B cells. Science 1993;260:1802–1805.

4   Romagnani S: Lymphokine production by human T cells in disease states. Annu Rev Immunol 1994;12:227–257.

5   Trinchieri G: Interleukin-12: A proinflammatory cytokine with immunoregulatory functions that bridge innate resistance and antigen-specific adaptive immunity. Annu Rev Immunol 1995;13:251–276.

6   Paul WE, Seder RA: Lymphocytes responses and cytokines. Cell 1994;76:241–251.

7   Constant S, Pfeiffer C, Woodard A, Pasqualini T, Bottomly K: Extent of T cell receptor ligation can determine the functional differentiation of naive CD4+ T cells. J Exp Med 1995;182:1591–1596.

8   Hosken NA, Shibuya K, Heath AW, Murphy KM, O'Garra A: The effect of antigen dose on CD4+ helper cell phenotype development in a T cell receptor-αβ-transgenic model. J Exp Med 1995;182:1579–1584.

9   Chen Y, Inobe J-I, Marks R, Gonnella P, Kuchroo VK, Weiner HL: Peripheral deletion of antigen-reactive T cells in oral tolerance. Nature 1995;376:177–180.

10   Guéry J-C, Galbiati F, Smiroldo S, Adorini L: Selective development of Th2 cells induced by continuous administration of low dose soluble proteins to normal and β2-microglobulin-deficient BALB/c mice. J Exp Med 1996;183:485–497.

11   Nicholson LB, Greer JM, Sobel RA, Lees MB, Kuchroo VK: An altered peptide ligand mediates immune deviation and prevents autoimmune encephalomyelitis. Immunity 1995;3:397–405.

12   Hsieh C-S, Macatonia SE, Tripp CS, Wolf SF, O'Garra A, Murphy KM: Development of Th1 CD4+ T cells through IL-12 produced by *Listeria*-induced macrophages. Science 1993;260:547–549.

13   Reiner SL, Locksley RM: The regulation of immunity to *Leishmania major*. Annu Rev Immunol 1995;13:151–177.

14   Openshaw P, Murphy EE, Hosken NA, Maino V, Davis K, Murphy K, O'Garra A: Heterogeneity of intracellular cytokine synthesis at the single-cell level in polarized T helper 1 and T helper 2 populations. J Exp Med 1995;182:1357–1367.

15   Mosmann TR, Sad S: The expanding universe of T-cell subsets: Th1, Th2 and more. Immunol Today 1996;17:138–146.

16   Pernis A, Gupta S, Gollob KJ, Garfein E, Coffman RL, Schindler C, Rothman P: Lack of interferon γ receptor β chain and the prevention of interferon γ signaling in Th1 cells. Science 1995;269:245–247.

17   Bach EA, Szabo S, Dighe AS, Ashkenazi A, Aguet M, Murphy KM, Schreiber RD: Ligand-induced autoregulation of IFN-γ receptor β chain expression in T helper cell subsets. Science 1995;270:1215–1218.

18   Szabo SJ, Jacobson AG, Gubler U, Murphy KM: Developmental commitment to the Th2 lineage by extinction of IL-12 signaling. Immunity 1995;2:665–675.

19   Rogge L, Barberis-Maino L, Biffi M, Passini N, Presky DH, Gubler U, Sinigaglia F: Selective expression of an interleukin-12 receptor component by human T helper 1 cells. J Exp Med 1997;185:825–831.

20   Szabo SJ, Dighe AS, Gubler U, Murphy KM: Th cell developmental commitment by regulation of the IL-12R β2 subunit. J Exp Med 1997;185:817–824.

21   Manetti R, Parronchi P, Giudizi MG, Piccinni M-P, Maggi E, Trinchieri G, Romagnani S: Natural killer cell stimulatory factor (interleukin 12, IL-12) induces T helper type 1 (Th1)-specific immune responses and inhibits the development of IL-4-producing Th cells. J Exp Med 1993;177:1199–1204.

22   Afonso LCC, Scharton TM, Vieira LQ, Wysocka M, Trinchieri G, Scott P: The adjuvant effect of interleukin-12 in a vaccine against *Leishmania major*. Science 1994;263:235–237.

23   Kiniwa M, Gately M, Gubler U, Chizzonite R, Fargeas C, Delespesse G: Recombinant interleukin-12 suppresses the synthesis of IgE by interleukin-4 stimulated human lymphocytes. J Clin Invest 1992;90:262–266.

24   Schmitt E, Hoehn P, Huels C, Goedert S, Palm N, Ruede E, Germann T: T helper type 1 development of naive CD4+ T cells requires the coordinate action of interleukin-12 and interferon-γ and is inhibited by transforming growth factor-β. Eur J Immunol 1994;24:793–798.

25 Gajewski TF, Fitch FW: Anti-proliferative effect of IFN-gamma in immune regulation. I. IFN-gamma inhibits the proliferation of Th2 but not Th1 murine helper T lymphocyte clones. J Immunol 1988;140:4245–4253.

26 Moore K, O'Garra A, de Waal Malefyt R, Vieira P, Mosmann TR: Interleukin-10. Annu Rev Immunol 1993;11:165–190.

27 D'Andrea A, Aste-Amezaga M, Valiante NM, Ma X, Kubin M, Trinchieri G: Interleukin-10 (IL-10) inhibits human lymphocyte interferon-γ production by suppressing natural killer cell stimulatory factor/IL-12 synthesis in accessory cells. J Exp Med 1993;178:1041–1048.

28 de Waal Malefyt R, Figdor CG, Huijbens R, Mohan-Peterson S, Bennett B, Culpepper J, Dang W, Zurawski G, de Vries JE: Effects of IL-13 on phenotype, cytokine production, and cytotoxic function of human monocytes. Comparison with IL-4 and modulation by IFN-γ or IL-10. J Immunol 1993;151:6370–6381.

29 Wang ZE, Zheng S, Corry DB, Dalton DK, Seder RA, Reiner SL, Locksley RM: Interferon gamma-independent effects of interleukin-12 administered during acute or established infection due to *Leishmania major*. Proc Natl Acad Sci USA 1994;91:12932–12936.

30 Lamont AG, Adorini L: IL-12: A key cytokine in immune regulation. Immunol Today 1996;17: 214–217.

31 Constant S, Schweitzer N, West J, Ranney P, Bottomly K: B lymphocytes can be competent antigen-presenting cells for priming CD4[+] T cells to protein antigens in vivo. J Immunol 1995;155:3734–3741.

32 Epstein MM, Di Rosa F, Jankovic D, Sher A, Matzinger P: Successful T cell priming in B cell-deficient mice. J Exp Med 1995;182:915–922.

33 Constant S, Sant'Angelo D, Pasqualini T, Taylor T, Levin D, Flavell R, Bottomly K: Peptide and protein antigen require distinct antigen-presenting cell subsets for the priming of CD4[+] T cells. J Immunol 1995;154:4915–4923.

34 Crowley MT, Inaba K, Steinman RM: Dendritic cells are the principal cells in mouse spleen bearing immunogenic fragments of foreign proteins. J Exp Med 1990;172:383–386.

35 Guéry J-C, Sette A, Leighton J, Dragomir A, Adorini L: Selective immunosuppression by administration of MHC class II-binding peptides. I. Evidence for in vivo MHC blockade preventing T cell activation. J Exp Med 1992;175:1345–1352.

36 Guéry J-C, Neagu M, Rodriguez-Tarduchy G, Adorini L: Selective immunosuppression by administration of major histocompatibility complex class II-binding peptides. II. Preventive inhibition of primary and secondary antibody responses. J Exp Med 1993;177:1461–1468.

37 Guéry JC, Ria F, Adorini L: Dendritic cells but not B cells present antigenic complexes to class II-restricted T cells following administration of protein in adjuvant. J Exp Med 1996;183:751–757.

38 Guéry J-C, Ria F, Galbiati F, Smiroldo S, Adorini L: The mode of protein antigen administration determines preferential presentation of peptide-class II complexes by lymph node dendritic or B cells. Int Immunol 1997;9:9–15.

39 Kobayashi M, Fitz L, Ryan M, Hewick RM, Clark SC, Chan S, Loudon R, Sherman F, Perussia B, Trinchieri G: Identification and purification of natural killer cell stimulatory factor, a cytokine with multiple biologic effects on human lymphocytes. J Exp Med 1989;170:827–845.

40 Stern AS, Podlaski FJ, Hulmes JD, Pan Y-CE, Quinn PM, Wolitzky AG, Familletti PC, Stremlo DL, Truitt T, Chizzonite R, Gately MK: Purification to homogeneity and partial characterization of cytotoxic lymphocyte maturation factor from human B-lymphoblastoid cells. Proc Natl Acad Sci USA 1990;87:6808–6812.

41 O'Garra A, Hosken N, Macatonia S, Wenner CA, Murphy K: The role of macrophage- and dendritic cell-derived IL-12 in Th1 phenotype development. Res Immunol 1995;146:466–472.

42 Maruo S, Oh-hora M, Ahn H-J, Wysocka M, Kaneko Y, Yagita H, Okumura K, Kikutani H, Kishimoto T, Kobayashi M, Hamaoka T, Trinchieri G, Fujiwara H: B cells regulate CD40 ligand-induced IL-12 production in antigen-presenting cells (APC) during T cell/APC interactions. J Immunol 1997;158:120–126.

43 D'Andrea A, Rengaraju M, Valiante NM, Chehimi J, Kubin M, Aste M, Chan SH, Kobayashi M, Young D, Nickbarg E, Chizzonite R, Wolf SF, Trinchieri G: Production of natural killer cell stimulatory factor (interleukin-12) by peripheral blood mononuclear cells. J Exp Med 1992;176: 1387–1398.

44   Macatonia SE, Hosken NA, Litton M, Vieira P, Hsieh C-S, Culpepper JA, Wysocka M, Trinchieri G, Murphy KM, O'Garra A: Dendritic cells produce IL-12 and direct the development of Th1 cells from naive CD4+ T cells. J Immunol 1995;154:5071–5079.

45   Heufler C, Koch F, Stanzl U, Topar G, Wysoka M, Trinchieri G, Enk A, Steinman RM, Romani N, Schuler G: Interleukin-12 is produced by dendritic cells and mediates T helper 1 development as well as interferon-γ production by T helper 1 cells. Eur J Immunol 1996;26:659–668.

46   Koch F, Stanzl U, Jennewein P, Janke K, Heufler C, Kaempgen E, Romani N, Schuler G: High level IL-12 production by murine dendritic cells: Upregulation via MHC class II and CD40 molecules and downregulation by IL-4 and IL-10. J Exp Med 1996;184:741–746.

47   Cella M, Scheidegger D, Palmer-Lehmann K, Lane P, Lanzavecchia A, Alber G: Ligation of CD40 on dendritic cells triggers production of high levels of interleukin-12 and enhances T cell stimulatory capacity: T-T help via APC activation. J Exp Med 1996;184:747–752.

48   Trembleau S, Penna G, Bosi E, Mortara A, Gately MK, Adorini L: IL-12 administration induces Th1 cells and accelerates autoimmune diabetes in NOD mice. J Exp Med 1995;181:817–821.

49   Trembleau S, Germann T, Gately MK, Adorini L: The role of IL-12 in the induction of organ-specific autoimmune diseases. Immunol Today 1995;16:383–386.

50   Ronchese F, Hausmann B: B lymphocytes in vivo fail to prime naive T cells but can stimulate antigen-experienced T lymphocytes. J Exp Med 1993;177:679–690.

51   Racke MK, Bonomo A, Scott DE, Cannella B, Levine A, Raine CS, Shevach EM, Roecken M: Cytokine-induced immune deviation as a therapy for inflammatory autoimmune disease. J Exp Med 1994;180:1961–1966.

52   Croft M, Swain SL: Recently activated naive CD4 T cells can help resting B cells, and can produce sufficient autocrine IL-4 to drive differentiation to secretion of T helper 2-type cytokines. J Immunol 1995;154:4269–4282.

53   Stockinger B, Zal T, Zal A, Gray D: B cells solicit their own help from T cells. J Exp Med 1996;183:891–899.

54   Day MJ, Tse AGD, Puklavec M, Simmonds SJ, Mason DW: Targeting autoantigen to B cells prevents the induction of a cell-mediated autoimmune disease in rats. J Exp Med 1992;175:655–659.

55   Saoudi A, Simmonds S, Huitinga I, Mason DW: Prevention of experimental allergic encephalomyelitis in rats by targeting autoantigen to B cells: Evidence that the protective mechanism depends on changes in the cytokine response and migratory properties of autoantigen-specific T cells. J Exp Med 1995;182:335–344.

56   Eynon EE, Parker DC: Small B cells as antigen-presenting cells in the induction of tolerance to soluble protein antigens. J Exp Med 1992;175:131–138.

57   Wolf SD, Dittel BN, Hardardottir F, Janeway CA: Experimental autoimmune encephalomyelitis induction in genetically B cell-deficient mice. J Exp Med 1996;184:2271–2278.

58   Degermann S, Pria E, Adorini L: Soluble protein but not peptide administration diverts the immune response of a clonal CD4+ T cell population to the T helper 2 pathway. J Immunol 1996;157:3260–3269.

59   Goodman RE, Nestle F, Naidu YM, Green JM, Thompson CB, Nickoloff BJ, Turka LA: Keratinocyte-derived T cell costimulation induces preferential production of IL-2 and IL-4 but not IFN-gamma. J Immunol 1994;152:5189–5198.

60   Becher B, Dodelet V, Fedorowicz V, Antel JP: Soluble tumor necrosis factor receptor inhibits interleukin-12 production by stimulated human adult microglial cells in vitro. J Clin Invest 1996;98:1539–1543.

61   Aloisi F, Penna G, Cerase J, Menendez Iglesias B, Adorini L: Astrocytes inhibit IL-12 production by central nervous system microglia. J Immunol 1997;159, in press.

62   Chan SH, Perussia B, Gupta JW, Kobayashi M, Pospisil M, Young HA, Wolf SF, Young D, Clark SC, Trinchieri G: Induction of interferon γ production by natural killer cell stimulatory factor: Characterization of the responder cells and synergy with other inducers. J Exp Med 1991;173:869–879.

63   Frei K, Siepl P, Groscurth P, Bodmer S, Schwerdel C, Fontana A: Antigen presentation and tumor cytotoxicity by interferon-γ-treated microglial cells. Eur J Immunol 1987;17:1271–1278.

64   Murphy EE, Terres G, Macatonia SE, Hsieh C-S, Mattson J, Lanier L, Wysocka M, Trinchieri G, Murphy K, O'Garra A: B7 and interleukin-12 cooperate for proliferation and interferon γ production by mouse T helper clones that are unresponsive to B7 costimulation. J Exp Med 1994;180:223–231.
65   Kubin M, Kamoun M, Trinchieri G: Interleukin-12 synergizes with B7/CD28 interaction in inducing efficient proliferation and cytokine production of human T cells. J Exp Med 1994;180:211–222.
66   Rott O, Fleisher B, Cash E: Interleukin-10 prevents experimental allergic encephalomyelitis in rats. Eur J Immunol 1994;24:1434–1440.
67   Issazadeh S, Ljungdahl A, Hoejeberg B, Mustafa M, Olsson T: Cytokine production in the central nervous system of Lewis rats with experimental autoimmune encephalomyelitis: Dynamics of mRNA expression for interleukin-10, interleukin-12, tumor necrosis factor α and tumor necrosis factor β. J Neuroimmunol 1995;61:205–212.
68   Hart MN, Fabry Z: CNS antigen presentation. Trends Neurosci 1995;18:475–481.
69   Powrie F, Coffmann RL: Cytokine regulation of T cell function: Potential for therapeutic intervention. Immunol Today 1993;14:270–274.
70   O'Garra A, Murphy K: T-cell subsets in autoimmunity. Curr Opin Immunol 1993;5:880–886.
71   Liblau RS, Singer SM, McDevitt HO: Th1 and Th2 CD4+ T cells in the pathogenesis of organ-specific autoimmune diseases. Immunol Today 1995;16:34–38.
72   Ando DG, Clayton J, Kong D, Urban JL, Sercarz EE: Encephalitogenic T cells in the B10.PL model of experimental allergic encephalomyelitis are of the Th1 lymphokine subtype. Cell Immunol 1989;124:132–143.
73   Haskins K, McDuffie M: Acceleration of diabetes in young NOD mice with a CD4+ islet-specific T cell clone. Science 1990;249:1433–1436.
74   Bergman B, Haskins K: Islet-specific T-cell clones from the NOD mouse respond to beta-granule antigen. Diabetes 1994;43:197–203.
75   Katz JD, Benoist C, Mathis D: T helper cell subsets in insulin-dependent diabetes. Science 1995; 268:1185–1188.
76   Yang X-D, Tisch R, Singer SM, Cao ZA, Liblau RS, Schreiber RD, McDevitt HO: Effect of tumor necrosis factor α on insulin-dependent diabetes mellitus in NOD mice. I. The early development of autoimmunity and the diabetogenic process. J Exp Med 1994;180:995–1004.
77   Wogesen L, Lee M-S, Sarvetnick N: Production of interleukin-10 by islet cells accelerates immune-mediated destruction of β cells in nonobese diabetic mice. J Exp Med 1994;179:1379–1384.
78   Anderson JT, Cornelius JG, Jarpe AJ, Winter WE, Peck AB: Insulin-dependent diabetes in the NOD mouse model. II. Beta cell destruction in autoimmune diabetes is a Th2 and not a Th1 mediated event. Autoimmunity 1993;15:113–122.
79   Akhtar I, Gold JP, Pan L-Y, Ferrara JL, Yang X-D, Kim JI, Tan K-N: CD4+ β islet cell-reactive T cell clones that suppress autoimmune diabetes in nonobese diabetic mice. J Exp Med 1995;182: 87–97.
80   Van der Veen RC, Stohlman SA: Encephalitogenic Th1 cells are inhibited by Th2 cells with related peptide specificity: Relative roles of interleukin (IL)-4 and IL-10. J Neuroimmunol 1993;48:213–220.
81   Khoury SJ, Hancock WW, Weiner HL: Oral tolerance to myelin basic protein and natural recovery from experimental autoimmune encephalomyelitis are associated with downregulation of inflammatory cytokines and differential upregulation of transforming growth factor β, interleukin-4, and prostaglandin E expression in the brain. J Exp Med 1992;176:1355–1364.
82   Rapoport MJ, Jaramillo A, Zipris D, Lazarus AH, Serreze DV, Leiter EH, Cyopick P, Danska JS, Delovitch TL: Interleukin-4 reverses T cell proliferative unresponsiveness and prevents the onset of diabetes in nonobese diabetic mice. J Exp Med 1993;178:87–99.
83   Pennline KJ, Roquegaffney E, Monahan M: Recombinant human IL-10 prevents the onset of diabetes in the nonobese diabetic mouse. Clin Immunol Immunopathol 1994;71:169–175.
84   Fowell D, Mason D: Evidence that the T cell repertoire of normal rats contains cells with the potential to cause diabetes. Characterization of the CD4+ T cell subset that inhibits this autoimmune potential. J Exp Med 1993;177:627–636.
85   Scott B, Liblau R, Degermann S, Marconi LA, Ogata L, Caton AJ, McDevitt HO, Lo D: A role for non-MHC genetic polymorphism in susceptibility to spontaneous autoimmunity. Immunity 1994;1:1–20.

86 Mueller R, Krahl T, Sarvetnick N: Pancreatic expression of interleukin-4 abrogates insulitis and autoimmune diabetes in nonobese diabetic mice. J Exp Med 1996;184:1093–1099.

87 Healey D, Ozegbe P, Arden S, Chandler P, Hutton J, Cooke A: In vivo activity and in vitro specificity of CD4+ Th1 and Th2 cells derived from the spleens of diabetic NOD mice. J Clin Invest 1995; 95:2979–2985.

88 Moritani M, Yoshimoto K, Tashiro F, Hashimoto C, Miyazaki J, Ii S, Kudo E, Izahana H, Hayashi Y, Sano T, Itakura M: Transgenic expression of IL-10 in pancreatic islet A cells accelerates autoimmune insulitis and diabetes in non-obese diabetic mice. Int Immunol 1994;6:1927–1936.

89 De Carli M, D'Elios M, Mariotti S, Marcocci C, Pinchera A, Ricci M, Romagnani S, Del Prete GF: Cytolytic T cells with Th1-like cytokine profile predominate in retroorbital lymphocytic infiltrates of Graves' ophthalmopathy. J Clin Endocrinol Metab 1993;77:1120–1124.

90 Brod SA, Benjamin D, Hafler DA: Restricted T cell expression of IL-2, IFN-γ mRNA in human inflammatory disease. J Immunol 1991;147:810–815.

91 Windhagen A, Newcombe J, Dangond F, Strand C, Woodroofe MN, Cuzner ML, Hafler DA: Expression of costimulatory molecules B7-1 (CD80) and B7-2 (CD86), and interleukin-12 cytokine in multiple sclerosis lesions. J Exp Med 1995;182:1985–1996.

92 Balashov KE, Smith DR, Khoury SJ, Hafler DA, Weiner HL: Increased interleukin-12 production in progressive multiple sclerosis: Induction by activated CD4+ T cells via CD40 ligand. Proc Natl Acad Sci USA 1997;94:599–603.

93 Foulis AK, McGill M, Farquahrson MA: Insulitis in type I (insulin-dependent) diabetes mellitus in man. Macrophages, lymphocytes and interferon-γ-containing cells. J Pathol 1991;165:97–103.

94 Miltenburg AM, van Laar JM, de Kuiper R, Daha MR, Breedveld FC: T cells cloned from human rheumatoid synovial membrane functionally represent the Th1 subset. Scand J Immunol 1992;35: 603–610.

95 De Carli M, D'Elios MM, Zancuoghi G, Romagnani S, Del Prete G: Human TH1 and TH2 cells: Functional properties, regulation of development and role in autoimmunity. Autoimmunity 1994; 18:301–308.

96 Simon AK, Seipelt E, Sieper J: Divergent T-cell cytokine patterns in inflammatory arthritis. Proc Natl Acad Sci USA 1994;91:8562–8566.

97 Wolf SF, Temple PA, Kobayashi M, Young D, Dicig M, Lowe L, Dzialo R, Fitz L, Ferenz D, Hewick RM, Kelleher H, Herrmann SH, Clark SC, Azzoni L, Chan SH, Trinchieri G, Perussia B: Cloning of cDNA for natural killer stimulatory factor, a heterodimeric cytokine with multiple biological effects on T and natural killer cells. J Immunol 1991;146:3074–3081.

98 Gubler U, Chua AO, Schoenhaut DS, Dwyer CM, McComas W, Motyka R, Nabavi N, Wolitzky AG, Quinn PM, Familletti PC, Gately MK: Coexpression of two distinct genes is required to generate secreted, bioactive cytotoxic lymphocyte maturation factor. Proc Natl Acad Sci USA 1991;88:4143–4147.

99 Cassatella MA, Meda L, Gasperini S, D'Andrea A, Ma X, Trinchieri G: Interleukin-12 production by human polymorphonuclear leukocytes. Eur J Immunol 1995;25:1–5.

100 Trinchieri G: Interleukin-12: A cytokine produced by antigen-presenting cells with immunoregulatory functions in the generation of T-helper cells type 1 and cytotoxic lymphocytes. Blood 1994; 84:4008–4027.

101 Germann T, Gately M, Schoenhaut DS, Lohoff M, Mattner F, Fischer S, Jin SC, Schmitt E, Rüde E: Interleukin-12/T cell stimulating factor, a cytokine with multiple effects on T helper type 1 (T$_h$1) but not on T$_h$2 cells. Eur J Immunol 1993;23:1762–1770.

102 O'Hara RM, Henderson SL: Interleukin-12 prevents the onset of diabetes in NOD mice. FASEB J 1995;9:5938.

103 Magram J, Connaughton S, Warrier R, Carvajal D, Wu C, Ferrante J, Stewart C, Sarmiento U, Faherty D, Gately MK: IL-12 deficient mice are defective in IFN-γ production and type 1 cytokine responses. Immunity 1996;4:471–482.

104 Santambrogio L, Crisi GM, Leu J, Hochwald GM, Ryan T, Thorbecke GJ: Tolerogenic forms of auto-antigens and cytokines in the induction of resistance to experimental allergic encephalomyelitis. J Neuroimmunol 1995;58:211–222.

105 Leonard JP, Waldburger KE, Goldman SJ: Prevention of experimental autoimmune encephalomyelitis by antibodies against interleukin-12. J Exp Med 1995;181:381–386.

106 Germann T, Szeliga J, Hess H, Stoerkel S, Podlaski FJ, Gately MK, Schmitt E, Ruede E: Administration of IL-12 in combination with type II collagen induces severe arthritis in DBA/1 mice. Proc Natl Acad Sci USA 1995;92:4823–4827.

107 McIntyre KW, Shuster DJ, Gillooly KM, Warrier RR, Connaughton SE, Hall RB, Arp LH, Gately MK, Magram J: Reduced incidence and severity of collagen-induced arthritis in interleukin-12-deficient mice. Eur J Immunol 1996;26:2933–2938.

108 Hess H, Gately MK, Ruede E, Schmitt E, Szeliga J, Germann T: High doses of interleukin-12 inhibit the development of joint disease in DBA/1 mice immunized with type II collagen in complete Freund's adjuvant. Eur J Immunol 1996;26:187–191.

109 Neurath MF, Fuss I, Kelsall BL, Stueber E, Strober W: Antibodies to interleukin-12 abrogate established experimental colitis in mice. J Exp Med 1995;182:1281–1290.

110 Stuber E, Strober W, Neurath M: Blocking the CD40L-CD40 interaction in vivo specifically prevents the priming of T helper 1 cells through the inhibition of interleukin-12 secretion. J Exp Med 1996; 183:693–698.

111 Neurath MF, Fuss I, Kelsall BL, Presky DH, Waegell W, Strober W: Experimental granulomatous colitis in mice is abrogated by induction of TGF-β-mediated oral tolerance. J Exp Med 1996;183: 2605–2616.

112 Mattner F, Fischer S, Guckes S, Jin S, Kaulen H, Schmitt E, Rüde E, Germann T: The interleukin-12 subunit p40 specifically inhibits effects of the interleukin-12 heterodimer. Eur J Immunol 1993; 23:2202–2208.

113 Gillessen S, Carvajal D, Ling P, Podlaski FJ, Stremlo DL, Familletti PC, Gubler U, Presky DH, Stern AS, Gately MK: Mouse interleukin-12 p40 homodimer: A potent IL-12 antagonist. Eur J Immunol 1995;25:200–206.

114 Ling P, Gately MK, Gubler U, Stern A, Lin P, Hollfelder K, Su C, Pan Y-CE, Hakimi J: Human IL-12 p40 homodimer binds to the IL-12 receptor but does not mediate biologic activity. J Immunol 1995;1995:116–127.

115 Podlaski FJ, Nanduri VB, Hulmes JD, Pan Y-CE, Levin W, Danho W, Chizzonite R, Gately MK, Stern AS: Molecular characterization of interleukin-12. Arch Biochem Biophys 1992;294:230–236.

116 Heinzel FP, Rerko RM, Ling P, Hakimi J, Schoenhaut DS: Interleukin-12 is produced in vivo during endotoxemia and stimulates synthesis of interferon-γ. Infect Immun 1994;62:4244–4249.

117 Wysoka M, Kubin M, Vieira LQ, Ozmen L, Garotta G, Scott P, Trinchieri G: Interleukin-12 is required for IFN-γ production and lethality in lipopolysaccharide-induced shock in mice. Eur J Immunol 1995;25:672–676.

118a Gately MK, Carvajal DM, Connaughton SE, Gillessen S, Warrier RR, Kolinsky KD, Wilkinson VL, Dwyer CM, Higgins GF, Podlaski FJ, Faherty DA, Familletti PC, Stern AS, Presky DH: IL-12 antagonist activity of mouse interleukin-12 p40 homodimer in vitro and in vivo. Ann NY Acad Sci 1996;795:1–12.

118b Trembleau S, Penna G, Gregori S, Gately MK, Adorini L: Deviation of pancreas-infiltrating cells to Th2 by IL-12 antagonist administration inhibits autoimmune diabetes. Eur J Immunol 1997;27, in press.

119 Rocken M, Shevach EM: Immune deviation – The third dimension of nondeletional T cell tolerance. Immunol Rev 1996;149:175–194.

120 Harrison LC: Islet cell autoantigens in insulin-dependent diabetes: Pandora's box re-visited. Immunol Today 1992;13:348–352.

121 Harrison LC, Honeyman MC, Trembleau S, Gallazzi F, Augstein P, Brusic V, Hammer J, Adorini L: A peptide-binding motif for I-A^{g7}, the class II MHC molecule of NOD and Biozzi AB/H mice. J Exp Med 1997;185:1013–1021.

122 Kaufman DL, Clare-Salzler M, Tian J, Forsthuber T, Ting GSP, Robinson P, Atkinson MA, Sercarz EE, Tobin AJ, Lehmann PV: Spontaneous loss of T-cell tolerance to glutamic acid decarboxylase in murine insulin-dependent diabetes. Nature 1993;366:69–72.

123 Tisch R, Yang X-D, Singer SM, Liblau RS, Fugger L, McDevitt HO: Immune response to glutamic acid decarboxylase correlates with insulitis in non-obese diabetic mice. Nature 1993;366: 72–75.

124 Tian J, Atkinson MA, Clare-Salzer M, Herschenfeld A, Forsthuber T, Lehmann PV, Kaufman DL: Nasal administration of glutamate decarboxylase (GAD65) peptides induces Th2 responses and prevents murine insulin-dependent diabetes. J Exp Med 1996;183:1561–1567.

125 Acha-Orbea H, Mitchell DJ, Timmermann L, Wraith DC, Tausch GS, Waldor MK, Zamvil SS, McDevitt HO, Steinman L: Limited heterogeneity of T cell receptors in experimental allergic encephalomyelitis. Cell 1988;54:263–273.

126 Waisman A, Ruiz PJ, Hirschenberg DL, Gelman A, Oskenberg JR, Brocke S, Mor F, Cohen IR, Steinman L: Suppressive vaccination with DNA encoding a variable region gene of the T-cell receptor prevents autoimmune encephalomyelitis and activates Th2 immunity. Nat Med 1996;2: 899–905.

127 Heinzel FP, Schoenhaut DS, Rerko RM, Rosser LE, Gately MK: Recombinant interleukin-12 cures mice infected with *Leishmania major*. J Exp Med 1993;177:1505–1509.

Luciano Adorini, Roche Milano Ricerche, Via Olgettina 58, I–20132 Milano (Italy)
Tel. (2) 2884816, Fax (2) 2153203, E-mail: Luciano.Adorini@Roche.com

Author Index

Subject Index

signal transduction pathways in Th cells 42, 43, 55

Interleukin-6, role in Th2 cell development 45

Interleukin-10
  Candida albicans response 114, 117–119
  neutrophil production in candidiasis 122, 123
  suppression of interleukin-12 expression 9, 15, 18

IP–10, antitumor activity with interleukin-12 164

Leishmania major
  interleukin-4 response and role 94, 97, 100–102, 105
  interleukin-12
    induction by parasite 4, 137, 138
    knockout mice susceptibility 90, 92, 93
    suppression as evasion mechanism 87, 88
    mouse model of parasitic disease 86, 87, 100
    signaling for T-cell activation 88, 89
    Th cell response
      antigen dose effects 97, 99
      development in absence of interleukin-12 94
      glycolipids responsible for induction 146
      resistant strains 87
      Th1 response in knockout mice 74

Lipopolysaccharide, mechanism of interleukin-12 induction 6–9, 11, 12, 17, 148

Lipoteichoic acid, interleukin-12 induction 148

Listeria monocytogenes, interleukin-12 induction 3

Macrophage, interleukin-12 expression 4
Mast cell, interleukin-12 expression 3
Measles, interleukin-12 induction 5
Microglia, astrocyte inhibition of interleukin-12 secretion 180, 181
Mucin, isolation from Trypanosoma cruzi and interleukin-12 induction 141, 142, 144, 145

Multiple sclerosis, Th cell role 183
Mycobacterium, interleukin-12 induction 3

Natural killer cell, antitumor activity of interleukin-12 154, 155
Neutrophil, candidiasis role
  ablation effects 121, 122
  interleukin-10 production 122, 123
  interleukin-12 production and effects 120–122, 129
Nitric oxide, antitumor activity with interleukin-12 165
Nuclear factor of activated T cells, role in Th cell differentiation 46
Nuclear factor-κB, role in Th cell differentiation 46, 47

p35
  dimerization with p40 1
  promoter structure and regulation 8, 9
p40
  antagonism of interleukin-12 receptor by dimer 31–33, 35, 186
  dimerization with p35 1
  induction by viruses 4, 5
  insulin-dependent diabetes mellitus inhibition by p40 dimer 186, 187, 189
  promoter structure and regulation 7
  suppression by Leishmania major 87, 88
Plasmodium falciparum, glycolipids responsible for interleukin-12 induction 147
Polymorphonuclear cell, interleukin-12 expression 2, 3

Receptor, interleukin-12
  antagonism by p40 dimer 31–33, 35, 186
  binding affinities 23, 24, 28–30
  cellular distribution 27, 28
  expression during Th cell development 40, 41
  gene induction 27
  human vs mouse characteristics 28–30, 35, 59–61
  recombinant receptor analysis 28–30

Receptor, interleukin-12 (continued)
  signal transduction
    differential signaling in Th1 and Th2
      cells 39, 40, 57, 58
    pathways 30, 31, 55
    Th cell differentiation 42, 43
    STAT1 requirement for β2 expression 59,
      65
  subunits
    amino acid sequences 26, 27
    cloning 23, 24
    knockout mice, β1 subunit analysis
      33–35
    structural features 24, 26
  tumor cells 155
Rheumatoid arthritis, Th cell role 183

Salmonella, interleukin-12 induction 3, 4
STAT1, role in interleukin-12 receptor
  expression 59
STAT4, regulation of interferon-γ gene 48,
  49, 57, 59
STAT6, regulation of interleukin-4 gene 48

Th0 cell, lymphokine secretion 38, 79,
  175
Th1 cell
  autoimmune disease role 182, 183, 186,
    190
  differentiation
    candidiasis 111–114, 116–119, 127, 128
    induction by interleukin-12 12–15, 55,
      56, 71–75, 137, 176
    interferon-γ role 43, 44, 55, 56, 71–74,
      82, 176
    interleukin-4 regulation 77–79, 82, 176
    regulation of interleukin-12 receptor β2
      subunit expression 42, 49
    signal transduction pathways 42, 43
    techniques in analysis 38, 39
    transcriptional events 45–47
    transforming growth factor-β
      regulation 75–77, 82
  genetic effects on development in mice
    62–64, 94
  interleukin-12 receptor expression during
    development 40, 41

lymphokine secretion 38, 47, 86,
  175
signal transduction
  interferon-γ 61, 62
  interleukin-12 39, 40, 57, 58
Th2 cell
  autoimmune disease role 182
  differentiation
    candidiasis 111–114, 116–119, 127,
      128
    induction by interleukin-4 12–15
    p40 dimer induction 186, 187, 189
    regulation of interleukin-12 receptor β2
      subunit expression 42
    signal transduction pathways 42, 43
    techniques in analysis 38, 39
    transcriptional events 45–47
  genetic effects on development in mice
    62–64, 94
  interleukin-6 role in development 45
  interleukin-12 receptor expression during
    Th cell development 40, 41
  lymphokine secretion 38, 47, 79, 86,
    175
  signal transduction
    interferon-γ 61, 62
    interleukin-12 39, 40, 57, 58
Toxoplasma gondii, interleukin-12 induction
  assay 138, 141
  cell-mediated immunity 4, 136, 137
  isolation of inducing glycolipids 143
  tachyzoites 138, 149
Transforming growth factor-β
  role in Th1 development 75–77
  suppression of interleukin-12 expression
    9, 10, 75–77
Trypanosoma brucei, glycolipids responsible
  for interleukin-12 induction 147
Trypanosoma cruzi
  interleukin-12 induction
    assay 138, 141
    cell-mediated immunity 136, 137
    GPI-mucins 144, 145
    isolation of inducing glycolipids 141,
      142
    trypomastigotes 138, 139, 149
  monokine stimulation 139